NEUROPATHOLOGY
Case Studies

NEUROPATHOLOGY
Case Studies

Second Edition

A Compilation of 70 Clinical Studies

By   **SYDNEY S. SCHOCHET, Jr., M.D.**
Professor of Pathology
Department of Pathology
University of Oklahoma Health Sciences Center
Oklahoma City, Oklahoma

and

WILLIAM F. McCORMICK, M.D.
*Professor of Pathology, Neurology
   and Surgery (Neurosurgery)*
Chief, Division of Neuropathology
University of Texas Medical Branch
Galveston, Texas

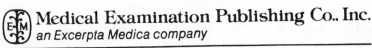 Medical Examination Publishing Co., Inc.
an Excerpta Medica company

969 Stewart Avenue   •   Garden City, New York 11530

SIMULTANEOUSLY PUBLISHED IN:

Europe   :   HANS HUBER PUBLISHERS
                              Bern, Switzerland

Japan   :   IGAKU-SHOIN Ltd.
                              Tokyo, Japan

South and East Asia   :   TOPPAN COMPANY (s) Pte. Ltd.
                              Singapore

United Kingdom   :   HENRY KIMPTON PUBLISHERS
                              London, England

Preface

In this second edition of *Neuropathology Case Studies*, we have expanded our coverage and updated our discussions and references. We have continued to select topics of general interest and to address areas of greatest confusion.

We extend special thanks to our secretary, Ms. Gail Stewart, for the job of typing and retyping the manuscript, and to Drs. Clyde Meyers and Charles Barnett, for reading our manuscript and making many helpful suggestions.

The Authors

Contents

notice

The editor(s) and/or author(s) and the publisher of this book have made every effort
to ensure that all therapeutic modalities
that are recommended are in accordance
with accepted standards at the time of pub-
lication.

The drugs specified within this book may
not have specific approval by the Food and
Drug Administration in regard to the indications and dosages that are recommended
by the editor(s) and/or author(s).   The
manufacturer's package insert is the best
source of current prescribing information.

NEUROPATHOLOGY

CASE 1: A Young Boy with Progressive Muscular Weakness and Pseudohypertrophy of Calves

CLINICAL DATA

This 5-year-old boy was the product of a normal pregnancy and delivery. He began to walk at the age of 15 months but has never been able to run. By the age of 3, he had difficulty climbing steps and fell frequently. In order to get up from the floor, he would assist himself by putting his hands on his knees. There was no family history of any neuromuscular disease.

On examination, he was found to have weakness of his shoulders, pelvic muscles and legs. His gait was unsteady and he could not hop on one foot. There was a mild lumbar lordosis. His deep tendon reflexes were decreased and he had minimal contractures of the Achilles tendons. There was considerable pseudohypertrophy of the calves. No myotonia could be elicited. Sensory examination was within normal limits.

Electromyography was suggestive of myopathy. Laboratory studies revealed a serum creatine phosphokinase (CPK) of 1,600 iu/l.

A biopsy of the quadriceps femoris was performed to confirm the clinical diagnosis.

QUESTIONS

1. The most likely clinical diagnosis is
    A. Duchenne muscular dystrophy
    B. limb-girdle muscular dystrophy
    C. myotonic dystrophy
    D. facioscapulohumeral muscular dystrophy

2. The pattern of inheritance in Duchenne muscular dystrophy is
    A. autosomal dominant
    B. autosomal recessive
    C. X-linked recessive
    D. variable

3. Good muscle biopsy technique includes
   A. selection of a moderately affected muscle
   B. avoidance of sites of previous injections, surgical
      incisions and punctures by EMG needles
   C. sharp dissection and use of an isometric clamp
   D. all of the above

4. Fig. 1.1 shows the histopathological changes in the muscle
   biopsy specimen. Which of the following morphological
   features are illustrated?
   A. Excessive random variation in myofiber size
   B. Degenerating myofibers
   C. Excessive endomysial connective tissues
   D. All of the above

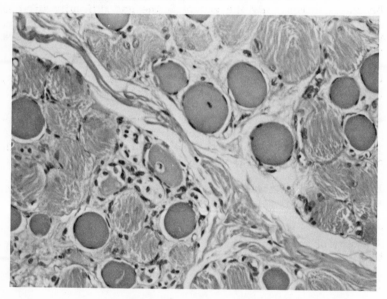

FIG. 1.1: Muscle biopsy specimen from the quadriceps of a patient with Duchenne muscular dystrophy.

5. A muscle biopsy from an older patient with Duchenne mus-
   cular dystrophy would be expected to show
   A. target fibers
   B. fascicles of atrophic myofibers
   C. severe endomysial fibrosis
   D. extensive adipose tissue

6.   Patients with Duchenne muscular dystrophy usually die
     during the second or third decades from
     A. myositis
     B. pulmonary disease
     C. cardiac involvement
     D. malignancies

7.   If this child's disease fails to progress, if he remains
     ambulatory past the age of 10 or 12 and if no electrocardio-
     graphic abnormalities appear, one would have to revise the
     diagnosis to
     A. limb-girdle muscular dystrophy
     B. myotonic dystrophy
     C. Becker muscular dystrophy
     D. none of these

8.   Younger male siblings with no overt clinical abnormalities
     may show
     A. histological evidence of active muscular dystrophy
     B. elevated serum muscle enzymes
     C. histological evidence of an abortive form of muscular
         dystrophy
     D. none of the above

9.   Which of the following are useful in determining whether
     the mother and any of her daughters are carriers?
     A. Muscle biopsy
     B. Serum muscle enzymes
     C. Electromyography
     D. All of these

10. The prevalence of Duchenne muscular dystrophy is
     A. 40/million
     B. 400/million
     C. 4/million
     D. 0.4/million

ANSWERS AND DISCUSSION

1.   (A) The clinical history, physical findings and creatine
phosphokinase level are typical of Duchenne muscular dystrophy. In this condition, the weakness usually becomes evident
when the child begins to walk and is manifested by a waddling
gait, frequent falls, inability to run and difficulty in climbing
steps. The severe involvement of the pelvic girdle results in
the Gowers' maneuver in which the child uses his stronger arm
and shoulder muscles to assist in rising from the floor. Pseudohypertrophy is a highly variable finding that gives the false

impression of normal or increased muscle development. This disease is relentlessly progressive leading to an inability to walk within ten years. Contractures and skeletal deformities occur with the passage of time. For unknown reasons, many of the patients show mild mental retardation. The marked elevation of the serum muscle enzymes, especially creatine phosphokinase (CPK), is characteristic of Duchenne muscular dystrophy.

Limb-girdle dystrophy usually has the onset of clinical symptoms during the second or third decades of life, the disease progresses slowly, and the patients remain ambulatory for many years. The serum muscle enzymes are nearly within normal ranges.

Facioscapulohumeral dystrophy usually begins during the second or third decades with weakness of facial muscles and progresses slowly to involve the shoulders and still later, the pelvic girdle. There are many abortive or mild cases. Serum muscle enzymes are usually normal or only slightly elevated.

Myotonic dystrophy is a relatively common muscular disorder. The clinical onset is generally during the second or third decades. The weakness is most pronounced in the facial muscles, neck flexors and distal muscles of the extremities. Myotonia can be demonstrated clinically and electromyographically. Associated systemic manifestations include mental retardation, cataracts, hypogonadism and cardiac abnormalities (See Case 5).

2. (C) Duchenne muscular dystrophy is inherited as an X-linked recessive trait. Males are affected with the disease while females are carriers. A female carrier will transmit the disease to one-half of her sons and will transmit the carrier state to one-half her daughters. Sporadic cases, i.e., the result of spontaneous mutations, are very common.

Facioscapulohumeral and myotonic dystrophies are inherited as autosomal dominant traits while limb-girdle and the congenital dystrophies are inherited as autosomal recessive traits.

3. (D) Muscle biopsy is a relatively simple technique yet one that is often done poorly. The clinical and electrodiagnostic findings must be considered in selecting an appropriate muscle to be biopsied. The muscle must be involved yet not so severely as to yield "end-stage" muscle in which case the

specimen is of little or no diagnostic value. Sites of recent injections, punctures by EMG needles and sites of previous surgical procedures must be carefully avoided. Care must be taken not to infiltrate the muscle specimen with the local anesthetic. Rarely is the use of general anesthesia justifiable. Sharp dissection and the use of an isometric clamp are important. The bulk of the muscle may limit the size of the specimen but a specimen measuring at least 1.0 x 0.5 x 0.5 cm can be obtained from most patients. The specimen, while still in the clamp, should be wrapped in gauze moistened with normal saline.

4. (D) Fig. 1.1 shows typical morphological features of active muscular dystrophy. Muscle normally shows some variation in myofiber size, however, in this specimen the variation is excessive and includes greatly enlarged myofibers. Many of the myofibers are degenerating and appear homogeneous or hyalinized. Fibers that have degenerated completely are replaced by clusters of macrophages within the sarcolemmal sheaths, so-called myophagocytosis. Still other fibers are regenerating and have amphophilic cytoplasm and vesicular nuclei. These fibers cannot be identified with certainty in the black and white photograph. Normally myofibers are surrounded by a very small amount of endomysial connective tissue that is barely perceptible with connective tissue stains. In this specimen, the endomysial connective tissue is readily evident and thus excessive. Other features that can be seen are the increased number of internal or central nuclei and fiber splitting.

5. (C, D) In an older patient, the muscle may be extensively replaced by adipose tissue. Sometimes only the presence of muscle spindles, which are remarkably persistent, indicates that the tissue was once a muscle. Remaining myofibers are usually surrounded by thick bands of endomysial fibrous tissue. Target fibers and fascicles of small atrophic myofibers are manifestations of denervation and would not be expected in a patient with muscular dystrophy.

6. (B, C) Patients with Duchenne muscular dystrophy usually die as the result of pneumonia or cardiac involvement. Even in young patients, tachycardia and electrocardiographic changes are commonly observed.

7. (C) Becker muscular dystrophy is a more benign variety of X-linked muscular dystrophy. The clinical manifestations and distribution of the weakness are similar but milder than in Duchenne muscular dystrophy. The patients usually remain

ambulatory for many years, have less cardiac involvement and may have a normal life span. Pseudohypertrophy may be even more pronounced than in Duchenne muscular dystrophy. Serum muscle enzymes are similarly elevated but may decline more slowly than in Duchenne dystrophy. The morphological findings on biopsy are milder than those found in patients with Duchenne muscular dystrophy and the fibrosis is somewhat less pronounced.

8. (A, B, D) If the mother is a carrier, she will transmit the disease to one-half of her sons. The affected sons have elevated serum muscle enzymes and histological evidence of active muscular dystrophy long before the clinical manifestations are overt. There are no partially affected or abortive cases of Duchenne muscular dystrophy.

9. (D) Serum muscle enzymes, especially creatine phosphokinase (CPK) and aldolase (Ald), are elevated in about 70% of the carriers. Electromyography also can detect about 50-70% of the carriers. Muscle biopsy specimens are morphologically abnormal in some carriers. Currently, the most satisfactory approach is a combination of these methods.

10. (A) Duchenne muscular dystrophy is the most common of the muscular dystrophies and has a prevalence of about 40/ million males. It is about 10 times as common as Becker dystrophy.

REFERENCES

1. Brooke MH: A Clinician's View of Neuromuscular Disease. Williams and Wilkins Co., Baltimore, 1977, pp. 95-124.

2. Dubowitz V: Muscle Disorders in Childhood. W. B. Saunders Co., London, 1978, pp. 19-69.

3. Dubowitz V and Brooke MH: Muscle Biopsy: A Modern Approach. W. B. Saunders Co., London, 1973, pp. 168-252.

4. Pickard NA, et al.: Systemic membrane defect in the proximal muscular dystrophies. N Eng J Med 299:841-846, 1978.

5. Ringel SP, et al.: The spectrum of mild X-linked recessive muscular dystrophy. Arch Neurol 34:408-416, 1977.

6. Rowland LP: Pathogenesis of muscular dystrophies. Arch Neurol 33:3, 5-321, 1976.

: :

CASE 2: A 41-Year-Old Woman with Dysphagia and Muscular
          Weakness and Tenderness

CLINICAL DATA

This 41-year-old woman was admitted to the hospital for evaluation of muscular weakness and dysphagia that began insidiously
and progressed gradually over a 4-month period.   By the time
of admission, she had quit her job as a checkout clerk in a gro-
cery store, curtailed her household chores and had difficulty
climbing steps.   In addition to the weakness, she had muscle
tenderness on the volar aspect of her forearms and the
anterior aspect of her thighs.   Dysphagia was especially
pronounced with solids such as meat and bread.   She denied
any sensory disturbances, anorexia, weight loss, skin rashes
or arthralgias.

General physical examination was normal. Neurological examination revealed intact cranial nerve function and sensory perception. Evaluation of motor function revealed weakness of the
biceps, triceps, arm abductors, hip flexors and quadriceps.
There were no joint abnormalities.   Laboratory studies revealed a normal hemogram and urinalysis. The erythrocyte
sedimentation rate was 56 mm/hr. The creatine phosphokinase
(CPK) was 1420 iu/l and the lactic dehydrogenase (LDH) was
800 iu/l.   Latex agglutinations for rheumatoid arthritis and
antinuclear antibody tests were negative.   Motor nerve conduction velocity in the right median nerve was normal. Electromyography revealed resting fibrillations and positive sharp
waves with increased polyphasic potentials.   Motor units were
reduced in amplitude.   The interference pattern was full but
reduced in amplitude.   Chest x-rays, an upper gastrointestinal
series, a barium enema and an intravenous pyelogram were
all normal.   A biopsy of the left vastus lateralis was performed.

QUESTIONS

1. The most likely clinical diagnosis is
    A. limb-girdle muscular dystrophy
    B. rheumatoid arthritis
    C. polymyositis
    D. trichinosis

2. Skin lesions are present in about 40% of patients with poly-
   myositis in which case the disease is called dermatomyo-
   sitis. The skin lesions include
   A. elevated red patches on elbows and proximal inter-
      phalangeal joints
   B. erythematous atrophic areas about nails and finger
      tips
   C. dusky, erythematous periorbital and malar eruptions
   D. dusky lilac suffusion of upper eyelids

3. Fig. 2.1 shows the histological findings in the muscle
   biopsy specimen. Morphological features of polymyositis
   that are illustrated include
   A. increased variation in the size of myofibers
   B. degenerating myofibers
   C. chronic inflammatory cell infiltration
   D. perifascicular atrophy

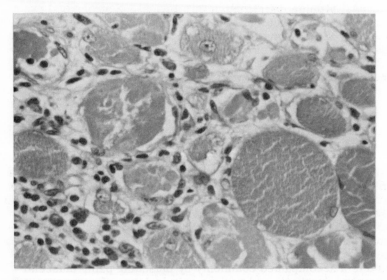

FIG. 2.1: Muscle biopsy specimen from a woman with poly-
         myositis.

4. The clinical evaluation of this patient included chest x-rays,
   upper and lower gastrointestinal series and a pyelogram.
   These were probably done because of
   A. signs and/or symptoms not included in the clinical
      abstract
   B. routine thorough examination of patients over age 40

    C. dysphagia suggesting additional disease of the gastro-
        intestinal system
    D. association between polymyositis and malignancies

5. Complications of polymyositis that are seen most often in
    children are
    A. calcinosis universalis
    B. gastrointestinal tract ulcerations
    C. hematuria
    D. epidermolysis

6. The prognosis for polymyositis is
    A. best among childhood cases
    B. best in adults with no latent neoplasm
    C. best in adults with resectable neoplasms
    D. equal in children and adults

7. The theories of pathogenesis include
    A. vitamin deficiency
    B. viral infection
    C. autoimmune phenomenon
    D. heavy metal intoxication

8. A granulomatous myositis is commonly encountered des-
    pite the absence of clinical manifestations implicating the
    muscles in
    A. Bornholm's disease
    B. cryptococcosis
    C. histoplasmosis
    D. sarcoidosis

ANSWERS AND DISCUSSION

1. (C) The clinical history, physical findings and results of
the laboratory studies are typical of polymyositis. This is a
diffuse inflammatory disease of skeletal muscle that causes
symmetrical, predominantly proximal, muscular weakness
and is a accompanied commonly by muscular pain, muscular
atrophy, dysphagia and various skin lesions. The disease
most commonly affects adult women but may occur at any age
in either sex. Skin lesions are often more pronounced in
children. The clinical course is variable. The serum muscle enzymes and erythrocyte sedimentation rate are generally
elevated. Electromyography may show both myopathic and
neurogenic features.

Limb-girdle dystrophy can cause the adult onset of weakness but would not be accompanied by the muscular pain, marked elevation in erythrocyte sedimentation rate and serum muscle enzymes. Rheumatoid arthritis would show more definite joint involvement and is commonly accompanied by positive latex agglutination test for the rheumatoid antibody. Trichinosis produces a more transient myositis.

2. (A, B, C, D) All of these skin lesions may be seen. The dusky lilac suffusion of the upper eyelids is called the "heliotrope rash" and is regarded by some workers as pathognomonic of dermatomyositis.

3. (A, B, C) The biopsy specimen shows changes that are typical of polymyositis. There is an increased variation in myofiber size but there are no excessively large myofibers as are seen in the muscular dystrophies. Myofiber degeneration is prominent and takes several forms including hyalinization, granular or floccular degeneration and occasionally vacuolar degeneration. Necrosis and myophagocytosis may be present. Regeneration, manifested by myofibers with amphophilic cytoplasm, is often prominent but is difficult to appreciate in the black and white photograph. Focal or diffuse inflammatory cell infiltrates are common and generally consist of lymphocytes, macrophages and plasma cells. Some specimens show myofiber atrophy that is especially prominent about the periphery of the fascicles. (Fig. 2.2) This is regarded as a significant histological feature but is not seen in all specimens.

4. (D) Malignant neoplasms are found in about 15% of all individuals with polymyositis and are present in nearly 50% of men who develop polymyositis when they are over 40 years old. Among the neoplasms are carcinomas of the lung, breast, colon and stomach. Removal of the malignancy may result in improvement in the myositis. Dysphagia is a common manifestation of the myositis due to involvement of the posterior pharyngeal and upper esophageal skeletal muscles and does not necessarily suggest additional gastrointestinal disease.

5. (A, B) Some children and young adults with dermatomyositis develop calcifications in the skin, subcutaneous tissues, skeletal muscles and periarticular structures. This usually occurs late in the course of the disease. Children occasionally have abdominal pain and gastrointestinal bleeding from ulcerations that are attributed to an associated inflammatory vasculitis.

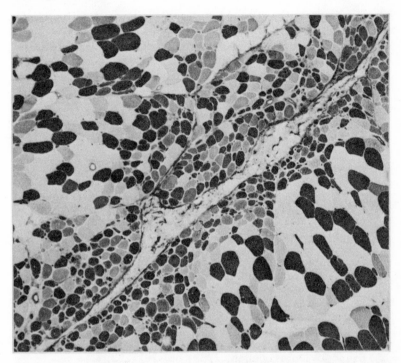

FIG. 2.2: Frozen section of muscle, stained by the ATP-ase
reaction at pH 4.3, showing perifascicular atrophy.

6. (A) It is generally agreed that the prognosis is better
among children than adults even when the patients with malignancies are excluded.

7. (B, C) The cause of polymyositis is unknown. Various
viral agents have been suspected but none have been proven to
be the etiological agent. Support for a viral pathogenesis was
provided by ultrastructural visualization of virus-like particles
in a few cases. However, no virus has actually been isolated.
An autoimmune basis has been suggested. Demonstration of
specific antibodies generally has been unsuccessful. Deposits
of globulins and complement have been demonstrated in the
walls of vessels, especially in children with dermatomyositis.
Experimentally cultured myocytes have been destroyed by
sensitized lymphocytes.

8. (D) Despite the absence of specific clinical manifestations, as many as 60% of patients with sarcoidosis have skeletal muscle involvement. The lesions are non-caseating granulomas that are often perivascular in location.

REFERENCES

1. Anonymous: Polymyositis and dermatomyositis. In: Primer on the rheumatic diseases. Rodnan GP (Ed.). JAMA 224:5 (Suppl): 717-719, 1973.

2. Bohnan A and Peter JB: Polymyositis and dermatomyositis. N Eng J Med 292:344-347, 403-407, 1975.

3. Brooke MH: A Clinician's View of Neuromuscular Diseases. Williams and Wilkins Co., Baltimore, 1977, pp. 138-152.

4. Carpenter S, et al.: The childhood type of dermatomyositis. Neurology 26:952-962, 1976.

5. Devere A and Bradley WG: Polymyositis: Its presentation, morbidity and mortality. Brain 98:637-666, 1975.

6. Dubowitz V: Muscle Disorders in Childhood. W.B. Saunders Co., London, 1978, pp. 202-222.

7. Dubowitz V and Brooke MH: Muscle Biopsy: A Modern Approach, W.B. Saunders Co., London, 1973, pp. 316-346.

: :

CASE 3: A 17-Year-Old with Severe Episodic Weakness and
         Paralysis

CLINICAL DATA

This 17-year-old boy was admitted to the hospital for evaluation
of an 18-month history of recurrent episodes of weakness and
paralysis. Since their onset, he had had about 15 episodes of
paralysis and numerous bouts of weakness. The attacks usually
occurred at night often following a day of strenuous exercise.
He would be awakened by aching of his arms and legs. This
was followed by weakness that often progressed to total paralysis except for speaking, swallowing and breathing. The paralysis would last up to 16 hours. This was followed by a gradual
return of strength accompanied by increased muscular pain.
During the attacks, sensation remained normal. There was no
family history of a similar disorder.

The initial physical examination was normal except for mild
muscular tenderness. All clinical laboratory determinations,
including thyroid function studies, were within normal limits.
While hospitalized, he experienced a spontaneous episode of
paralysis during which time reflexes were absent. Myotonia
could not be elicited. A serum potassium level measured during the attack was 2.2 mEq/l. The electrocardiogram showed
changes consistent with hypokalemia. An electromyogram
showed electrical silence in the still paralyzed muscles.

Subsequently, a muscle biopsy was performed during a period
of mild weakness induced with glucose and insulin.

QUESTIONS

1. The most appropriate diagnosis in this case is
    A. myasthenia gravis
    B. hysteria
    C. hypokalemic periodic paralysis
    D. McArdle's syndrome

2. Fig. 3.1 shows the histological alterations encountered in
    the muscle biopsy specimen. Which of the following changes
    are illustrated?
    A. Target fibers
    B. Nemaline bodies
    C. Vacuolization of myofibers
    D. Fascicular atrophy

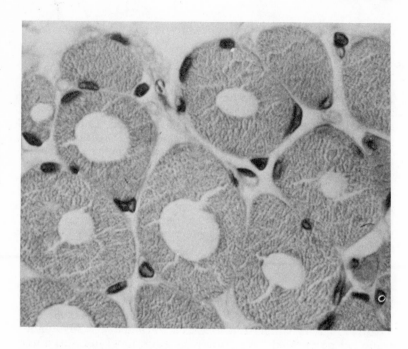

FIG. 3.1: Transverse section of the muscle biopsy specimen stained with hematoxylin and eosin.

3. FIG. 3.2 is an electron micrograph prepared from the same biopsy specimen. Which of the following changes are illustrated?
    A. Vacuolization of the myofiber
    B. Continuity of the vacuole with the T-tubules
    C. Dilatation of the sarcoplasmic reticulum
    D. Excessive glycogen deposits

4. Which of the following characterize hyperkalemic periodic paralysis?
    A. Onset during rest following exercise
    B. Elevated serum potassium during the attacks
    C. Myotonia
    D. Rapid onset, short duration and rapid abatement of the weakness

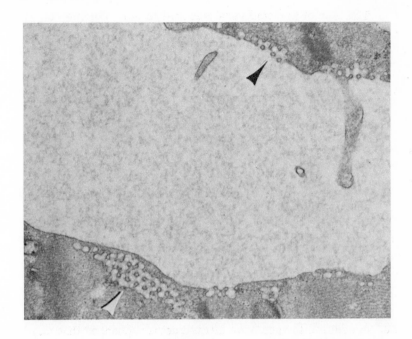

FIG. 3.2: Electron micrograph prepared from the muscle biopsy specimen. Note the large vacuole, the so-called
"honeycomb" arrays of tubules (white arrow) and the
continuity between the "honeycomb" array and the
vacuole (black arrow).

5. Which of the following characterize the periodic paralysis
   associated with thyrotoxicosis?
   A. Serum potassium is reduced during attacks
   B. Strong family history
   C. More common among Japanese
   D. Disappears with correction of thyroid activity

6. A patient with hypokalemic periodic paralysis may
   A. have fewer attacks with the passage of time
   B. develop a permanent myopathy
   C. die during an attack
   D. develop hyperkalemic periodic paralysis

7. The type of periodic paralysis that is most common is
   A. normokalemic periodic paralysis
   B. hyperkalemic periodic paralysis
   C. familial hypokalemic periodic paralysis
   D. periodic paralysis associated with hyperthyroidism

8. Hypokalemic periodic paralysis is currently regarded as
   the result of
   A. adrenocortical hypersecretion
   B. a disorder of carbohydrate metabolism
   C. a disorder of myofiber organelles
   D. a disorder of hypothalamic electrolyte regulation

9. The roles of the sarcoplasmic reticulum in the contraction
   and relaxation muscle are to
   A. take up calcium from the surrounding medium in the
      presence of ATP
   B. release calcium in response to action potentials trans-
      mitted by the T-system
   C. interact with myosin to produce shortening of the
      myofibers
   D. generate ATP

10. In addition to vacuoles, ultrastructural changes that may
    be encountered in muscle biopsy specimens from patients
    with hyperkalemic periodic paralysis include
    A. nemaline bodies
    B. aggregates of elongated straight tubules
    C. aggregates of filaments
    D. lysis of thin filaments

ANSWERS AND DISCUSSION

1. (C) The periodic paralyses are characterized by recurrent
episodes of weakness and paralysis. In hypokalemic periodic
paralysis, the attacks are accompanied by a decrease in the
serum potassium level and electrocardiographic evidence of
hypokalemia. The condition is usually familial, inherited as
an autosomal dominant trait. This patient was one of the less
common sporadic cases. The symptoms usually become manifested during the second decade. In a typical attack, the muscles of the trunk and extremities become weak or paralyzed
while speech, swallowing and respiration are relatively spared.
The paralyzed muscles are electrically silent. The attacks
usually begin at night or during a prolonged period of rest following strenuous exercise or after a high carbohydrate meal.

During the attacks, urine output is often reduced and is followed
by diuresis during recovery. Most patients are normal between
attacks but some show a progressive myopathy after repeated
episodes.

Patients suspected of having hypokalemic periodic paralysis
must be examined for thyrotoxicosis and for aldosteronism or
renal tubular acidosis which may produce secondary hypokalemic periodic paralysis. Some patients with periodic paralysis
initially have been labeled erroneously as hysterical. This can
be avoided by observing the attacks and obtaining appropriate
laboratory studies during the paralytic episodes. Myasthenia
gravis commonly presents with involvement of the extraocular
and bulbar muscles. Characteristically, the weakness is
greatest in the evening after exercise and improves with rest.
Tendon reflexes tend to be preserved. The diagnosis can be
substantiated with a Tensilon test. McArdle's syndrome is
characterized by muscular weakness and cramping following
moderately severe muscular exertion. The diagnosis can be
supported by demonstration of an unchanged venous lactate
level during an ischemic exercise test.

2.   (C) The photograph shows marked vacuolization of myofibers. This change is typically seen in muscle biopsy specimens from patients with hypokalemic periodic paralysis and
in the periodic paralysis associated with thyrotoxicosis. The
vacuolization may be more florid if the biopsy is performed
during an episode of weakness. Hyperkalemic and normokalemic periodic paralyses usually show far fewer vacuoles.
The vacuoles tend to be centrally located and extend for a considerable distance along the length of the myofiber. Unfortunately vacuoles are by no means pathognomonic of the periodic
paralyses. Among the other disorders that must be included
in the differential diagnosis of a vacuolar myopathy are glycogenoses type II, III, V and VII, paroxysmal myoglobinuria,
lipid storage myopathy and myositis associated with collagen
vascular diseases.

The illustrated myofibers show only the normal variation in
diameter; there are no groups of small angular myofibers,
i.e., fascicular atrophy. Target fibers are not seen but are
rather poorly demonstrated by the hematoxylin and eosin
stain and may be overlooked unless the trichrome or phosphotungstic acid-hematoxylin (P.T.A.H.) stains are also
utilized. When present these two alterations are indicative of
denervation.

Nemaline bodies are rod-like structures that are in continuity with and composed of Z-disc material. They may appear as eosinophilic structures with hematoxylin and eosin but are better demonstrated with the P.T.A.H. stain. When numerous, they are a manifestation of nemaline myopathy, a rare congenital myopathy.

3.   (A, B) The electron micrograph illustrates a large vacuole within a myofiber. The vacuole communicates with an elaborate tubular network (black arrow) that is derived from the T-tubules. According to Engel's work, the vacuoles in hypokalemic periodic paralysis begin as dilatations of the sarcoplasmic reticulum. Subsequently, the membranes of the T-system proliferate and trap the evolving vacuoles. The mature vacuoles limited by membranes derived from the T-tubules are in continuity with the honeycomb arrays derived from the T-tubules. Excess glycogen particles are not present. The finely granular material within the vacuole may be a proteinaceous precipitate.

4.   (A, B, C, D) The attacks of hyperkalemic periodic paralysis typically begin during a period of rest following strenuous exercise, but are not precipitated by high carbohydrate meals. The attacks are accompanied by mild elevation of the serum potassium and may be induced by ingestion of potassium compounds. The paralysis is less severe, tends to develop more rapidly, lasts for a shorter period of time and abates more rapidly than in hypokalemic periodic paralysis. Many of the patients display myotonia, demonstrable by physical examination or electromyography.

5.   (A, C, D) The attack of periodic paralysis in thyrotoxicosis is precipitated by rest after exercise or excess carbohydrates and is accompanied by a decline in the serum potassium. The periodic paralysis associated with hyperthyroidism is never familial, tends to be more common among the Japanese and disappears with correction of the thyroid hyperactivity.

6.   (A, B, C) The attacks tend to be most frequent during early adult life. In many patients, especially women, they become progressively less frequent and eventually disappear. On the other hand, some patients develop permanent myopathic weakness and a few, about 10%, die during an attack.

7.   (C) Familial hypokalemic periodic paralysis is the most common type of periodic paralysis. Hyperkalemic and normokalemic periodic paralyses are quite rare. Periodic paralysis associated with hyperthyroidism is encountered predominantly among the Japanese.

8. (C) Many theories have been proposed regarding the pathogenesis of hypokalemic periodic paralysis. Intermittent hypersecretion of aldosterone has been suggested; however, there is
no consistent relation between the paralysis and retention of
sodium. The precipitation of attacks by high carbohydrate
meals has led to the suggestion that this disorder may be due
to a defect in carbohydrate metabolism. This hypothesis has
not been confirmed. Many workers now feel that the basic abnormality is within the myofiber, possibly dysfunction of the
sarcoplasmic reticulum.

9. (A, B) In response to an action potential transmitted by the
T-tubule, the sarcoplasmic reticulum releases calcium into the
sarcoplasm. There the calcium is bound to troponin, a component of the thin filaments and induces contraction of the myofiber.
Relaxation is achieved at least in part, by the removal of the calcium by the sarcoplasmic reticulum in the presence of ATP.

10. (B, C) Aggregates of elongated straight tubules and aggregates of filaments, the so-called filamentous bodies have
been observed in a number of cases of hyperkalemic periodic paralysis. Neither of these structures is unique to this disorder.

REFERENCES

1. Engel AG: Vacuolar Myopathies: Multiple Etiologies and
   Sequential Structural Studies. In: The Striated Muscle.
   Pearson CM and Mostofi FK (Eds.). Williams and Wilkins
   Co., Baltimore, 1973, pp. 301-341.

2. Engel AG: Hypokalemic and Hyperkalemic Periodic Paralyses. In: Scientific Approaches to Clinical Neurology.
   Goldensohn ES and Appel SH (Eds.). Lea and Febiger,
   1977, pp. 1742-1765.

3. Ionasescu V, et al.: Biochemical abnormalities of muscle
   ribosomes during attacks of hyperkalemic period paralysis.
   J Neurol Sci 19:389-398, 1973.

4. Ionasescu V, et al.: Hypokalemic periodic paralysis. J
   Neurol Sci 21:419-429, 1974.

5. Pearson CM: The Periodic Paralyses. In: Handbook of
   Clinical Neurology. Vinken PJ and Bruyn GW (Eds.).
   North-Holland, Amsterdam, 1976, Vol. 28, pp. 581-601.

6. Pearson CM and Kalyanaraman K: The Periodic Paralyses.
   In: The Metabolic Basis of Inherited Disease. Stanbury JB,
   et al. (Eds.). McGraw-Hill, New York, 1972, pp. 1181-1203.
: :

CASE 4: A Weak, Hypotonic Infant with Normal Serum Muscle
Enzymes

CLINICAL DATA

This 2-week-old male infant was the product of a full term gestation and an uncomplicated delivery. However, during the last
two months of her pregnancy, the mother had no longer felt fetal
movements. At birth, the child weighed six pounds, was pro-
foundly limp and had a poor cry. He could not suck well and had
to be fed by gavage.

When examined, the child seemed normally alert but was extremely limp, symmetrically weak and diffusely areflexic. His
legs assumed a frog-like posture but there were no joint contractures. He cried appropriately upon painful stimulation but
the cry was weak and accompanied by minimal facial movements. He exhibited a full range of extraocular movements
and normal pupillary reactions. The remainder of the physical
examination was normal except for occasional scattered rales.
All clinical laboratory determinations were within normal
limits. An electromyogram and nerve conduction studies were
interpreted as consistent with denervation due to anterior horn
cell disease. A muscle biopsy was performed to confirm the
clinical impression.

QUESTIONS

1. The most appropriate clinical diagnosis is
    A. Werdnig-Hoffmann's disease
    B. Zellweger's syndrome
    C. Pompe's disease
    D. centronuclear myopathy

2. The histological characteristics of muscle biopsy specimens
    from patients with Werdnig-Hoffmann's disease include
    A. angular atrophic myofibers
    B. rounded atrophic myofibers
    C. occasional hypertrophied myofibers
    D. increased endomysial connective tissue

3. Which of the following are the histochemical character-
    istics of muscle biopsy specimens from patients with
    Werdnig-Hoffmann's disease?
    A. Atrophic myofibers are both type 1 and type 2
    B. Atrophic myofibers are type 1 only

C. Atrophic myofibers are type 2 only
D. Hypertrophied myofibers are generally type 1

4. The histopathological changes in the central nervous system of patients with Werdnig-Hoffmann's disease include
    A. loss of motor neurons from the anterior horns of the spinal cord
    B. loss of motor neurons from the hypoglossal nucleus
    C. demyelination of the corticospinal tracts
    D. atrophy of the dorsal spinal roots

5. The incidence of Werdnig-Hoffmann's disease is approximately
    A. 400/100,000
    B. 40/100,000
    C. 4/100,000
    D. 0.4/100,000

6. Kugelberg-Welander's disease is
    A. a slowly progressive form of spinal muscular atrophy
    B. a congenital variant of Werdnig-Hoffmann's disease
    C. characterized histologically by group atrophy with rounded and angular myofibers
    D. a milder form of sex-linked muscular dystrophy

ANSWERS AND DISCUSSION

1. (A) The most appropriate clinical diagnosis is Werdnig-Hoffmann's disease. Weakness and hypotonia in infancy, the so-called "floppy infant" syndrome can result from numerous disorders of the central nervous system, the peripheral nervous system or the muscles or it can be a manifestation of certain systemic diseases. Infants with both profound weakness and hypotonia are more likely to have a neuromuscular disorder than infants in whom hypotonia is out of proportion to the weakness. Among the neuromuscular disorders with an early onset, Werdnig-Hoffmann's disease is the most common. This is an autosomal recessive form of spinal muscular atrophy. The disorder begins prenatally, as in the present case, or during the first few years of life. The weakness initially affects the legs, subsequently involves the back, neck, shoulders and arms and finally extends to the muscles of deglutition. The diaphragm is relatively spared. Muscular atrophy and fasciculations may be obscured by the subcutaneous fat. The disease progresses relentlessly and the patients die of respiratory complications within a few months of onset.

Zellweger's syndrome (see Case 66) is characterized by profound hypotonia, hyporeflexia, weakness and seizures. These
neurological manifestations are accompanied by a distinctive
craniofacial configuration, hepatosplenomegaly and a bleeding
diathesis.

Pompe's disease may produce weakness and hypotonia but
cardiomegaly, hepatomegaly and congestive heart failure are
concomitant manifestations.

Centronuclear myopathy has been regarded as one of the so-
called "congenital myopathies." In about two-thirds of the
cases, hypotonia becomes manifested during the neonatal period. The course of the disease is variable with most of the
patients showing slow, insidious progression of muscular
weakness. Ptosis, external ophthalmoplegia, facial diplegia
and weakness of masticatory muscle are common features.
Electromyography is inconclusive. This rare condition can
be diagnosed with certainty only by muscle biopsy. The biopsy
specimen shows centrally placed nuclei accompanied by a perinuclear clear zone in the majority of the myofibers. The condition is genetically heterogeneous.

2. (B, C) Histologically, Werdnig-Hoffmann's disease is characterized by numerous fascicles of severely atrophic myofibers
(Fig. 4.1). Unlike other forms of neurogenic atrophy, however,
the atrophic myofibers are rounded rather than angular. Occasional large hypertrophied fibers are seen scattered among the
atrophic fibers. Target fibers are not present. The endomysial connective tissue is not significantly increased in
quantity but the paramysial connective tissue appears more
abundant.

3. (A, D) Histochemical evaluation of muscle biopsy specimens from patients with Werdnig-Hoffmann's disease has shown
that the atrophic myofibers are both type 1 and type 2 fibers.
The scattered hypertrophied myofibers are generally type 1
fibers; however, some authors have also described hypertrophied type 2 fibers.

Preferential atrophy of type 1 fibers in the adult is associated
with myotonic dystrophy. In some patients with centronuclear
myopathy, "hypotrophy" of type 1 fibers has been described.
Preferential atrophy of type 2 fibers in the adult is correlated
with disuse atrophy.

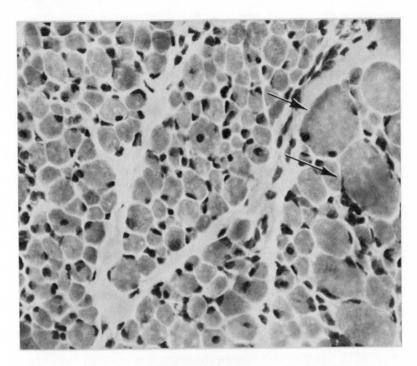

FIG. 4.1: Frozen section of muscle biopsy specimen showing small rounded myofibers and scattered hypertrophied myofibers (arrows).

4. (A, B) Histopathological study of the central nervous system from patients with Werdnig-Hoffmann disease has disclosed changes in the spinal cord and brain stem. In the spinal cord, these changes consist of loss of motor neurons from the anterior horns especially in the lumbar and cervical enlargements. Comparison with age-matched control sections of corresponding levels facilitates recognition of these losses. The remaining motor neurons in the anterior horns have been described as chromatolytic, ballooned or shrunken, however, these changes are usually inconspicuous. The anterior horns may become gliotic and contain a few scattered macrophages. The ventral roots usually become obviously shrunken while the dorsal or posterior roots remain unaltered. The long tracts within the spinal cord such as the corticospinal tracts remain unaffected. Within the brain stem loss of motor neurons can

be detected in various cranial nerve nuclei including the hypoglossal nucleus. An electron microscopic study by Chou and
Fakadej has demonstrated glial hyperplasia in anterior spinal
and cranial nerve roots. These authors suggested that glial
proliferation in the nerve roots was the basic pathological process in Werdnig-Hoffmann's disease. Others have considered
degeneration of the motor neurons as the primary process.

5.   (C) Epidemiologists use the terms incidence and prevalence in a precisely defined fashion. Incidence means the number of new cases per 100,000 people per year. Prevalence
means the number of cases per 100,000 people on a given day.
The incidence of Werdnig-Hoffmann's disease is approximately
4/100,000.

6.   (A, C) Kugelberg-Welander's disease is a juvenile, slowly
progressive form of spinal muscular atrophy. The weakness
mainly affects the proximal muscles of the lower limbs. The
condition is genetically heterogeneous with most cases inherited
as an autosomal recessive trait but others inherited as an autosomal dominant trait. Histologically, the muscle shows group
atrophy with both rounded and angular myofibers. The hypertrophied fibers characteristic of Werdnig-Hoffmann's disease
are not found in this condition.

REFERENCES

1.   Brooke MH: A Clinician's View of Neuromuscular Dis-
     eases. Williams and Wilkins Co., Baltimore, 1977,
     pp. 34-44.

2.   Chou SM and Fakadej AV: Ultrastructure of chromato-
     lytic motorneurons and anterior spinal roots in a case of
     Werdnig-Hoffmann's disease. J Neuropath Exp Neurol
     30:368-379, 1971.

3.   Dubowitz V and Brooke MH: Muscle Biopsy: A Modern
     Approach. W.B. Saunders Co., London, 1973, pp. 148-
     167.

4.   Schochet SS Jr, et al.: Centronuclear myopathy: Disease
     entity or a syndrome? J Neurol Sci 16:215-228, 1972.

: :

CASE 5: A 34-Year-Old Farmer with Difficulty Performing
his Chores

CLINICAL DATA

This 34-year-old farmer was admitted for evaluation of the
complaint that he was now having more difficulty performing
his chores than a year ago. He complained of stiffness in his
hands, especially in cold weather. However, he could drink
cold liquids and eat ice cream without adverse effects. The
family history was significant in that the patient's father has
myotonic dystrophy and was unable to walk at the age of
59.

Physical examination revealed a cooperative man with a high
school education. Frontal baldness was pronounced. His face
was mask-like with hollow temples and cheeks. The masseter
and temporalis muscles were moderately atrophic. No myotonia was noted on eye closure and no lid lag was evident. The
extraocular movements, tongue movements, swallowing and
palatal movements were normal. He walked, climbed stairs
and hopped without difficulty. Strength and reflexes in the
lower extremities were normal. His deltoid muscles were
slightly atrophic, but he had normal strength in his biceps and
triceps. There was mild weakness of the forearm extensors
and his grip was weak with delayed relaxation. The greatest
weakness was noted in the neck flexors. The remainder of the
physical examination was normal. An electrocardiogram was
normal. Slit lamp examination revealed posterior subcapsu-
lar opacities. Electromyography of the right first dorsal in-
terosseous muscle revealed increased insertional activity and
myotonic discharges. Motor nerve conduction velocities were
normal. Serum immunoelectrophoresis was normal. Creatine
phosphokinase and aldolase levels were normal. The right
deltoid muscle was biopsied in order to confirm the clinical
diagnosis.

QUESTIONS

1. The most appropriate clinical diagnosis for this patient is
    A. myasthenia gravis
    B. myotonic dystrophy
    C. oculopharyngeal dystrophy
    D. facioscapulohumeral dystrophy

2. Myotonic dystrophy is inherited
   A. as an autosomal recessive trait
   B. as an autosomal dominant trait
   C. as an X-linked recessive trait
   D. variably in different kindred

3. Fig. 5.1 is a photograph of a section prepared from the muscle biopsy specimen. It shows
   A. excessive variation in myofiber size
   B. clumps of pycnotic nuclei
   C. myofiber splitting
   D. excessive internal nuclei

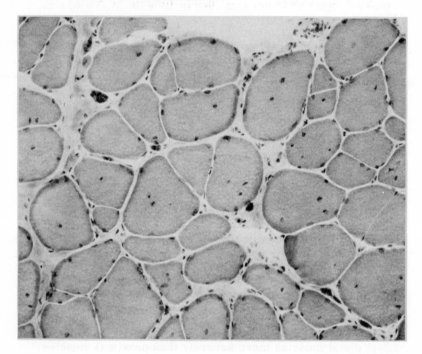

FIG. 5.1: Frozen section of the deltoid muscle biopsy specimen.

4. Features commonly observed by electron microscopy in muscle biopsy specimens from patients with myotonic dystrophy include
   A. sarcoplasmic masses
   B. internal nuclei
   C. "honeycomb" tubular arrays
   D. nemaline rods

5. Clinical laboratory procedures that may reveal abnormal-
    ities in patients with myotonic dystrophy include
    A. determination of serum muscle enzymes
    B. serum immunoelectrophoresis
    C. determination of serum electrolytes
    D. glucose tolerance test

6. Patients with myotonic dystrophy are prone to
    A. cardiac arrhythmias
    B. untoward reactions to anesthetics
    C. dislocation of the lens
    D. rupture of aortic aneurysms

7. The pathophysiological basis for myotonic dystrophy is
    A. an abnormality of nerve conduction
    B. an abnormality of neuromuscular transmission
    C. an abnormality of muscular contraction
    D. unknown

8. Infantile myotonic dystrophy is characterized by
    A. difficulty in sucking and swallowing
    B. facial diplegia
    C. generalized hypotonia
    D. talipes equinovarus

ANSWERS AND DISCUSSION

1. (B) The history, physical findings and the results of the
laboratory studies are indicative of myotonic dystrophy. This
is an hereditary myopathy that is characterized by slowly progressive muscular weakness, wasting and mytonia and is accompanied by a wide variety of associated lesions involving
multiple organ systems. The weakness and atrophy tend to be
most pronounced in the muscles of the head and neck such as
the temporales, masseters, and neck flexors. Involvement of
the oropharyngeal muscles may produce dysarthria and dysphagia. The weakness and atrophy in the extremities tend to
affect distal muscles more severely than proximal muscles.
This is in contrast to the pattern usually seen with true dystrophies. The weakness and atrophy are slowly progressive
and may severely incapacitate the patient during late adult life.

The myotonia is usually less of a handicap for the patient but is
an important diagnostic feature. Involvement of the hand and
forearm muscles permit the astute clinician to diagnose the
condition while shaking hands with his patient. It can also be
demonstrated as an inability to fully open tightly closed eyelids

and as a lid-lag on sudden eye movements. Percussion myotonia
can be demonstrated by percussing the tongue or muscles of the
extremities.

The associated lesions are numerous. The myocardium is affected in about 75% of the patients and is manifested as dys-
rhythmias or other electrocardiographic abnormalities. Cataracts can be demonstrated by slit-lamp examination in virtually
every patient. They may be the first or only manifestation of
the disorder. Frontal baldness is common and along with the
muscular atrophy and weakness, contribute to the characteristic facial appearance. This has been described as "hatchet
faced." The mouth often hangs open and the lips form an in-
verted "V." A number of endocrine abnormalities are commonly encountered. Hypogonadism is manifested by testicular
atrophy in men and by menstrual abnormalities in women.
Both sexes show diminished fertility. Thyroid function is often
depressed. Low intelligence and deviant behavior are common
among these patients.

A similar facial appearance can be found in patients with oculo-
pharyngeal and facioscapulohumeral dystrophies but these conditions lack the myotonia. Myasthenia gravis may also produce a similar facial appearance but shows a characteristic
progressive muscular fatiguing and responds to anticholinesterase compounds.

2. (B) Myotonic dystrophy is inherited as an autosomal dominant trait. There is marked variation in severity and many
cases are subclinical unless carefully studied. Cataracts,
demonstrable only by slit-lamp examination, may be the only
manifestation of the disease.

3. (A, B, C, D) This muscle biopsy specimen is characteristic
of myotonic dystrophy. It shows marked variation in myofiber
size, numerous internal nuclei, fiber splitting and some clumps
of pycnotic nuclei. Histochemical evaluation showed preferential atrophy of the type 1 myofibers.

The histopathological findings in muscle biopsy specimens from
patients with myotonic dystrophy vary with the duration and the
severity of the disease. Preferential atrophy of the type 1 myofibers may be the most conspicuous feature in specimens from
children and young adults with this disease. The mildly atrophic type 1 myofibers often contain internal nuclei, even before
they are conspicuously increased in the type 2 fibers. As the

disease progresses, fiber splitting, small angular myofibers
and clumps of pycnotic nuclei become more pronounced. Type
2 fibers may hypertrophy and accentuate the variation in myofiber size. Additional features that may be seen include ring
fibers and sarcoplasmic pads. Ring fibers result from peripheral myofibrils that are oriented perpendicular to the long
axis of the myofiber. They are common in, but not specific
for myotonic dystrophy. Sarcoplasmic pads are pale areas that
appear to be devoid of myofibrils.

Late in the course of the disease, endomysial fibrosis and adipose replacement may become prominent. It has been reported
that muscle spindles from patients with myotonic dystrophy contain an excessive number of intrafusal fibers.

4.   (A, B, C) Electron microscopy of muscle biopsy specimens from patients with myotonic dystrophy confirms changes
noted by light microscopy such as the internal nuclei and ring
fibers. The sarcoplasmic pads or masses are subsarcolemmal areas in which these are collections of glycogen granules,
mitochondria and lysosomes. The myofibrils are fragmented
or absent in these areas. Elsewhere in the myofibers, "honeycomb" arrays of tubules derived from the T-tubules may be
conspicuous. None of these changes are pathognomonic.

5.   (A, B, D) Serum muscle enzymes are normal in the majority of patients with myotonic dystrophy. Only rarely are
they significantly elevated. Serum immunoelectrophoresis
often shows decreases in the globulins, especially IgG. This
reduction is attributed to an accelerated catabolism of the globulins. Glucose tolerance tests are occasionally abnormal.
Serum electrolytes are unaffected.

6.   (A, B) The heart is involved in over 50% of patients with
myotonic dystrophy. This involvement can be detected by
electrocardiography and may lead to arrhythmias or sudden
death. Patients with myotonic dystrophy often react unpre-
dictably toward anesthetic agents. Even a history of tolerating
a previous anesthetic does not indicate that a future exposure
will be tolerated. Local anesthetics should be used whenever
possible.

7.   (D) The pathophysiological basis for myotonic dystrophy
is unknown. The selective atrophy of type 1 myofibers, the
occurrence of small angular myofibers and abnormalities in
nerve terminals demonstrated by supravital staining are among
the features on which a defect in neural control has been

postulated by some authors. The fact that curare does not affect the myotonia suggests that there is also a defect in the
myofiber itself. The disease is clearly quite unlike the usual
muscular dystrophies and the designation "myotonic atrophy"
is probably more desirable than "myotonic dystrophy." The
pathogenetic mechanism must also account for the numerous
non-muscular aberrations encountered in this disease.

8. (A, B, C, D) Infantile myotonic dystrophy shows a number
of features that are somewhat different from myotonic dystrophy in the adult. Prominent manifestations in the infantile
cases are generalized hypotonia, facial diplegia, difficulties
with sucking and swallowing and talipes equinovarus. The hypotonia may be quite severe and the disease must be considered
among the causes of the "floppy infant syndrome." Myotonia
and the usual morphological manifestations of myotonic dystrophy may not be evident for several years. Virtually all
cases of infantile myotonic dystrophy have a mother who is affected with myotonic dystrophy. The basis for this sex link-
age is unknown.

REFERENCES

1. Brooke MH: A Clinician's View of Neuromuscular Diseases. Williams and Wilkins Co., Baltimore, 1977, pp.
   126-134.

2. Drachman, DB and Fambrough DM: Are muscle fibers
   denervated in myotonic dystrophy? Arch Neurol 33:485-
   488, 1976.

3. Dubowitz V and Brooke MH: Muscle Biopsy: A Modern
   Approach. W.B. Saunders Co., London, 1973, pp.
   213-230.

4. Karpati G, et al.: Infantile mytonic dystrophy. Neurology
   23:1066-1077, 1973.

5. Zellweger H and Ionasescu V: Myotonic dystrophy and its
   differential diagnosis. Acta Neurol Scand (Suppl 55)
   49:1-28, 1973.

: :

CASE 6: A Young Woman with Weakness, Ophthalmoplegia
         and Heart Block

CLINICAL DATA

This 18-year-old woman was admitted to the hospital for evaluation of ophthalmoplegia and progressive muscular weakness.
At the age of six, she was noted to squint and was given glasses.
At seven, she complained of double vision that gradually resolved spontaneously. She did reasonably well until her
early teens when she found herself unable to compete with
other children at play or in physical education.   Approximately one year prior to this hospital admission, double
vision recurred but again spontaneously improved. For the
past six months she complained of progressive generalized
weakness and has difficulty rising from a seated to standing
position.

Physical examination revealed a short young woman with ptosis
and paucity of spontaneous facial expressions. Eye movements
were virtually absent in all directions. The pupils responded
to light. The visual fields were full to confrontation but her
visual acuity was reduced even with correction. Her fundi
showed pigmentary degeneration. No cataracts were present.
Hearing was normal and her sensory perception was intact.
There was questionable cerebellar ataxia. Weakness was most
pronounced in the neck muscles and in the proximal leg muscles. The deep tendon reflexes were reduced. No myotonia
could be elicited by percussion or detected by electromyography. There was no response to a Tensilon test. An
electrocardiogram demonstrated incomplete heart block. Serum
muscle enzymes were within normal limits. Thyroid function studies revealed no abnormalities. A muscle biopsy
was performed.

QUESTIONS

1. The clinical data are consistent with a diagnosis of
    A. myasthenia gravis
    B. Kearns-Shy syndrome
    C. Graves' disease
    D. centronuclear myopathy

2. Muscle biopsy specimens from patients with this disorder
    show few or no conspicuous abnormalities when paraffin
    embedded sections are examined. However, frozen sec-
    tions stained with the modified trichrome stain show
    A. nemaline bodies
    B. "ragged-red" fibers
    C. abundant internal nuclei
    D. central cores

3. Ultrastructural findings in muscle biopsy specimens from
    patients with this condition include
    A. vacuoles derived from the T-tubules
    B. increased glycogen
    C. Z-disc streaming
    D. Intramitochondrial paracrystalline inclusions

4. Paracrystalline mitochondrial inclusions are
    A. pathognomonic of the Kearns-Shy syndrome
    B. confined to skeletal muscle
    C. found in a wide variety of neuromuscular disorders
    D. found only in adults

5. The reported cases of the Kearns-Shy syndrome suggest
    that the disorder occurs
    A. sporadically
    B. as an autosomal dominant trait
    C. as a sex-linked recessive trait
    D. as an autosomal recessive trait

ANSWERS AND DISCUSSION

1. (B) The clinical data are consistent with a diagnosis of the
Kearns-Shy syndrome. Karpati et al. introduced this eponym
to designate an ill-defined syndrome that is characterized most
often by ptosis, extraocular muscle weakness or ophthalmoplegia, pigmentary degeneration of the retina, heart block and
ataxia. Variable features include muscle weakness, deafness,
small stature and mental retardation. The clinical onset of the
disorder varies from childhood to adult life. Clinical laboratory studies reveal a normal to moderately elevated cerebrospinal fluid protein level and normal to mildly elevated serum
muscle enzymes.

Myasthenia gravis is reasonably eliminated by the lack of response to a Tensilon test. Graves' disease can be eliminated
by adequate tests of thyroid function. Centronuclear myopathy
is not accompanied by the pigmentary degeneration of the retina
or the cardiac conduction defects. Myotonic dystrophy is eliminated from consideration by the absence of myotonia.

2. (B) In frozen sections stained with the modified trichrome stain, the so-called "ragged-red" fibers can be seen in muscle biopsy specimens from patients with the Kearns-Shy syndrome. The "ragged-red" fibers are characterized by subsarcolemmal and intermyofibrillar deposits of red staining granular material that stand out in contrast to the green myofibers. The abnormal myofibers vary in number from few (1%) to many (25%). By the use of serial sections, the "ragged-red" fibers have been shown to be predominantly type 1 myofibers. The abnormal fibers contain increased quantities of lipid as shown by staining with oil-red-O. This myofiber alteration is characteristic but not pathognomonic of the Kearns-Shy syndrome since occasional "ragged-red" fibers can be encountered in a variety of other conditions. In the paraffin-embedded sections, the "ragged-red" fibers are generally not detectable. Occasionally the fibers may appear somewhat granular and basophilic with hematoxylin-eosin or irregularly stained about the periphery with a modified phosphotungstic acid hematoxylin stain (P. T. A. H.) (Fig. 6.1).

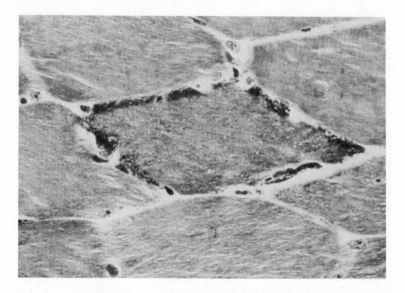

FIG. 6. 1: Paraffin-embedded muscle from a patient with Kearns-Shy syndrome. The section has been stained with a modified phosphotungstic acid hematoxylin technique. Note the dark-stained granular material about the periphery of the muscle fiber in the center of the photograph.

With the modified trichrome stain on frozen sections, nemaline bodies appear as red-staining rods arising from the Z-discs. In paraffin-embedded sections, nemaline rods are best demonstrated with P. T. A. H. stains. They are characteristic of nemaline myopathy, a slowly or non-progressive myopathy that results in weakness and hypotonia. Occasional nemaline bodies can be seen in other conditions such as denervation. Central cores when numerous are characteristic of central core disease, another slowly or non-progressive myopathy. They are readily demonstrated by oxidative enzyme stains on frozen sections or by the trichrome stain on paraffin-embedded sections. Internal nuclei can be seen in a wide variety of circumstances. An occasional internal nucleus can be encountered in normal muscle. When more abundant, they are suggestive of a myopathy and when very abundant and in long chains, are suggestive of myotonic dystrophy. It must also be remembered that internal nuclei are normally abundant adjacent to fascial or tendinous insertions.

3.   (B, D) The most striking ultrastructural abnormalities in this disorder involve the mitochondria. Some of the mitochondria are enlarged, some have concentrically oriented cristae and characteristically, some contain distinctive paracrystalline inclusions (Fig. 6.2). The paracrystalline inclusions vary in appearance depending upon the plane of section. When seen in longitudinal section, they appear as sets of four parallel lines with small projections about every 10 nm. When seen on end, they again appear as four parallel lines with small projections. These lines have been interpreted by Karpati et al. as the boundaries of parallel plates with alternating surface projections. Collections of abnormal mitochondria are most often encountered just beneath the sarcolemma. In addition to the paracrystalline inclusions, the abnormal myofibers contain increased numbers of lipid droplets and glycogen granules.

4.   (C) Occasional paracrystalline mitochondrial inclusions have been found in a wide variety of unrelated neuromuscular disorders including muscular dystrophy, amyotrophic lateral sclerosis, polymyositis, myotonic dystrophy, periodic paralysis, steroid myopathy, thyroid myopathy, and certain congenital myopathies. The paracrystalline inclusions alone are not pathognomonic for the Kearns-Shy syndrome but are highly significant when considered in conjunction with the clinical and histological data. Furthermore, in the Kearns-Shy syndrome, the paracrystalline mitochondrial inclusions are not confined to skeletal muscle. They have also been demonstrated

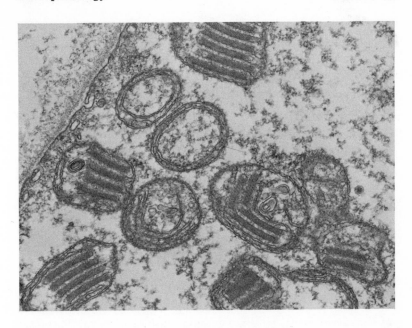

FIG. 6. 2: Electron micrograph prepared from the muscle biopsy specimen.

in eccrine sweat glands, cerebellum and liver. Their presence in several different tissues supports the concept that the Kearns-Shy syndrome is a multisystem disorder involving mitochondrial metabolism. The presence of similar mitochondrial inclusions in other conditions is unexplained.

5. (A, B) The majority of the cases of the Kearns-Shy syndrome have been isolated sporadic cases.

REFERENCES

1. Adachi M, et al.: Electron microscopic and enzyme histochemical studies of cerebellum, ocular and skeletal muscles in chronic progressive ophthalmoplegia with cerebellar ataxia. Acta Neuropath 23:300-312, 1973.

2. Berenberg RA, et al.: Lumping or splitting? "Ophthalmoplegia-plus" or Kearns-Sayre syndrome? Ann Neurol 1:37-54, 1977.

3. DiMauro S, et al.: Mitochondrial Myopathies: Which and
    How Many? In: Exploratory Concepts in Muscular Dys-
    trophy II. Milhorat AT (Ed.). Excerpta Medica,
    Amsterdam, 1973, pp. 506-515.

4. Karpati G, et al.: The Kearns-Shy syndrome. J Neurol
    Sci 19:133-151, 1973.

5. Olson W, et al.: Oculocraniosomatic neuromuscular dis-
    ease with "ragged-red" fibers. Arch Neurol 26:193-211,
    1972.

: :

CASE 7: A 24-Year-Old Woman with Weakness and Double
         Vision

CLINICAL DATA

About 5 years ago, this 24-year-old woman had sought medical
attention because of generalized weakness. She had also noted
drooping of her eyelids and double vision, especially late in the
day. She was treated effectively with anticholinesterase agents
and did well for about 3-1/2 years. Following a divorce, she
complained of further weakness and blurred vision despite progressive increases in the dosage of her medication.

On examination, there was ptosis of both eyelids and weakness
of all extraocular muscles. No dysphagia or dysarthria was
evident. Sensory examination was entirely normal. The patient
had generalized weakness that was more marked in the upper
than lower limbs and more pronounced in proximal than distal
muscles. She had a swinging gait and performed heel and toe
walking with difficulty. The deep tendon reflexes were hyperactive.

Routine laboratory studies were within normal limits. A chest
x-ray was interpreted as normal.

The dosage of her anticholinesterase agent was gradually decreased and steroids were begun in preparation for an operation.

QUESTIONS

1. The clinical data are most consistent with a diagnosis of
    A. amyotrophic lateral sclerosis
    B. myasthenia gravis
    C. polymyositis
    D. chronic inflammatory polyneuropathy

2. Fig. 7.1 illustrates the histopathology of the surgical
    specimen. It shows
    A. thymus with lymphoid hyperplasia
    B. thymoma
    C. metastatic carcinoma in a lymph node
    D. Hodgkin's disease

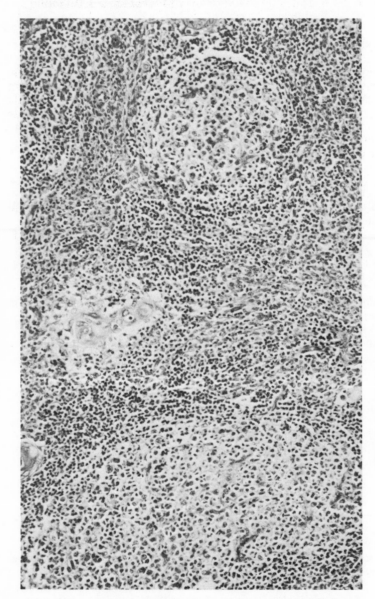

FIG. 7.1: Photomicrograph of the surgical specimen.

3. The lesions found most commonly in muscle biopsy speci-
   mens from patients with myasthenia gravis are
   A. lymphorrhages
   B. atrophy of type 2 myofibers
   C. mildly atrophic myofibers of both fiber types
   D. nemaline rods

4. Current views regarding the pathogenesis of myasthenia
   gravis emphasize the significance of
   A. decreased release of acetylcholine
   B. antibodies directed against motor nerve terminals
   C. antibodies directed against myofiber A-band proteins
   D. antibodies directed against neuromuscular acetylcholine
      receptor sites

5. Neonatal myasthenia gravis is attributed to
   A. a congenital thymoma
   B. transplacental passage of IgM antibodies
   C. transplacental passage of IgG antibodies
   D. anticholinesterase intoxication

6. The Eaton-Lambert syndrome is
   A. associated with certain malignant neoplasms
   B. characterized by weakness predominantly of the extra-
      ocular muscles
   C. due to impaired release of acetylcholine
   D. diagnosed most readily by a muscle biopsy

ANSWERS AND DISCUSSION

1. (B) The clinical data are most consistent with a diagnosis
of myasthenia gravis. This is a relatively common neurological disorder with a prevalence estimated to be 2-10 per 100,000.
The onset of clinical manifestations is commonly in the third
or fourth decade. Women are affected twice as frequently as
men. Among the older patients with thymomas, the sexes are
affected nearly equally.

The disease is characterized by weakness that is exacerbated
by activity and relieved by rest. The distribution of the weakness is variable but almost always involves cranial muscles
such as the eyelids, extraocular muscles and bulbar muscles.
Ptosis and diplopia are common initial manifestations and in a
few patients, the weakness may be restricted to the eye muscles, so-called ocular myasthenia. Limb muscle involvement
tends to be more pronounced proximally but varies, reflecting,
in part, activity. Muscular atrophy may develop in some patients. Sensation remains intact.

Electrophysiological studies show a characteristic decremental
response to repetitive nerve stimulation in the vast majority of
patients. The diagnosis is generally confirmed by pharmaco-
logic tests, e.g. response to edrophonium (Tensilon).

The course of the illness is variable. About 25% of patients
with myasthenia gravis have a partial or complete remission
after a few years; others remain unchanged or get progressively
worse. Emotional crises and intercurrent infections often precipitate exacerbations. Some patients show dramatic improvement following thymectomy, even in the absence of a thymoma.
Controversy still exists regarding the indications, timing and
response with this mode of therapy. Deaths are now rarely
directly attributable to myasthenia gravis but may result from
aspiration or less commonly, respiratory failure.

2. (A) About 75% of patients with myasthenia gravis have
morphologically demonstrable, thymic abnormalities. The most
common of these, as in the present case, is lymphoid hyperplasia of the thymus. This is characterized by the presence of
germinal follicles in the medulla where they are normally not
found. The weight of the thymus may be within normal limits
for the age of the patient.

About 10-15% of patients with myasthenia gravis, especially
those over 30 years of age, have a thymoma. These neoplasms
are generally benign or only locally invasive. Even in patients
with thymomas, the adjacent non-neoplastic thymic tissue often
shows lymphoid hyperplasia.

Still other patients with myasthenia gravis have no morphologically demonstrable thymic abnormalities.

3. (B, C) Traditionally, the presence of lymphorrhages, lymphocytic infiltrates about degenerating or necrotic myofibers,
has been emphasized in muscle specimens from patients with
myasthenia gravis. However, these are relatively uncommon
and are found in only 10-20% of the patients. More commonly,
the muscle biopsy specimens show patchy type 2 myofiber atrophy, mild denervation with atrophy of both types, or they may
even appear histologically normal. Ultrastructural studies
have shown alterations in the myoneural junctions. The primary
clefts are widened and contain osmiophilic dense granules. The
second clefts are reduced in number and are shallow.

4. (D) Over 80% of patients with myasthenia gravis have antibodies directed against the neuromuscular acetylcholine receptors.

Recently, Engel, et al., have demonstrated morphologically
the presence of IgG and complement on the receptor sites in
muscle from patients with myasthenia. This may inhibit access
by acetylcholine, accelerate the degradation of the receptor
sites, or decrease the resynthesis of the receptor sites.
Current evidence favors the first two processes.

An experimental allergic myasthenia gravis has been produced
in rabbits immunized with receptor from electric eels.   This
experimental model shares many clinical, electrophysiological
and ultrastructural features with the naturally occurring human
disease.

The thymic lymphoid hyperplasia and the increased prevalence
in association with various autoimmune disorders, such as
rheumatoid arthritis, lupus erythematosus, thyroiditis, etc.,
provide additional support for the immunological pathogenesis
of myasthenia gravis. However, there is little evidence that
the antimuscle antibodies that bind to the A-bands have any role
in the development of this disease.

5.   (C) About 12% of infants born to myasthenic women are
afflicted with transient weakness. This is manifested by weak
sucking and crying, feeble limb movements and occasionally,
respiratory difficulties. The weakness usually lasts no more
than a few weeks, after which the infant is apparently entirely
normal. The condition is attributed to the effects of maternal
IgG antibodies that cross the placenta and enter the fetal circulation.

6.   (A, C) The Eaton-Lambert syndrome is a disorder of
neuromuscular transmission that is associated with malignant
neoplasms, often oat cell carcinomas. The syndrome is characterized by weakness of the trunk and leg muscles, with relative sparing of the cranial musculature. The diagnosis is
established electrophysiologically. There is an incrementing
response with rapid nerve stimulation. The condition has been
attributed to impaired release of acetylcholine from nerve terminals.

REFERENCES

1.   Drachman DB: Myasthenia gravis. N Eng J Med 298:
     136-142, 186-193, 1978.

2.   Engel AG, et al.: Immune complexes (IgG and C3) at the
     motor end-plate in myasthenia gravis. Mayo Clin Proc
     52:267-280, 1977.

3. Fenichel GM: Clinical syndromes of myasthenia in infancy and childhood. Arch Neurol 35:97-103, 1978.

4. Rowland LP: Myasthenia gravis. In: Scientific Approaches to Clinical Neurology. Goldensohn ES and Appel SH (Eds.). Lea and Febiger, Philadelphia, 1977, pp. 1518-1554.

5. Simpson JA: Myasthenia gravis: A personal view of pathogenesis and mechanism. Muscle Nerve 1:45-56, 151-156, 1978.

: :

CASE 8: A 39-Year-Old Farmer with Ataxia and Numbness
         and Weakness in Hands and Feet

CLINICAL DATA

This 39-year-old farmer was admitted to the hospital complaining of tingling, numbness and weakness in his hands and feet.
About 2-1/2 months prior to admission, he had developed
"shingles" on his right shoulder and neck. Six weeks prior to
admission, the tingling and numbness began in the distal phalanges of his hands and feet and, over a two-week period, progressed to above his wrists and above his knees. He also
complained of anorexia and a 10-pound weight loss.

Physical examination revealed scars from the herpetic lesions
in the C_2, C_3 and C_4 dermatomes on the right. His gait was
ataxic but finger to nose and alternating rapid movement tests
were performed appropriately. His grip was slightly weakened
and the deep tendon reflexes were slightly decreased. A lumbar puncture yielded cerebrospinal fluid with a protein content
of 66 mg/dl and a glucose of 75 mg/dl. Transverse white lines
(Aldrich-Mees lines) were noted on his hands (Fig. 8.1). A
sural nerve biopsy was performed and samples of hair and
urine were obtained for arsenic determinations. The hair was
found to contain 18 μ g/g and the urine 3,000 μ g/1 of arsenic.
Further questioning revealed that the patient had multiple ex-
posures to various agricultural chemicals over the past six
months.

QUESTIONS

1.   The most appropriate diagnosis is
     A. arsenical neuropathy
     B. thallium intoxication
     C. herpes zoster
     D. Guillain-Barre disease

2.   Fig. 8.2 is a photograph of a section prepared from the
     sural nerve biopsy specimen. The pathological changes
     that are demonstrated include
     A. decreased number of myelinated fibers
     B. reactive axonal swellings
     C. phagocytosis of myelin debris by Schwann cells and
         macrophages
     D. "onion bulb" formations

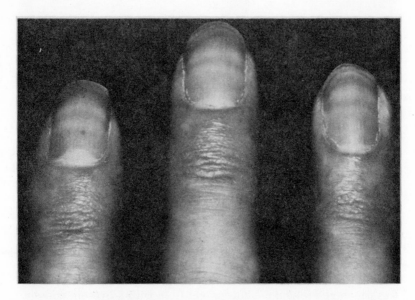

FIG. 8. 1: Photograph of the patient's fingers showing the
Aldrich-Mees lines.

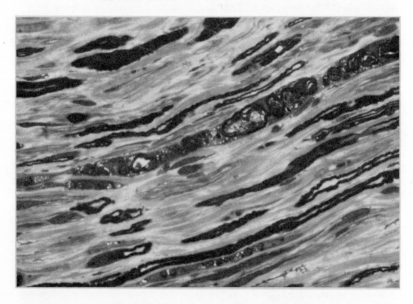

FIG. 8. 2: An epoxy-embedded section of the sural nerve biopsy specimen.

3. The biochemical lesion in arsenical neuropathy is
    A. inhibition of cytochrome oxidase
    B. interference with pyruvate oxidase system
    C. interference with glycogen synthesis
    D. inhibition of succinic dehydrogenase

4. Other metals that can produce a peripheral neuropathy
    include
    A. thallium
    B. lead
    C. silver
    D. iron

5. Herpes zoster occasionally accompanies chronic arsenic
    intoxication. Herpes zoster is due to
    A. the same virus that causes varicella
    B. recrudescence of a latent viral infection
    C. primary infection of an adult by a virus that is usually
        encountered initially during childhood
    D. infection by a papovavirus in an immunologically com-
        promised host

6. Neuropathological features observed in dorsal root ganglia
    involved by herpes zoster include
    A. hemorrhagic ganglionitis
    B. Cowdry type A inclusions in dorsal root ganglion cells
    C. Cowdry type A inclusions in the dorsal root satellite
        cells
    D. degeneration of the dorsal root ganglion and satellite
        cells

7. The Ramsay Hunt syndrome is due to
    A. otitis media
    B. trigeminal ganglionitis
    C. labrynthitis
    D. geniculate ganglionitis and facial neuritis

8. A metal intoxication that can produce a hemorrhagic
    ganglionitis in experimental animals is
    A. lead
    B. bismuth
    C. cobalt
    D. cadmium

9.   Varicella-zoster encephalomyelitis is due to
     A. an autoimmune reaction following acute ganglionitis
     B. invasion of the central nervous system by the varicella-
         zoster virus
     C. symbiotic action of the varicella-zoster virus and an
         unidentified papovavirus
     D. a vasculitis caused by the varicella-zoster virus

ANSWERS AND DISCUSSION

1.   (A) The history, physical findings and results of the laboratory studies support a diagnosis of arsenical polyneuropathy.
Arsenic poisoning can follow excessive exposure to various arsenic containing agricultural chemicals that are used as fruit
sprays, weed killers and pesticides.   The onset of polyneuropathy appears 2-8 weeks after the epigastric pain, vomiting
and diarrhea associated with acute arsenic ingestion or may be
further delayed in cases of chronic arsenic poisoning. Initially,
the neuritic symptoms consist of numbness and tingling, especially in the legs. Pain and paresthesia may persist for several
days or weeks before the onset of weakness.   The weakness
may progress to flaccid paralysis and generally affects the
lower extremities earlier and more severely than the upper
extremities.   Sensation is impaired or lost in a "stocking and
glove" distribution. Vibration is the most vulnerable modality.
Transverse white lines on the nails (Aldrich-Mees lines) are
strong clinical evidence of arsenic intoxication that usually appear 40-60 days after the arsenic ingestion. They are not pathognomonic however and may be seen with some other intoxications
such as thallium.   The diagnosis of arsenical polyneuropathy is
confirmed by the elevated arsenic content of the hair and urine.
Hair can absorb arsenic externally and the level may be spurious
if the patient is subject to external contamination.   Levels in
excess of 0.1 mg/100g of hair are indicative of excessive
ingestion or external contamination.   Urine normally contains
less than 0.1 mg/24 hour specimen.

Herpes zoster or "shingles" may follow ingestion of arsenic
but occurs more commonly in association with systemic infections, lymphomas, or other malignancies. This disorder
usually begins with neuralgia in the distribution of the affected
nerve roots and is followed by the appearance of cutaneous
vesicles.   These become covered with scabs which desquamate
and are then followed by pigmented scars. Rarely, involvement of cervical or lumbar nerve roots may be accompanied by
weakness. Post-herpetic neuralgia is most common in elderly,
debilitated patients and consists of persistent lancinating pains.

2.   (A, C) The illustration shows a decreased number of normally myelinated nerve fibers and numerous myelinated nerve
fibers that are undergoing active axonal degeneration. This is
manifested by fragmentation of axons and the formation of myelin ovoids in Schwann cells. Some of the myelin debris is transferred subsequently from the Schwann cells to macrophages.
In addition, a few fibers may show segmental demyelination.

3.   (B) Arsenic compounds exert their toxic effects by react-
ing with sulfhydryl groups and thus inhibiting essential enzyme
systems. The pyruvate oxidase system is especially susceptible due to the reaction between the arsenic and the sulfhydryl
groups of reduced lipoamide, an essential co-factor. For this
reason, there are similarities between arsenical polyneuropathy and the neuropathy that accompanies thiamine deficiency.

4.   (A, B) Acute thallium intoxication is manifested by a gas-
troenteritis, tachycardia and various neurological symptoms
such as delirium, convulsions and coma. Chronic intoxication
with smaller doses may produce a polyneuropathy and blindness. Alopecia generally occurs after ten days to two weeks
and is often the first manifestation that suggests the correct
clinical diagnosis. Limited morphological studies have suggested that the peripheral neuropathy is due to both segmental
demyelination and Wallerian degeneration.

Lead intoxication in the adult produces a motor neuropathy that
has a predilection for the extensor muscles of the wrist and
fingers. The neuropathy is usually accompanied by anemia and
stippling of erythrocytes. The diagnosis is established by
demonstration of elevated urinary coproporphyrins and lead
content. Morphologic studies have demonstrated segmental demyelination.

There is no evidence that silver produces a neuropathy. Iron,
often as ferrous sulfate, produces gastric ulceration, vascular
collapse and hepatic necrosis but does not produce a polyneuropathy.

5.   (A, B) Herpes zoster is produced by herpes varicellae, the
same virus that produces varicella in childhood. The virus remains latent in dorsal root or other sensory ganglia. In response to a variety of stimuli later in life, the virus spreads
along the peripheral nerves and produces the painful cutaneous
vesicles in the dermatomes subserved by the affected ganglia.

6.   (A, B, C, D) During an attack of herpes zoster, the dorsal root ganglia corresponding to the affected dermatomes show a wide range of pathological changes. These include hemorrhagic necrosis, inflammatory cell infiltrates and occasionally prominent intranuclear (Cowdry type A) inclusions in both the satellite and ganglion cells.

7.   (D) The Ramsay Hunt syndrome is a cephalic form of herpes zoster in which there is a vesicular eruption on the tympanic membrane and external auditory canal and an associated facial paralysis.   The syndrome is due to reactivation of a herpes zoster infection in the geniculate ganglion and spread along the facial nerve.   The morphological changes in the geniculate ganglion range from minimal inflammation to hemorrhagic necrosis.

8.   (D) Acute cadmium intoxication in rodents produces a hemorrhagic ganglionitis that is most conspicuous in the trigeminal and dorsal root ganglia. The relation of this lesion to the pain in human cadmium intoxication is currently unclear.

9.   (B) In a small number of patients recrudescence of a latent varicella-zoster infection produces a generalized varicella-like eruption rather than the usual zoster lesions. Multiple organs may be involved including the central nervous system. In these cases, the brain and spinal cord show perivascular inflammation and scattered foci of necrosis.   Intranuclear inclusion bodies are rarely encountered. Recently, the varicella-zoster virus has been observed ultrastructurally and has been isolated from the central nervous system indicating that the condition is due to direct invasion by the virus rather than merely an auto-immune phenomenon.

REFERENCES

1.   Aleksic SN, et al.: Herpes zoster oticus and facial paralysis (Ramsay Hunt syndrome). J Neurol Sci 20:149-159, 1973.

2.   Gabbiani G, et al.: Cadmium-induced selective lesions of sensory ganglia. J Neuropath Exp Neurol 26:498-506, 1967.

3.   Ghatak N and Zimmerman HM: Spinal ganglion in herpes zoster. Arch Path 95:411-415, 1973.

4. Goldstein NP, et al.: Metal Neuropathy. In: Peripheral
    Neuropathy. Dyck PJ, et al. (Eds.). W. B. Saunders
    Co., Philadelphia, 1975, pp. 1227-1262.

5. Jenkins RB: Inorganic arsenic and the nervous system.
    Brain 89:479-498, 1966.

6. Ludwig G: Arsenical Poisoning. In: Scientific Approaches
    to Clinical Neurology. Goldensohn ES and Appel SH (Eds.).
    Lea and Febiger, Philadelphia, 1977, pp. 1374-1479.

7. McCormick WF, et al.: Varicella-zoster encephalo-
    myelitis. Arch Neurol 21:559-570.

: :

CASE 9: A 50-Year-Old Woman with Weakness Following an
           Acute Gastrointestinal Disorder

CLINICAL DATA

This 50-year-old woman developed fever and diarrhea.   These
complaints resolved over a 3-day period with the use of only
home remedies.   About 1 week later, she noted numbness and
tingling in her hands and feet and developed progressive weakness of her feet and legs.   Examination at that time revealed
normal cranial nerve functions.   There were symmetrical
motor weakness and depressed deep tendon reflexes in all four
limbs, but no sensory deficits.   Over the next 48 hours, she
became weaker, developed slurred speech and became somnolent.   A lumbar puncture yielded cerebrospinal fluid with an
elevated protein content but a normal cell count.   Because of
progressive respiratory difficulties, a tracheostomy was performed and she was placed on a respirator.   She was then
transferred to the university hospital.

On arrival, she was afebrile with a pulse of 102 and a blood
pressure of 94/70 mm Hg.   Extraocular muscle movements,
pupillary reactions and ocular fundi were normal.   She had bilateral facial weakness.   There was flaccid paralysis of all
limbs, except for slight flexion of the wrists and fingers.
Deep tendon reflexes were absent. Electrical studies revealed
minimally depressed motor conduction velocities.

Two days later, the patient became febrile and developed pulmonary infiltrates.   Despite vigorous antibiotic therapy, the
patient's condition continued to deteriorate and she died of
respiratory complications.

QUESTIONS

1. The most appropriate clinical diagnosis is
    A. myasthenia gravis
    B. Guillain-Barre syndrome
    C. poliomyelitis
    D. carotid artery thrombosis

2. Typically, the cerebrospinal fluid from patients with the
    Guillain-Barre syndrome contains
    A. polymorphonuclear leukocytes
    B. numerous lymphocytes
    C. increased protein
    D. increased measles antibodies

3. The Guillain-Barre syndrome is generally considered to be due to
    A. persistent infection by the agent causing the antecedent illness
    B. reactivation of a latent virus infection
    C. immunological mechanisms directed against neuronal fibrous proteins
    D. immunological mechanisms directed against peripheral nerve myelin sheaths

4. The histopathological findings in peripheral nerve specimens from patients with the Guillain-Barre syndrome include
    A. perivascular and endoneurial mononuclear inflammatory cell infiltrates
    B. segmental demyelination
    C. Wallerian degeneration
    D. preferential loss of unmyelinated nerve fibers

5. Chronic inflammatory polyradiculoneuropathy is characterized by
    A. motor weakness
    B. areflexia
    C. reduced nerve conduction velocity
    D. reduced numbers of large, heavily myelinated nerve fibers

ANSWERS AND DISCUSSION

1. (B) The most appropriate clinical diagnosis is the Guillain-Barre syndrome. This is an acute or subacute polyradiculo-neuropathy of variable severity. In most instances, weakness begins in the legs and may progress to total quadriplegia and respiratory paralysis. The deep tendon reflexes are generally depressed or abolished, even when the weakness is minimal. Facial weakness develops in over 50% of the cases and may be uni- or bilateral. Other cranial nerves may be affected, especially in severe cases. Involvement of sphincters is infrequent with urinary incontinence more common than fecal incontinence. Although subjective sensory complaints are common, evidence of objective sensory loss is minimal to absent. Autonomic function is frequently abnormal and manifested by tachycardia, hypotension and anhidrosis.

In over 50% of cases, an acute viral illness precedes the onset of the paralytic disease by 1-3 weeks. Other types of antecedent illnesses and associated conditions have been described; these include: bacterial and mycoplasmal infections, collagen vascular diseases, certain malignant neoplasms, immunizations, surgery and organ transplantation. The paralytic disease generally evolves over a period of 1-3 weeks and is followed by recovery in most cases, although this may be slow, and some cases may have permanent residua. Death occurs in only a small number of cases, 5 to 10%, and is generally due to respiratory complications.

2. (C) The cerebrospinal fluid from patients with Guillain-Barre syndrome typically contains an increased level of protein. This may not be apparent early in the course of the disease since the maximal values are not attained until 4-6 weeks after the onset of clinical symptoms. The elevation in the protein content has been attributed to the involvement of nerve roots.

In most cases, the cell count remains disproportionately low, the so-called "albuminocytologic dissociation." The cells that are present are predominantly lymphocytes.

3. (D) The Guillain-Barre syndrome is generally considered to be a demyelinating disease, caused by immunological mechanisms directed against the myelin sheaths of peripheral nerves. The specific antigens and precise immunological mechanisms involved in this disease remain unknown. Evidence of participation of both humoral and cell-mediated mechanisms have been reported. Recently, Lisak, et al, have suggested that partial and even transient episodes of immunosuppression might contribute to the pathogenesis of Guillain-Barre syndrome.

4. (A, B, C) The histopathological changes associated with Guillain-Barre syndrome are distributed very unevenly throughout the peripheral nervous system. Affected nerves contain areas of perivascular and endoneurial mononuclear inflammatory cell infiltrates. These infiltrates range from highly cellular to sparsely cellular. Patients who have been treated with corticosteroids generally have sparsely cellular infiltrates (Fig. 9.1). The infiltrates contain lymphocytes, plasma cells, macrophages and occasional polymorphonuclear leukocytes. The affected nerves contain foci of mild to severe segmental demyelination and with recovery, remyelination. In severe cases, the nerves also show Wallerian degeneration. This has been attributed to axonal disruption in foci of exceptionally intense inflammation and Wallerian degeneration in the distal segments (Fig. 9.2). The perivascular and endoneurial inflammatory cell infiltrates may extend beyond the distal terminations of motor nerves, and involve the endomysial connective tissue of skeletal muscles.

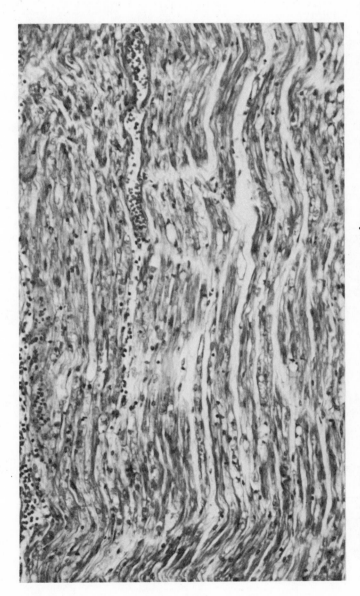

FIG. 9.1: Peripheral nerve from a fatal case of Guillain-Barré disease. Note the sparse perivascular mononuclear inflammatory cell infiltrate.

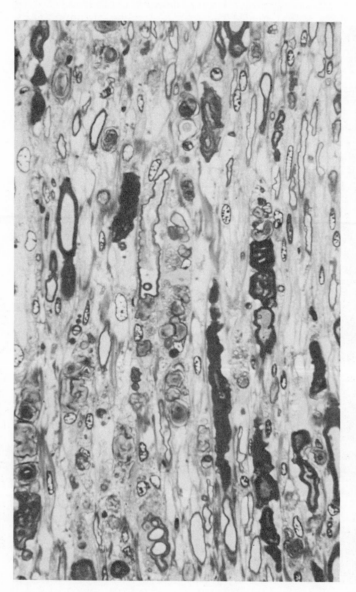

FIG. 9.2: Epoxy-embedded section prepared from the posterior tibial nerve of a patient who died from Guillain-Barré syndrome. Note the Wallerian degeneration.

Dorsal root ganglia may show loss of neurons and inflammatory cell infiltrates. The spinal cord may show meningeal inflammatory cells and chromatolysis of motor neurons in the anterior horns of the spinal cord. The axons of these chromatolytic neurons, presumably, are ones that have undergone Wallerian degeneration.

5. (A, B, C, D) Chronic inflammatory polyradiculoneuropathy is a chronic progressive or relapsing neuropathy characterized by motor weakness (often greater proximally than distally), areflexia and minimal sensory deficits. Patients have severely reduced nerve conduction velocities and often have an elevated cerebrospinal fluid protein content. Histologically, sural nerve biopsy specimens are characterized by a reduced number of myelinated nerve fibers, segmental demyelination, thinly invested remyelinated fibers and variable degrees of endoneurial edema, perivascular and endoneurial inflammation, and onion bulb formations.

As in Guillain-Barre syndrome, this disorder is thought to have an immunological pathogenesis.

REFERENCES

1.   Arnason BGW: Inflammatory Polyradiculoneuropathies. In: Peripheral Neuropathy. Dyck PJ, et al. (Eds.). W.B. Saunders Co., Philadelphia, 1975, pp. 1110-1148.

2.   Dyck PJ, et al.: Chronic inflammatory polyradiculoneuropathy. Mayo Clin Proc 50:621-637, 1975.

3.   Lisak RP, et al.: Guillain-Barre syndrome and Hodgkin's disease: Three cases with immunological studies. Ann Neurol 1:72-78, 1977.

4.   Prineas JW and McLeod JG: Chronic relapsing polyneuritis. J Neurol Sci 27:427-458, 1976.

: :

CASE 10: A 40-Year-Old Man with Difficulty Walking and
          Palpable Nerves

CLINICAL DATA

This 40-year-old man has had difficulty walking and running
since he was a teenager. More recently, he has been unable
to fully straighten his fingers. He claims that other members
of his family have "trouble with their feet."

Physical examination revealed intact cranial nerves and normal ocular fundi. There was weakness and atrophy of the intrinsic foot and peroneal muscles. Pes cavus and hammer toe
deformities were noted. There was also weakness and atrophy
of the intrinsic hand muscles, with claw hand deformities.
Sensory examination revealed a mild loss of sensation over the
toes. Deep tendon reflexes could not be elicited at the ankles
or knees. Peripheral nerves, especially the peroneal and ulnar nerves, were slightly enlarged to palpation.

Routine laboratory studies were normal. The nerve conduction
velocity in the median nerve was only 18.0 m/sec. A sural
nerve biopsy was performed to confirm the clinical diagnosis.

QUESTIONS

1. The clinical data are most consistent with a diagnosis of
    A. hypertrophic Charcot-Marie-Tooth disease
    B. neuronal Charcot-Marie-Tooth disease
    C. Dejerine-Sottas disease
    D. Refsum's disease

2. The pattern of inheritance in hypertrophic Charcot-Marie-
    Tooth disease is
    A. autosomal recessive
    B. autosomal dominant
    C. X-linked recessive
    D. unknown

3. For optimal evaluation of peripheral nerve biopsy specimens,
    which of the following morphological techniques should be
    employed?
    A. light microscopy of paraffin-embedded tissue
    B. light microscopy of epoxy-embedded tissue
    C. "teased" nerve preparations
    D. electron microscopy

4. Fig. 10.1 was prepared from an epoxy-embedded section
    of the sural nerve biopsy specimen. It shows
    A. giant axonal enlargements
    B. endoneurial amyloid deposits
    C. onion bulb formations
    D. Renaut's bodies

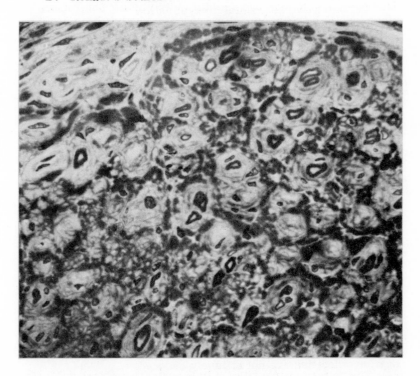

FIG. 10. 1: Epoxy-embedded sections prepared from the sural
            nerve biopsy specimen.

5. Other neuropathies in which onion bulb formations may be
    conspicuous include
    A. Dejerine-Sottas disease
    B. Refsum's disease
    C. porphyric neuropathy
    D. diabetic symmetrical polyneuropathy

6. The histopathological changes expected in a sural nerve
    biopsy specimen from a patient with neuronal Charcot-
    Marie-Tooth disease (hereditary motor sensory neuro-
    pathy type II of Dyck, et al) would include
    A. increased transverse fascicular area
    B. loss of large myelinated nerve fibers
    C. extensive segmental demyelination
    D. onion bulb formations

ANSWERS AND DISCUSSION

1. (A) The clinical data are consistent with a diagnosis of
hypertrophic Charcot-Marie-Tooth disease (hereditary motor
sensory neuropathy type I of Dyck, et al.). This disease becomes manifested during the second to fourth decade and is
characterized by an abnormal gait, weakness and atrophy of
foot and peroneal muscles, and foot deformities such as pes
cavus and hammer toes. Weakness and atrophy of hand and
forearm muscles may develop later. Sensory impairment is
usually mild. Characteristically, there is marked reduction
of both motor and sensory nerve conduction velocities in all
nerves. Only about 25% of the cases have palpably enlarged
peripheral nerves, as does this patient. The disease progresses very slowly and some cases remain nearly asymptomatic.

Neuronal Charcot-Marie-Tooth disease (hereditary motor sensory neuropathy type II of Dyck, et al.) generally has a later
onset, usually after the age of 40. Although the foot and leg
weakness may be more severe and accompanied by more pronounced sensory deficits, the hands and forearms are less involved. Peripheral nerves are not palpably enlarged and conduction velocities are not diffusely reduced.

Dejerine-Sottas disease (hereditary motor sensory neuropathy
type III of Dyck, et al.) becomes manifested in infancy or early
childhood and is characterized by delayed motor development
and progressive gait impairment. Symmetrical, distal sensory involvement is prominent. The peripheral nerves are often markedly enlarged and may have a gelatinous consistency.
Pupillary abnormalities are frequently observed.

Refsum's disease is a slowly progressive hypertrophic polyneuropathy that is accompanied by night blindness, retinitis
pigmentosa, deafness, ataxia and ichthyosis. This disease is
due to impaired degradation of phytanic acid derived from
dietary sources.

2. (B) Both the hypertrophic and neuronal types of Charcot-Marie-Tooth disease are inherited as autosomal dominant traits; sporadic cases may also occur.

By contrast, Dejerine-Sottas disease and Refsum's disease are inherited as autosomal recessive traits.

3. (A, B, C, D) For optimal evaluation of peripheral nerve biopsy specimens, a variety of morphological techniques should be employed. Good quality sections of paraffin-embedded peripheral nerve specimens are relatively difficult to prepare, frequently display prominant fixation artifacts and require the use of multiple special stains, e.g., trichrome, myelin, silver, Congo Red, etc. These sections permit examination of a relatively large volume of tissue and are especially suitable for detection of inflammatory processes, vasculitides and amyloid deposits.

Although the sections are much smaller and the use of special stains sharply limited, light microscopy of epoxy-embedded sections usually provides far more information than the paraffin-embedded sections. It is probably the single most useful technique for the examination of peripheral nerve biopsy specimens.

"Teased" nerve preparations are technically difficult and tedious to prepare but provide valuable diagnostic information. For this purpose, a segment of nerve, 1 cm or longer, is fixed in formalin or glutaraldehyde, post-fixed in osmium tetroxide solution and soaked in glycerine. After removal of the epineurium and perineurium, nerve fascicles can be pulled apart ("teased") under a dissecting microscope until individual fibers are obtained. Examination of "teased" nerve fibers is the most effective means of detecting segmental demyelination and remyelination. Even the examination of incompletely "teased" nerve fascicles can be informative.

Electron microscopy is frequently performed on peripheral nerve specimens. It is the only means for accurately evaluating the small unmyelinated nerve fibers and detecting certain axoplasmic changes, certain deposits in Schwann cells, clusters of denervated Schwann cell processes and basement membrane thickening. Electron microscopy is generally done only after the other studies have been completed. Blocks, suitable for electron microscopy, should be carefully selected by meticulous light microscopy of the thick epoxy-embedded sections.

4. (C) The histopathology of hypertrophic Charcot-Marie-Tooth disease has been studied extensively. The enlargement of the nerves is reflected by an increased transverse fascicular area. In addition, there is a decrease in the total number of myelinated nerve fibers due to preferential loss of both the very large and very small myelinated fibers. Teased nerve preparations show segmental demyelination and remyelination. Onion bulb formations, as shown in Fig. 10.1, result from segmental demyelination and remyelination. Ultrastructurally, they are composed of concentrically laminated Schwann cell processes and longitudinal nerve fibers (Fig. 10.2). In hypertrophic Charcot-Marie-Tooth disease, the segmental demyelination is regarded to be secondary to axonal atrophy.

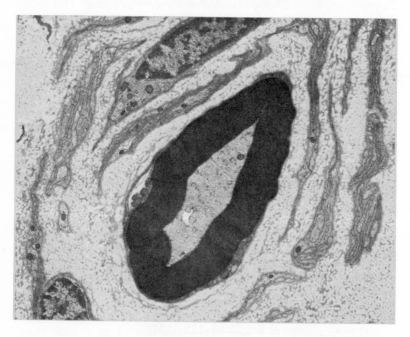

FIG. 10.2: Electron micrograph showing an onion bulb formation composed of concentrically laminated Schwann cell processes and longitudinally oriented collagen fibers surrounding a myelinated nerve fiber.

Renaut's bodies are fusiform, subperineurial collections of fibroblasts, collagen, thin fibrils and mucopolysaccharide.

They are normal structures of unknown significance and are found in greatest numbers where nerves are normally subject to compression.

5.   (A, B, D) As discussed, onion bulb formations are a manifestation of repeated episodes of segmental demyelination and remyelination.   Therefore they may be encountered in many different neuropathies.   They are especially conspicuous in hypertrophic Charcot-Marie-Tooth disease, Dejerine-Sottas disease and Refsum's disease and may be prominent in some cases of diabetic polyneuropathy and chronic inflammatory polyradiculoneuropathy.

6.   (B) Sural nerve biopsy specimens from patients with neuronal Charcot-Marie-Tooth disease are characterized by nearly normal transverse fascicular areas and loss of large myelinated nerve fibers.   There is minimal to no segmental demyelination and virtually no onion bulb formations.

REFERENCES

1.   Behse F and Buchthal F: Peroneal muscular atrophy (PMA) and related disorders. II: Histological findings in sural nerves. Brain 100:67-85, 1977.

2.   Buchthal F and Behse F: Peroneal muscular atrophy (PMA) and related disorders. I: Clinical manifestations as related to biopsy findings, nerve conduction and electromyography. Brain 100:41-66, 1977.

3.   Dyck PJ: Inherited Neuronal Degeneration and Atrophy Affecting Peripheral Motor, Sensory, and Autonomic Neurons. In: Peripheral Neuropathy. Dyck PJ, et al. (Eds.). W.B. Saunders Co., Philadelphia, 1975, pp. 825-867.

4.   Low PA, et al.: Hypertrophic Charcot-Marie-Tooth disease. Light and electron microscope studies of the sural nerve. J Neurol Sci 35:93-115, 1978.

: :

CASE 11: A 70-Year-Old Man with Slowly Progressive Weakness, Decreased Pain Perception, Constipation and Diarrhea

CLINICAL DATA

This 70-year-old man developed progressive numbness, tingling and weakness of his arms and legs over a 1-1/2 year period. At the time of evaluation, he required a walker for ambulation. He also complained of frequent episodes of constipation and more recently, diarrhea. There was no history of dietary deficiency, alcohol abuse or exposure to known toxins.

On examination, he was found to have intact cranial nerves and normal ocular fundi. There was weakness of distal limb muscles and depression of the deep tendon reflexes. Sensation, especially pain perception, was decreased distal to the midforearms and below the knees. The remainder of the physical examination was unremarkable.

Chest x-rays, a gastrointestinal series and a proctoscopic examination were all normal. A lumbar puncture yielded normal cerebrospinal fluid. The blood urea nitrogen was mildly elevated but the fasting blood sugar and glucose tolerance test were normal. The urine contained a small amount of protein. Assays for heavy metals were within normal limits. Serum electrophoresis revealed mildly elevated gamma globulin but normal total protein. Bone marrow aspiration revealed no abnormalities. A sural nerve biopsy was performed.

QUESTIONS

1. Fig. 11.1 shows a microscopic section stained with hematoxylin and eosin that was prepared from the nerve biopsy specimen. The findings are consistent with
    A. carcinomatous neuropathy
    B. chronic inflammatory polyradiculoneuropathy
    C. amyloid neuropathy
    D. giant axonal neuropathy

2. Morphological studies that would confirm this diagnosis are
    A. staining with Congo Red followed by examination with polarized light
    B. staining with a myelin stain such as luxol fast blue
    C. staining with an axonal stain such as Bodian silver
    D. examination by electron microscopy

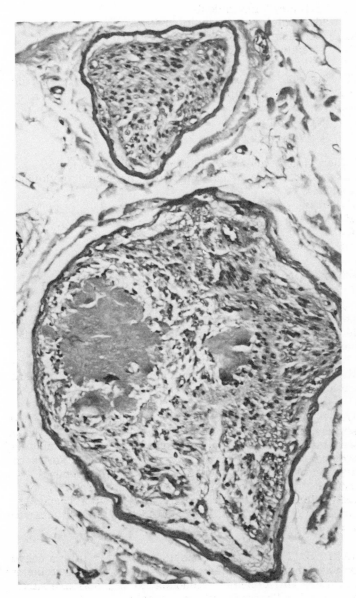

FIG. 11.1: Microscopic section stained with hematoxylin and eosin, prepared from the nerve biopsy specimen.

3. The presence of amyloid within a nerve biopsy specimen is
    consistent with
    A. "primary" amyloidosis
    B. "dysproteinemic" amyloidosis
    C. "secondary" amyloidosis
    D. hereditary amyloidosis

4. The amyloid in "primary" amyloidosis is derived from
    A. immunoglobulin light chains
    B. "A"-protein
    C. hormone peptides
    D. polysaccharides

5. Other structures that commonly harbor extensive
    amyloid deposits in patients with "primary" amyloidosis
    include
    A. brain
    B. heart
    C. kidneys
    D. dorsal root and autonomic ganglia

ANSWERS AND DISCUSSION

1. (C) The histopathological findings are consistent with a
diagnosis of amyloid neuropathy.   There are conspicuous deposits of a hyalin material in the endoneurium and about the
endoneurial blood vessels. Other changes that are also present, but less evident from the photograph, include preferential loss of small myelinated and unmyelinated nerve fibers
and axonal degeneration.

2. (A, D) Amyloid is preferentially stained with Congo Red
and shows a distinctive apple-green birefringence color when
the sections are examined with polarized light. Unfortunately,
collagen can assume a similar appearance if the stain is excessive and the polarizing lenses are optically imperfect. For
this reason, the diagnosis is confirmed most reliably by
electron microscopy. Ultrastructurally, amyloid deposits
appear as a feltwork of stiff fibrils, 7 to 10 nm in diameter
(Fig. 11.2).

3. (A, B, D) The presence of amyloid deposits within a nerve
biopsy specimen is consistent with "primary," "dysproteinemic"
or hereditary amyloidosis.   Endoneurial deposits are rarely,
if ever, found in "secondary" amyloidosis.

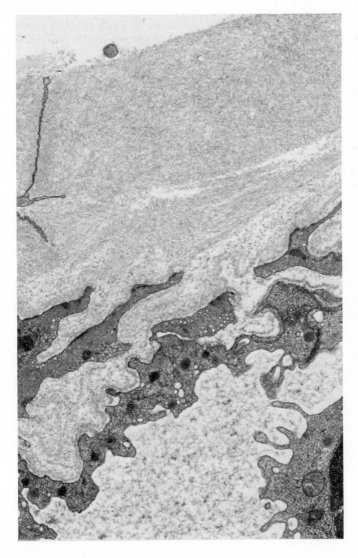

FIG. 11.2: Electron micrograph of amyloid deposited about a small blood vessel. Note the characteristic fibrillar ultrastructure of the amyloid.

4. (A) "Primary" amyloidosis is characterized by the absence of overt concurrent or antecedent disease but is probably always associated with a minor plasma cell dyscrasia.
"Dysproteinemic" amyloidosis is essentially the same as "primary" amyloidosis except for the presence of multiple myeloma
or other overt plasma cell dyscrasias. The amyloid deposits
in these two forms of amyloidosis are derived principally from
immunoglobulin light chains.

"Secondary" amyloidosis is characteristically associated with
chronic inflammatory disorders such as rheumatoid arthritis,
tuberculosis, osteomyelitis or leprosy. The amyloid deposits
in this form of amyloidosis are derived principally from a unique
serum protein ("A"-protein) that is not an immunoglobulin and
to a lesser extent, from light chain material.

The hereditary amyloid neuropathies are a heterogeneous group
of relatively rare diseases that are classified according to the
distribution of the amyloid deposits.   The derivation of the
amyloid in these conditions is currently unknown.   Apparently,
neither immunoglobulin light chain material nor the "A"-pro-
tein is involved.

5. (B, C, D) Patients with "primary" amyloidosis commonly
have amyloid deposits in the heart, small blood vessels, gastrointestinal tract, skeletal muscles (especially the tongue), peripheral nerves and kidneys. Renal and cardiac involvement are
major causes of death in "primary" amyloidosis.

Dorsal root and autonomic ganglia often harbor extensive deposits of amyloid in patients with "primary" amyloidosis. The
involvement of these structures is reflected by the prominent
sensory signs and symptoms and the autonomic dysfunction that
are characteristically found in amyloid neuropathy.

Occasionally, amyloid deposits in the flexor retinaculum can
give rise to a compressive neuropathy, i.e., carpal tunnel
syndrome.

The central nervous system is very rarely involved in the generalized systemic amyloidoses but is affected somewhat more
commonly in some of the hereditary amyloid neuropathies.
When involved, the deposits are predominantly in subpial and
subependymal locations.

Amyloidosis of cerebral blood vessels is a common but incon-
sistent finding in patients with Alzheimer's disease and other

degenerative conditions. Similar vascular lesions also occur in a small number of elderly individuals with no apparent neurological disorders. Two patterns of vascular involvement have been described. In the so-called "congophile angiopathy of Pantelakis," the amyloid is found predominantly in the media of leptomeningeal arterioles and to a lesser extent, in cortical arterioles. In the so-called "drusige Entartung of Scholz," the amyloid is found in cortical arterioles and in stellate perivascular deposits. Both of these forms of cerebral vascular amyloidosis predominantly affect the occipital lobes. Rarely, cerebral hemorrhages have been attributed to cerebral vascular amyloid deposits.

Senile plaques contain amyloid but arise independently of the systemic or hereditary amyloidosis (see Case 67, Alzheimer's disease, for further discussion).

REFERENCES

1. Cohen AS and Benson MD: Amyloid Neuropathy. In: Peripheral Neuropathy. Dyck PJ et al., (Eds.). W.B. Saunders Co., Philadelphia, 1975, pp. 1067-1091.

2. Glenner GG and Page DL: Amyloid, amyloidosis and amyloidogenesis. Int Rev Exp Path 15:1-92, 1976.

3. Lee S-S and Stemmermann GN: Congophilic angiopathy and cerebral hemorrhage. Arch Pathol Lab Med 102: 317-321, 1978.

4. Trotter JL, et al.: Amyloidosis with plasma cell dyscrasia: An overlooked cause of adult sensorimotor neuropathy. Arch Neurol 34:209-214, 1977.

: :

CASE 12: A 49-Year-Old Man with a Progressive Neuropathy
of 6-8 Months Duration

CLINICAL DATA

This 49-year-old man had experienced progressive, distal limb
numbness and weakness over the past 6-8 months. When evaluated, he was having difficulty walking, writing and feeding himself. The patient had no prior neurological problems and there
was no family history of neurological disease. He denied use of
alcohol or drugs, glue-sniffing or contact with toxic chemicals.

Physical examination disclosed intact cranial nerve functions.
There was marked distal weakness in all limbs and atrophy in
the lower legs, feet and hands. Sensory examination revealed
decreased perception of pain, temperature and touch in a
"stocking and glove" distribution. Vibratory sensation was absent in all limbs. He had bilateral foot drop and was unable to
rise on his toes or heels. The deep tendon reflexes were absent at the ankles and decreased in the upper limbs.

Electromyography revealed diffuse denervation. Motor nerve
conduction velocities in the median and ulnar nerves were normal. Sensory action potentials were unobtainable.

Routine clinical laboratory studies were normal. Assays for
heavy metals were normal. The vitamin B_{12} level was 190 pg/
ml, the Schilling test, part I, was 3.87% and the Schilling test,
part II, was 3.04%. These data were interpreted as a vitamin
B_{12} deficiency due to malabsorption.

A sural nerve biopsy was performed.

QUESTIONS

1.   Figs. 12.1 and 12.2 illustrate the findings in the sural
     nerve biopsy specimen as seen by light and electron
     microscopy. The most appropriate morphological diag-
     nosis is
     A. giant axonal neuropathy
     B. hypertrophic neuropathy
     C. amyloid neuropathy
     D. tomaculous neuropathy

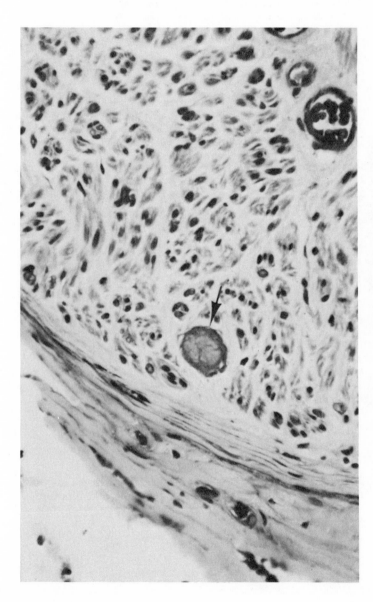

FIG. 12.1: Light micrograph of sural nerve biopsy specimen.

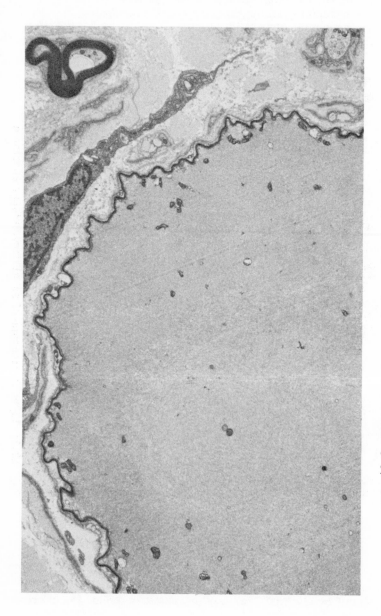

FIG. 12.2: Electron micrograph of sural nerve biopsy specimen.

2. Disorders characterized by the presence of giant axonal enlargements in peripheral nerves include
   A. hereditary childhood giant axonal neuropathy
   B. porphyric neuropathy
   C. lead neuropathy
   D. "glue-sniffing" neuropathy

3. Patients with hereditary childhood giant axonal neuropathy commonly have
   A. kinky hair
   B. pili torti
   C. ataxia
   D. nystagmus

4. Adults with giant axonal neuropathy commonly have
   A. kinky hair
   B. a history of exposure to certain hydrocarbons
   C. palpably enlarged peripheral nerves
   D. decreased motor nerve conduction velocities

5. Neuropathological findings in vitamin B_{12} deficiency may include
   A. degeneration of dorsal and lateral columns of the spinal cord
   B. petechial hemorrhages in the mammillary bodies
   C. atrophy of the optic nerves
   D. foci of perivascular demyelination in the cerebral white matter

ANSWERS AND DISCUSSION

1. (A) The figures illustrate giant axonal enlargements. By light microscopy (see Fig. 12.1), cross-sections of the abnormal axonal enlargements appear as roughly oval profiles with homogeneous to finely fibrillar contents. In longitudinal sections, the axonal enlargements are usually fusiform in shape and are often paranodal in location. Some appear to involve both sides of a node of Ranvier. The abnormally enlarged axons are generally surrounded by markedly thinned or no myelin sheaths.

Fig. 12.2 illustrates a portion of one axonal enlargement as seen by electron microscopy. The axoplasm is filled with myriads of closely packed neurofilaments arranged in interwoven bundles. Small aggregates of osmiophilic granular or coarsely fibrillar material may be scattered among the neurofilaments. Other axoplasmic organelles, e.g., microtubules, mitochondria and cisterns of smooth endoplasmic reticulum, are largely confined to subaxolemmal or internal channels. The myelin sheaths surrounding the larger axonal enlarge- ments are often thinned, uneven in thickness or even focally absent.   Some normal sized or only slightly enlarged myeli- nated axons and some of the unmyelinated axons show the same axoplasmic alterations.

2.   (A, D) As originally described, giant axonal enlargements are characteristically encountered in peripheral nerves in chil- dren with hereditary giant axonal neuropathy, a distinct form of slowly progressive sensory-motor neuropathy.

In addition, morphologically similar axonal enlargements have been encountered in adults with certain toxic neuropathies due especially to exposure to n-hexane (glue-sniffing neuropathy), methyl butyl ketone or acrylamide.   These and related com- pounds have been used to reproduce these lesions in various experimental animals, where they have been studied exhaustively. The occurrence of giant axonal enlargements in other conditions such as in this patient with B_{12} malabsorption, has been studied less extensively. The full spectrum of disorders in which these lesions may be encountered remains to be determined.

3.   (A, C, D) Childhood giant axonal neuropathy is a rare pro- gressive polyneuropathy, with onset of clinical manifestation before the age of 3. It is thought to be an autosomal recessive disorder.   Most of the patients have had ataxia and nystagmus and several have had impaired speech and mild to moderate mental retardation.   Most cases have had abnormally kinky hair and in several, the hair color was abnormally light. How- ever, the hairs do not show pili torti, the hair shaft abnormal- ity seen in Menkes' disease otherwise known as "kinky hair" disease or trichopoliodystrophy.

In all of the reported cases, the giant axonal enlargements have contained prominent osmiophilic granular and/or fibrillary deposits scattered among the neurofilaments.   In at least 4 cases, there was also filamentous hyperplasia in Schwann cells, fibroblasts and endothelial cells.   This involvement of diverse cells has led to the suggestion that this disease is a generalized disorder of filament production. However, this feature has not been observed in all reported cases.

4.   (B, D) Most adults with giant axonal neuropathy have a history of glue-sniffing or occupational exposure to n-hexane, methyl butyl ketone or acrylamide.   The disorder is a mixed

motor and sensory neuropathy and may be accompanied by clinical evidence of central nervous system involvement.   The patients often show marked slowing of motor nerve conduction
velocities.   This has been attributed to the paranodal myelin
retraction that occurs with this predominantly axonal lesion.

Ultrastructurally, the axonal enlargements are similar to those
occurring in the hereditary, childhood giant axonal neuropathy,
although the presence of osmiophilic granular and fibrillary
dense bodies have not been emphasized in the published reports.
Furthermore, there is no mention of filamentous hyperplasia in
structures other than axons.

Spencer and Schaumburg have interpreted this entity as an
example of a central-peripheral distal axonopathy and have
emphasized the distal, though not necessarily terminal, involvement of axons in both the central and peripheral nervous systems.   Recently, it has been suggested that inhibition of glyco-
lysis may be involved in the evolution of this lesion.

5.   (A, C, D) Subacute combined degeneration of the spinal
cord is the lesion classically associated with severe vitamin
B_{12} deficiency and pernicious anemia. Both the dorsal columns
and the pyramidal tracts in the lateral columns show demyelination and to a lesser extent, axonal degeneration. The lesions
are usually most severe in the thoracic portion of the spinal
cord. The affected areas typically show prominent sponginess
and contain numerous lipid-laden macrophages. Gliosis tends
to be relatively sparse.

Small foci of perivascular demyelination, so-called Lichtheim
plaques, may be present in the cerebral white matter of some
patients. Demyelination and atrophy of the optic nerves have
also been observed.

Pallis and Lewis regard peripheral neuropathy as the most common neurological complication of vitamin B_{12} deficiency. The
histopathology of the neuropathy has not been investigated as
extensively as other lesions in this condition. Some of the older
reports described the peripheral nerves as normal, while others
reported a decreased number of myelinated fibers. More recent
studies have disclosed axonal degeneration. The prevalence of
giant axonal neuropathy in association with vitamin B_{12} deficiency, as in the present case, remains to be determined.

REFERENCES

1. Asbury AK and Johnson PC: Pathology of Peripheral
    Nerve. W. B. Saunders Co., Philadelphia, 1978, pp.
    88-90, 178-180.

2. Pallis CA and Lewis PD: The Neurology of Gastroin-
    testinal Disease. W. B. Saunders Co., London, 1974,
    pp. 30-97.

3. Sabri MI, et al.: Towards the metabolic basis of hexa-
    carbon distal (dying-back) axonopathy. J Neuropath Exp
    Neurol 37:684, 1978.

4. Schochet SS Jr and Chesson AL Jr: Giant axonal neuro-
    pathy: Possibly secondary to vitamin B_{12} malabsorption.
    Acta Neuropath 40:79-83, 1977.

5. Spencer PS and Schaumburg HH: Central - Peripheral
    Distal Axonopathy - The Pathology of Dying-Back Poly-
    neuropathies. In: Progress in Neuropathology.
    Zimmerman HM (Ed.). Grune and Stratton, New York,
    Vol. III, 1976, pp. 253-295.

: :

CASE 13: A Newborn Child with a Meningomyelocele and Enlarging Head

CLINICAL DATA

The patient was the product of an uncomplicated delivery and a normal pregnancy in a 20-year-old woman. The patient weighed 7 lbs, 8 oz, and had an Apgar of 2 at birth and of 5 at 5 minutes. The child had a lumbosacral meningomyelocele that measured 4 x 5 cm. He had no anal tone, a thoracic sensory level and was unable to move his legs. The left hip was dislocated and both feet had talipes equinovarus malformations. The head circumference was 40 cm and the anterior fontanelle was widened. An intravenous pyelogram revealed bilateral hydronephrosis and hydroureters. An air and Pantopaque ventriculogram revealed non-communicating hydrocephalus. A ventriculo-peritoneal shunt was performed. Subsequently, the child was readmitted on several occasions because of leaking of the meningomyelocele, progressive head enlargement and recurrent infections. The child died at the age of four months.

QUESTIONS

1. Fig. 13.1 illustrates the meningomyelocele. The use of this term indicates that there is
   A. a skeletal defect in the posterior aspect of the vertebral canal
   B. an externally visible sac that extends through a skeletal defect and contains meninges and cerebrospinal fluid
   C. an externally visible sac that extends through a skeletal defect and contains meninges, neural tissue including nerve roots and cerebrospinal fluid
   D. cystic dilatation of the central canal of the spinal cord

2. Dissection of a meningomyelocele will reveal
   A. nerve roots extending dorsally from a ventrally situated dysplastic neural plate
   B. nerve roots extending ventrally from a dorsally situated dysplastic neural plate
   C. dorsally and ventrally situated lamina of dysplastic neural plates with nerve roots between the laminae
   D. nerve roots extending dorsally and ventrally from a ventrally situated dysplastic neural plate

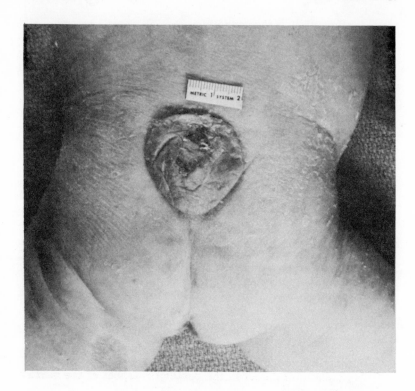

FIG. 13.1: Back of child showing the meningomyelocele.

3. Meningomyeloceles are most commonly located in the
   A. cervical region
   B. thoracic region
   C. lumbar region
   D. lumbosacral region

4. Most patients with meningomyeloceles also have
   A. hydrocephalus
   B. a Dandy-Walker malformation
   C. an Arnold-Chiari malformation
   D. hydromyelia

5. Components of the Arnold-Chiari malformation include
   A. elongated tongues of cerebellar tissue located along
      the dorsolateral aspects of the medulla and cervical
      spinal cord

   B. elongation of the medulla with "Z"-shaped cervico-
       medullary junction
   C. elongation of the pons
   D. a "beak"-shaped malformation of the mesencephalic
       tectum

6. The basis for development of the Arnold-Chiari malfor-
    mation is
   A. traction on the spinal cord due to tethering by the
       meningomyelocele
   B. caudal herniation secondary to hydrocephalus
   C. overgrowth of posterior fossa contents
   D. unknown

7. Current surgical therapy, i.e., closure of the meningo-
    myelocele with or without shunting procedures for the
    associated hydrocephalus yields
   A. uniformly good results
   B. good results in most patients
   C. good results in some patients
   D. poor results in most patients

8. A spinal cord malformation that may be found in some pa-
    tients with spina bifida is
   A. myelomalacia
   B. diastematomyelia
   C. hematomyelia
   D. cysts of the filum terminale

ANSWERS AND DISCUSSION

1. (C) A number of different terms are applied to midline defects to indicate the severity of the defect and the composition
of the lesion. A midline skeletal defect in the spine is called
spina bifida. If the osseous defect is not visible from the ex-
terior, the lesion is referred to as spina bifida occulta. This
is a common lesion but is usually clinically asymptomatic. If
a sac protrudes through the skeletal defect and is visible externally, the lesion can be referred to as spina bifida cystica.
When the cyst contains anomalous meninges and spinal fluid but
no neural elements, the lesion is correctly referred to as a
meningocele. This is a relatively rare lesion. When the sac
contains nerve roots or other neural tissue in addition to the
meninges and spinal fluid, the lesion is designated as a
meningomyelocele. This is the common form of spina bifida
cystica. Cystic dilatation of the central canal of the spinal
cord is referred to as hydromyelia. This lesion is often found
in the spinal cord rostral to a meningomyelocele.

2. (B) Dissection of a meningomyelocele will demonstrate continuity between the spinal cord and the rostral end of the sac. Within the dome of the sac are the remnants of the dysplastic spinal cord. The sac is covered to a variable degree by epithelium growing centripetally from the margins of the meningomyelocele sac. Most of the interior of the sac corresponds to an enlargement of the subarachnoid space that would have been situated ventral and lateral to the spinal cord had normal development occurred. This space is traversed by nerve roots extending ventrally from the degenerated dysplastic remnants of the neural plate. The meninges and blood vessels in and about the sac are also dysplastic.

3. (D) The vast majority of meningomyeloceles are lumbosacral in location. Only a few are pure lumbar, thoracolumbar or in some other location. Very rarely the defects and sacs are multiple.

4. (A, C, D) Almost all patients with a meningomyelocele have an Arnold-Chiari malformation and some degree of hydrocephalus. The converse association does not seem to be as constant; a few patients have the Arnold-Chiari malformation without a meningomyelocele. Hydromyelia, dilatation of the central canal of the spinal cord, is very commonly found in patients with meningomyeloceles (Fig. 13.2). This lesion is distinguished from a syrinx by having an ependymal lining derived from the central canal.

5. (A, B, C, D) The Arnold-Chiari malformation is a complex malformation with numerous components (Fig. 13.3). Elongated tongues of gliotic, "dysmorphic" cerebellar tissue extend caudally along the dorsolateral aspects of the medulla and cervical spinal cord. These tongues of tissue are often incorrectly referred to as the cerebellar "tonsils." The medulla is elongated and displaced downward. Often the caudal end of the medulla is wider than the rostral end. The dorsal aspect of the medulla is elongated more than the ventral aspect producing a "Z"-shaped cervicomedullary junction. The pons is also elongated and flattened. In association with the pontine and medullary deformities, the fourth ventricle is elongated, flattened and displaced caudally. The cerebellum is often hypoplastic, the posterior fossa small and the foramen magnum large. The mesencephalic tectum is not differentiated into distinct superior and inferior colliculi but remains as a single "beak"-shaped mass. The aqueduct is usually stenotic and may be the component of the malformation responsible for the hydrocephalus. The massa intermedia is often quite large. The cerebral hemispheres have an excessively complex convolutional pattern often referred to as polymicrogyria. Heterotopias may be present along the ventricular surfaces.

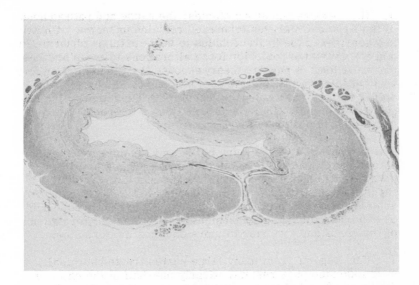

FIG. 13. 2: Transverse section of the spinal cord showing hydromyelia. Note the ependymal lining.

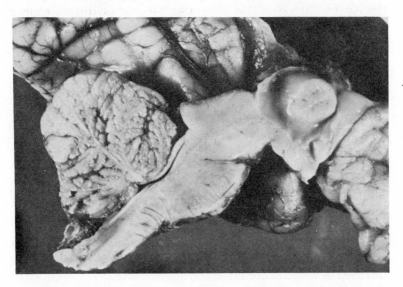

FIG. 13. 3: Sagittal section of the brain showing components of the Arnold-Chiari malformation.

6. (D) Despite numerous studies, the cause and pathogenesis of the Arnold-Chiari malformation remains unknown. Chiari had considered the hydrocephalus to be the primary abnormality and attributed the posterior fossa alterations to complications of herniation. A popular theory espoused by a number of authors was based on traction of the neuraxis due to tethering of the spinal cord by the meningomyelocele. Other authors have re-garded the Arnold-Chiari malformation as the result of over-growth of the posterior fossa contents.

The pathogenesis of the spina bifida and meningomyelocele is also disputed. Most of the older reports suggested failure of neural tube closure. However, Padget has interpreted the de-fects in the neural tube as being due to cleft formation (neuro-schisis) rather than failure of closure. Other changes, such as abnormal folding and adhesions, may follow the formation of the clefts and give rise to more complex malformations.

7. (D) Reports from many large series treated surgically have indicated poor results. Nearly one-half of the children die by age 2 and of the survivors, most have severe multisys-tem physical handicaps.

8. (B) Diastematomyelia is division of the spinal cord into two halves often on either side of an osseous or fibrous septum. The lesion is commonly associated with some degree of spina bifida. The two halves of the spinal cord tend to rotate so that the ventral horns are directed medially. Each half has anterior and posterior nerve roots. Hematomyelia is hemorrhage into the spinal cord and is not a malformation. Similarly, myelo-malacia is softening of the spinal cord due to any cause. Cysts of the filum terminale are commonly found as remnants of the partially obliterated central canal and are not especially asso-ciated with spina bifida.

REFERENCES

1. Bell WE and McCormick WF: Increased Intracranial Pres-sure in Children. W. B. Saunders Co., Philadelphia, 1978, pp. 132-215.

2. Lorber J: Spina bifida cystica, results of treatment of 270 consecutive cases with criteria for selection for the future. Arch Dis Child 47:854-873, 1972.

3. Padget DH: Neuroschisis and human embryonic mal-
    development: New evidence on anencephaly, spina bifida
    and diverse mammalian defects. J Neuropath Exp Neurol
    29:192-216, 1970.

4. Peach B: Arnold-Chiari malformation. Anatomic features
    of 20 cases. Arch Neurol 12:613-621, 1965.

5. Warkany J: Congenital Malformations. Year Book Medi-
    cal Publishers, Chicago, 1971, pp. 272-292, 217-231.

: :

CASE 14: A 19-Month-Old Girl With Hydrocephalus and an
          Elevated Inion

CLINICAL DATA

This 19-month-old girl was the product of a normal pregnancy
and delivery.   At the age of 3 months, she had been evaluated
at another hospital for increasing head size. At that time, subdural taps yielded no subdural fluid.   Pneumoencephalography
failed to produce ventricular filling. A right ventriculo-atrial
shunt was inserted. The patient was able to walk by the age of
13 months and spoke a few words.

The child was hospitalized because of a one-day history of
vomiting, lethargy and opisthotonic posturing.   Physical examination revealed a pulse of 112/minute, a temperature of
38.3°C and a head circumference of 52 cm. The child's pupils
were equal and reactive to light and funduscopic examination
revealed no abnormalities. Marked nuchal rigidity was present. The deep tendon reflexes were normal. The ventriculo-
atrial shunt was thought to be functioning normally. A lumbar puncture yielded spinal fluid with a pressure of 88 mm
water containing 15 WBC's/cmm, a glucose of 65 mg/dl, and
a protein of 129 mg/dl. Intravenous fluids and antibiotics were
started. The child became afebrile and her neck became less
stiff after three days of treatment. A ventricular tap revealed
clear, colorless ventricular fluid with a pressure of 250 mm
of water.   The pressure would not decrease due to non-func-
tion of the shunt. Two days later, the ventricular tap was repeated and revealed a pressure of 380 mm of water. The child
continued to maintain an arched posture. Seven days after admission, she developed respiratory difficulties and died.

QUESTIONS

1.   Fig. 14.1 illustrates the base of the child's brain and
     Fig. 14.2 illustrates the cerebellum. This lesion is
     called
     A. the Arnold-Chiari malformation
     B. the Dandy-Walker malformation
     C. hydranencephaly
     D. porencephaly

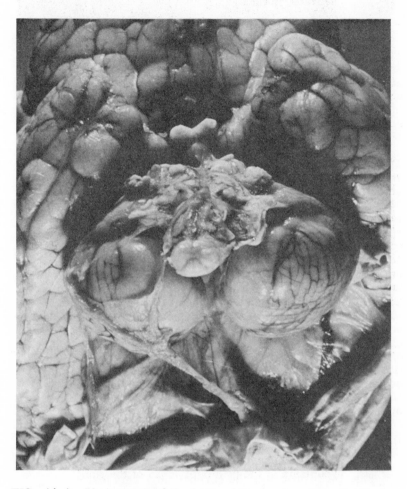

FIG. 14. 1: Photograph of the base of the brain. Note the large
posterior fossa cyst that has been partially torn
during removal of the brain.

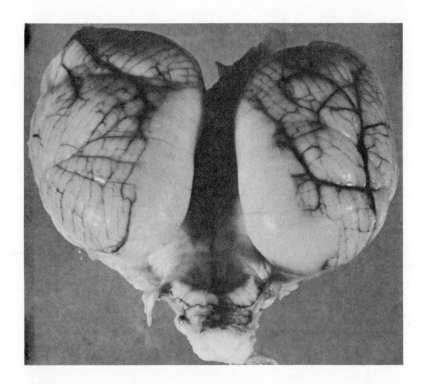

FIG. 14. 2: Photograph of the inferior surface of the cerebellum
showing the abnormalities of the vermis and cerebellar hemispheres.

2.   The major components of this malformation include
     A.   agenesis of the cerebellar vermis
     B.   cystic dilatation of the fourth ventricle
     C.   lateral displacement of the cerebellar hemispheres
     D.   hypoplasia of the posterior fossa of the skull

3.   The wall of the posterior fossa cyst is composed of
     A.   ependyma only
     B.   arachnoid only
     C.   ependyma and choroid plexus
     D.   ependyma and leptomeninges

4. The Dandy-Walker malformation has been interpreted as
    A. cystic dilatation of the fourth ventricle due to atresia
        of the foramina of Luschka and Magendie
    B. failure of the normal regressive changes in the
        posterior medullary vellum
    C. cystic dilatation of the fourth ventricle due to hydro-
        cephalus before the foramina of the fourth ventricle
        normally open
    D. all of the above

5. Brain anomalies that have been found in association with
    the Dandy-Walker malformation include
    A. agenesis of the corpus callosum
    B. cerebral heterotopias
    C. cerebellar heterotopias
    D. malformations of the inferior olivary nuclei

6. Clinical findings in a patient with hydrocephalus suggestive
    of the Dandy-Walker malformation include
    A. head enlargement
    B. prominence of the occipital region
    C. elevated inion
    D. elevated position of transverse sinuses

7. Complications associated with ventriculoatrial shunts
    include
    A. obstruction of the shunt
    B. septicemia
    C. pulmonary thromboembolism
    D. perforation of the heart

8. Porencephaly is characterized by
    A. a skull defect with herniation of cerebral parenchyma
        and ventricular system
    B. cystic dilatation of a single ventricle
    C. cysts at the sites of the anterior and posterior neuro-
        pores
    D. a cerebral defect that extends from the ventricular
        system to the subarachnoid space

9. Hydranencephaly is characterized by
    A. thin-walled sacs in place of the cerebral hemispheres
    B. a single large ventricle resulting from failure of
        development of the prosencephalon
    C. subdural sacs filled with cerebrospinal fluid
    D. a head that can be transilluminated

10. Hydranencephaly results from
    A. agenesis of the cerebral hemispheres
    B. incomplete differentiation of the prosencephalon
    C. intrauterine destruction of the cerebral hemispheres
    D. arrested hydrocephalus

ANSWERS AND DISCUSSION

1. (B) These photographs illustrate a brain with hydrocephalus
due to the Dandy-Walker malformation.

2. (B, C) The major components of the Dandy-Walker malformation include cystic dilatation of the fourth ventricle, lateral
displacement of the cerebellar hemispheres by the abnormally
enlarged fourth ventricle and malformation of the cerebellar
vermis. The anterior portion of the vermis is displaced rostrally while the inferior portion of the vermis is reduced to the
abnormal white matter on the medial surfaces of the cerebellar
hemispheres. Thus, there is severe malformation but not true
agenesis of the cerebellar vermis. The cystic dilatation of the
fourth ventricle results in an abnormally large posterior fossa.
Other central nervous system anomalies are also present in
over half of the patients.

3. (D) The wall of the posterior fossa cyst is composed of
ependyma and leptomeninges. The ependymal lining is evidence
that the cyst results from dilatation of the fourth ventricle and
is not merely an arachnoidal cyst within the posterior fossa.

4. (D) The pathogenesis of the Dandy-Walker malformation is
unknown despite the numerous hypotheses including those cited
in A, B, and C. The high incidence of associated cerebral malformations (over 50%) suggests the posterior fossa lesions are
merely components of a more general central nervous system
malformation that is established before the foramina of Luschka
and Magendie normally open. Furthermore, these foramina
appear to be patent in some of the patients with the Dandy-Walker malformation.

5. (A, B, C, D) Some of the more common anomalies that have
been described in association with the Dandy-Walker malformation include agenesis of the corpus callosum, cerebral and
cerebellar heterotopias and malformations of the inferior olivary nuclei.

6. (B, C, D) Head enlargement can result from many causes.
The marked enlargement of the posterior fossa is especially

characteristic of the Dandy-Walker malformation and can be
appreciated by several indirect findings. The occipital region
becomes quite prominent and the distance from the ear to the
occiput is relatively great. The inion can be palpated in an
abnormally high position on the back of the head. In older children, the abnormally elevated position of the transverse sinuses
can be demonstrated by plain skull x-rays.

7. (A, B, C, D) Shunts can become occluded at the proximal
end by choroid plexus, inflammatory exudate or by burrowing
into the cerebral parenchyma. The distal end of the shunt can
become thrombosed, or if the shunt tip is above the atrium,
the superior vena cava can become thrombosed. Perforation
of the heart is rare but has been reported. A very significant
problem is septicemia from bacterial colonization of the shunt.
Thromboembolism of the pulmonary vessels is commonly encountered but is often clinically asymptomatic.

8. (D) The term porencephaly is applied to cerebral defects
that extend from the ventricular system to the subarachnoid
space. Schizencephaly is a rare form of porencephaly that results from bilaterally symmetrical areas of agenesis or neuro-
schisis in the developing cerebral hemispheres. The more
common type of porencephaly, encephaloclastic porencephaly,
results from localized areas of destruction in the cerebral
hemispheres. The destruction is usually due to prenatal vascular or infectious disease.

9. (A, D) Hydranencephaly is a condition characterized by a
normal or mildly enlarged skull containing thin-walled sacs
filled with cerebrospinal fluid in place of the cerebral hemispheres. The basal ganglia, brain stem and cerebellum are
usually present but may show abnormalities. The thin-walled
sacs consist predominantly of glial tissue that is adherent to
the overlying leptomeninges. The ependyma is characteristically
destroyed. A head with hydranencephaly will transilluminate
but this phenomenon is not specific for hydranencephaly and
can be observed with advanced hydrocephalus, subdural hygromas, and some cases of porencephaly.

10. (C) Hydranencephaly is the result of massive destruction
of the cerebral hemispheres. This usually occurs in utero some
time after the 12th week of gestation. Rarely, it may occur
during the perinatal or neonatal period. There are multiple
causes including vascular, infectious and traumatic disorders.

REFERENCES

1. Bell WE and McCormick WF: Increased Intracranial
    Pressure in Children. W. B. Saunders Co., Philadelphia,
    1978, pp. 132-215.

2. Brown Jr: The Dandy-Walker Syndrome. In: Handbook
    of Clinical Neurology. Vinken PJ and Bruyn GW (Eds.).
    North-Holland, Amsterdam, 1977, Vol. 30, pp. 623-
    646.

3. Gardner E, et al.: The Dandy-Walker and Arnold-Chiari
    malformations. Arch Neurol 32:393-407, 1975.

4. Halsey JH, et al.: Hydrancephaly. In: Handbook of
    Clinical Neurology. Vinken PJ and Bruyn GW (Eds.).
    North-Holland, Amsterdam, 1977, Vol. 30, pp. 661-
    680.

5. Hart MN, et al.: The Dandy-Walker syndrome.
    Neurology 22:771-780, 1972.

: :

CASE 15: A 2-Day-Old Child with Hypotelorism, Micro-
          ophthalmia and Cleft Palate

CLINICAL DATA

This 2-day-old male infant was admitted to the hospital for evaluation of multiple congenital anomalies. He was the product of
a 40-week gestation in a gravida 5, para 5, 30-year-old woman.
During the pregancy, the mother had no illnesses and took no
medications. She did not regard this pregnancy as having been
different from her previous ones. There was no family history
of congenital anomalies and the other children were living and
well.   The labor and delivery were normal and at birth, the
child weighed 2,600 grams.

On physical examination, the head circumference was found to
be 29.5 cm, and there was a "scabbed abrasion" over the posterior fontanelle.   There was marked hypotelorism and the
child was thought to have severe microphthalmia or anophthalmia. The ears were low-set and had an abnormal configuration
with fusion of the helices bilaterally.   There were bilateral
lateral cleft lips and a cleft palate.   A systolic ejection murmur was heard along the right sternal border and radiated to
the axilla and the back.   The hands were markedly abnormal
with polydactyly, disproportionate finger lengths and simian
creases.

Chest x-rays demonstrated a normal-sized heart but increased
pulmonary vascular markings.   Skull x-rays were normal except for hypotelorism and microcephaly. Blood was submitted
for chromosomal analysis.   The child died ten days after admission to the hospital.

QUESTIONS

1.   From the description of the child's face, one would pre-
     dict that the brain is
     A. normal
     B. malformed, with a malformation belonging to the
         holoprosencephaly series
     C. malformed, with a malformation belonging to the
         lissencephaly-pachygyria series
     D. malformed, with a malformation belonging to the
         cranioschisis-rachischisis series

2. Figs. 15.1 and 15.2 are dorsal and ventral views of this
    child's brain. The malformation is best described as
    A. alobar holoprosencephaly
    B. lobar holoprosencephaly
    C. arhinencephaly
    D. hydranencephaly

3. Holoprosencephaly has been interpreted as a malformation
    involving
    A. closure of the neural tube
    B. migration of cortical neuroblasts
    C. diverticulation of the prosencephalon
    D. differentiation of the rhinencephalon

4. Individuals with holoprosencephaly may have
    A. trisomy 21
    B. Philadelphia chromosomes
    C. D trisomy
    D. normal karyotypes

5. One can expect the D (13-15) trisomy in those cases of
    holoprosencephaly that
    A. have microcephaly
    B. have microphthalmia
    C. have absence of the olfactory bulbs
    D. have multiple extracranial anomalies

6. Among the more common extracranial anomalies are
    A. polydactyly of hands and/or feet
    B. cardiac malformations
    C. renal agenesis
    D. hepatic cysts

7. The ocular abnormality that is most characteristic of the
    D (13-15) trisomy is
    A. coloboma
    B. microphthalmia
    C. retinal detachment
    D. intraocular cartilage

8. The usual prognosis for patients with the D (13-15) trisomy
    is
    A. death by 2 years of age
    B. severe mental retardation but a normal life span
    C. moderate mental retardation and a moderately
        shortened life
    D. severe mental retardation and a moderately shortened
        life

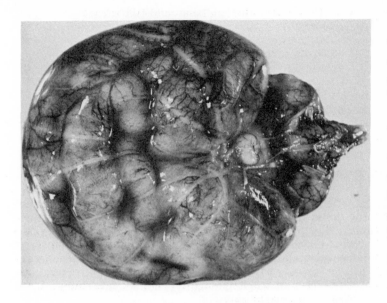

FIG. 15.2: Ventral surface of the brain.

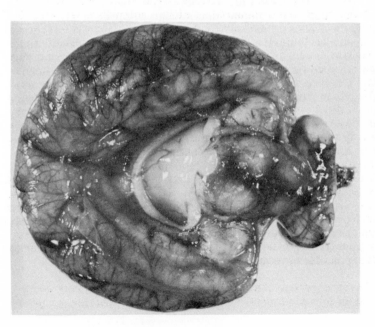

FIG. 15.1: Dorsal surface of the brain.

9. The D (13-15) trisomy has been associated with
   A. maternal x-rays
   B. older maternal age
   C. aberrant maternal diet
   D. eclampsia

10. Infants with trisomy 18 often show
    A. a low brain weight
    B. cerebral heterotopias
    C. hypoplasia of the cerebellar vermis
    D. malformations of the inferior olivary nuclei

ANSWERS AND DISCUSSION

1. (B) DeMyer, et al., have studied extensively the relation
between facial configurations and underlying cerebral malformations. They feel that cyclopia, ethmocephaly, cebocephaly,
and median clefts with hypotelorism are invariably accompanied
by a cerebral malformation belonging to the holoprosencephaly
series. Individuals with bilateral lateral cleft lips, orbital hypotelorism and microcephaly usually, but not invariably, have
some form of holoprosencephaly.

2. (A) The term holoprosencephaly is applied to a spectrum
of related cerebral malformations. The most severely abnormal examples are designated as alobar holoprosencephaly. In
these specimens, lobes are not demarcated and the cerebrum
is monoventricular. The specimens may be relatively flat
("pancake type") or cup-shaped ("cup type") with the dorsal surface covered by a thin membrane derived from the tela choroi-
dea. Others, like the present case, have cortex over the dorsal surface ("ball type"). There is no interhemispheric fissure
and no third ventricle dividing the thalamic mass. No olfactory
bulbs or tracts are present. Other rhinencephalic structures
such as the hippocampi are present although abnormally situated.
Cytoarchitectural studies by Yakovlev have shown that the
anterior median portion of the holosphere consists of giganto-
pyramidal cortex. The brain is thus homologous to the normal
hemispheres caudal to the motor cortex. The anterior portions
of the frontal lobes are absent. The optic nerves and eyes show
varying degrees of malformation. The brain stem and cerebellum are relatively normal except that the pyramidal tracts
are absent. This is reflected in the medulla where the inferior
olivary nuclei have an unusually ventral position.

A lesser degree of malformation is found in specimens designated as lobar holoprosencephaly. In these specimens, lobes

are partly demarcated and an interhemispheric fissure divides
the posterior portion of the cerebrum into hemispheres. Olfactory bulbs and tracts are usually absent.

The least malformed brains belonging to this series show normal development except for agenesis or hypoplasia of the olfactory bulbs and tracts. Only these specimens should be
designated as arhinencephaly. Yakovlev objects to any use of
this term since not all rhinencephalic structures are absent,
i.e., hippocampi, etc., are present.

3. (C) This spectrum of malformation has been regarded as
disorders of the diverticulation of the prosencephalon. The
telencephalic vesicles, optic bulbs and olfactory bulbs are
among the structures that can be regarded as normal diverti-
cula of the prosencephalon. Aberration in the diverticulation
of the telencephalic vesicles results in the undivided ventricular cavity or holosphere and the undivided striatum. When the
telencephalon fails to divide into hemispheres, the two olfactory bulbs fail to develop. Abnormal development of the optic
bulbs from the diencephalon results in varying degrees of ocular malformation ranging from anophthalmia to colobomas.
The malformation occurs between the 21st and 25th day of gestation.

4. (C, D) Individuals with holoprosencephaly usually have a
normal karyotype or a D (13-15) trisomy. A few cases have
been reported with other chromosomal anomalies such as partial deletion of chromosome 18.

5. (D) An abnormal karyotype, most often the D (13-15) trisomy, is usually found in patients with holoprosencephaly who
have multiple extracranial anomalies. The present case was
an example of the D trisomy.

6. (A, B) Among the common extracranial anomalies are polydactyly, curved overlapping fingers, cardiac malformations of
various types, genital abnormalities, and a single umbilical
artery. Other less common extracranial anomalies include
gastrointestinal abnormalities, polycystic kidneys, and splenic
abnormalities.

7. (D) Many ocular anomalies ranging from anophthalmia to
colobomas have been described in association with holoprosencephaly. The presence of intraglobal cartilage, however, is
characteristic of the D (13-15) trisomy.

8. (A) About 50% of these individuals die within the first month, and about 80% die within the first year. Almost all die within two years. Many of the fetuses with the D trisomy are aborted.

9. (B) Older maternal age may be a significant factor in the development of this chromosomal aberration. An average maternal age of 30.9 years has been reported. Other cases have been reported in association with maternal diabetes, syphilis, and toxoplasmosis, but these are probably coincidental associations. Holoprosencephaly was regarded as a hereditary condition in sheep but this was later attributed to the consumption of certain toxic plants. Similar exogenous toxins seem to be of no significance in man.

10. (A, B, C, D) A wide variety of brain malformations have been described in patients with trisomy 18. In general, they tend to be less severe than those found in association with trisomy 13-15. The brain weight is generally lower than expected for the patient's age or body weight. Gyral abnormalities, often rather subtle ones, are consistently present. Cerebral periventricular heterotopias are commonly encountered and considered highly characteristic by some authors. The cerebellum is frequently abnormal with hypoplasia of the vermis, heterotopias and dysplastic folia. The inferior olivary nuclei show increased cellularity and thickened, simplified convolutions.

REFERENCES

1. DeMyer W: Holoprosencephaly (Cyclopia-arhinencephaly). In: Handbook of Clinical Neurology. Vinken PJ and Bruyn GW (Eds.). North-Holland, Amsterdam, 1977, Vol. 30, pp. 431-478.

2. Mottet NK and Jensen H: The anomalous embryonic development associated with trisomy 13-15. Am J Clin Path 43:334-346, 1965.

3. Sumi SM: Brain malformations in the trisomy 18 syndrome. Brain 93:821-830, 1970.

4. Terplan KL, et al.: Histologic structural anomalies in the brain in trisomy 18 syndrome. Amer J Dis Child 119:228-235, 1970.

5. Yakovlev PI: Pathoarchitectonic studies of cerebral malformations, III, arrhinencephalies (holotelencephalies). J Neuropath Exp Neurol 18:22-55, 1959.

: :

CASE 16: A Premature Infant with Subarachnoid Hemorrhage

CLINICAL DATA

This infant girl was born approximately two months prematurely
according to menstrual history. The mother was a gravida 6,
para 3, 28-year-old woman who had received no prenatal care.
The child's birth weight was 2 lbs, 7 oz, and the head circumference was 25 cm.   The child was meconium stained and
had Apgar scores of 5 at 1 and 5 minutes. The temperature was
97.4°F and the pulse was 160/min. Respirations were slow and
grunting. The child developed cyanosis of the face and neck and
her temperature dropped to 95.6°F. A spinal tap yielded bloody
cerebrospinal fluid. A blood culture was obtained and antibiotics
were instituted. Recurrent apneic spells occurred and the child
died at 24 hours of age.

At the time of autopsy, the child's brain appeared immature
and there was a small amount of subarachnoid hemorrhage,
especially about the foramina of Luschka and Magendie.

QUESTIONS

1.   Fig. 16.1 is a photograph of a coronal section of the brain.
     The pathological changes that are illustrated include
     A. demyelination of the centrum semiovale
     B. intraventricular hemorrhage
     C. subependymal matrix hemorrhage
     D. periventricular leukomalacia

2.   Fig. 16.2 is a photograph of a macrosection from the
     brain of a fetus. The dark-colored areas in the lateral
     ventricles are the subependymal germinal matrix tissue.
     In the course of normal development, the cells of the
     subependymal germinal matrix
     A. undergo necrosis
     B. differentiate into neurons
     C. differentiate into glial cells
     D. give rise to the choroid plexi

3.   The subependymal germinal matrix layer disappears by the
     A. sixth postnatal month
     B. first postnatal month
     C. end of gestation
     D. ninth fetal month

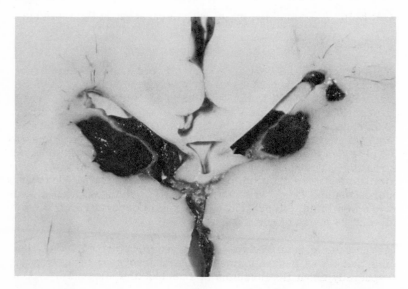

FIG. 16.1: Coronal section of the premature infant's brain.

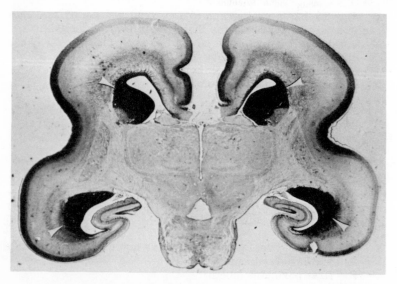

FIG. 16.2: Macrosection of the brain of a fetus. Note the dark staining subependymal matrix about the lateral ventricles (arrows).

4. Subependymal germinal matrix hemorrhages are currently regarded as manifestations of
    A. the difference between intrauterine and atmospheric pressure encountered at the time of delivery
    B. excessive molding of the head during parturition
    C. hypoxic damage between the 35th and 40th week of gestation
    D. hypoxic damage between the 25th and 35th week of gestation

5. Subependymal matrix cysts (Fig. 16.3)
    A. are due to toxoplasmosis
    B. may be sequela of subependymal matrix hemorrhages
    C. may result from subependymal germinolysis
    D. are more common than subependymal matrix hemorrhages

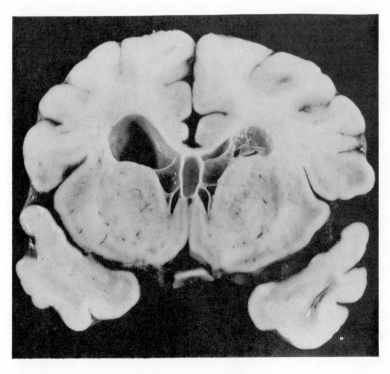

FIG. 16.3: Coronal section of an infant's brain showing subependymal matrix cysts.

6. Cerebral hypoxia in the term infant tends to be manifested by
   A. cerebral cortical necrosis
   B. periventricular necrosis
   C. subependymal matrix hemorrhages
   D. status marmoratus

7. Periventricular leukomalacia refers to
   A. massive demyelination of the central white matter
   B. necrosis of white matter commissures, e.g., corpus callosum, anterior commissure, etc.
   C. focal areas of necrosis in the deep periventricular white matter
   D. hypermyelination of the corpus striatum

8. Status marmoratus is
   A. a term used to describe a streaked or marbled appearance of the corpus striatum and thalamus
   B. hypermyelination of axons in congenitally malformed areas of the corpus striatum
   C. often associated with anoxia
   D. a pattern of glial scarring in which astrocytic processes are surrounded by myelin lamellae

9. Fig. 16.4 illustrates the appearance of Obersteiner's layer. This is a manifestation of
   A. the age of the patient
   B. intrauterine infection
   C. intrauterine anoxia
   D. maternal X-radiation

10. Normally the external granular cell layer is no longer evident after
    A. the eighth fetal month
    B. parturition
    C. the first postnatal month
    D. the ninth postnatal month

ANSWERS AND DISCUSSION

1. (B, C) The poor demarcation between the grey matter and white matter is due to a paucity of myelin. This reflects the immaturity of the brain and is not due to demyelination. Myelination in the brain begins in the medial longitudinal fasciculus during the fourth fetal month and progresses in an orderly and predictable fashion. The brain appears grossly myelinated by the sixth postnatal month but it is not completed until puberty.

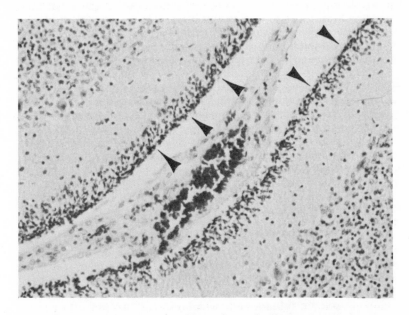

FIG. 16.4: Microscopic section of cerebellum showing an external layer of Obersteiner (arrows).

There are areas of hemorrhage and hemorrhagic necrosis in the floor of the lateral ventricles involving the subependymal matrix. The hemorrhage has ruptured into the ventricular system and was the source of the subarachnoid hemorrhage described externally about the foramina of Luschka and Magendie.

2.   (B, C) The subependymal germinal matrix is a derivative of the mantle layer and consists of immature multipotential cells. These migrate outward and differentiate into neurons and glial cells.

3.   (A) The subependymal germinal matrix is especially prominent during the sixth to eighth fetal months. The cells undergo progressive migration and maturation. The remnants of the subependymal germinal matrix have disappeared by the sixth postnatal month in full-term infants. They persist longer in premature infants.

4.   (D) Formerly the intraventricular hemorrhages in infants were attributed to the difference between the intrauterine and

atmospheric pressure or excessive molding of the head encountered at the time of parturition. More recent studies,
especially by Towbin, have indicated that subependymal matrix
hemorrhage and hemorrhagic necrosis result from cerebral
hypoxia between the 25th and 35th week of gestation.

5. (B, C) Subependymal matrix cysts are much less commonly
encountered than subependymal matrix hemorrhages. Many of
the cysts are residua of subependymal matrix hemorrhages from
which the blood, blood pigments and necrotic tissue have been
largely removed. Occasionally, subependymal matrix cysts
are encountered in which there is absolutely no evidence of an
antecedent hemorrhage. At least some of these are the result
of destruction of the subependymal matrix cells by viruses.
This process has been termed subependymal germinolysis.
Rubella and cytomegalovirus have been reported to cause such
lesions.

6. (A) In the older fetus and term infant, the cerebral cortex
suffers more severely than the periventricular structures from
anoxia. The cortical damage can vary from focal to diffuse
cortical necrosis. Subependymal matrix hemorrhages are uncommon in term infants and, when present, are usually regarded as evidence of earlier intrauterine hypoxia.

7. (C) The term periventricular leukomalacia is used to describe focal areas of necrosis in the deep periventricular white
matter. These are commonly encountered in premature infants
and have been variously attributed to hypoxia, acidosis, or circulatory insufficiency. Banker and Larroche emphasized their
occurrence in the borders between the perfusion zones of the
anterior, middle and posterior cerebral arteries while DeReuck,
et al, emphasized their occurrence in the border zones between
ventriculopetal and ventriculofugal arteries.

8. (A, C, D) The terms status marmoratus and etat marbre
are used to describe a peculiar marbled or streaked appearance
of the corpus striatum and thalamus. These areas stain heavily
with both myelin and glial stains. Formerly, they were interpreted as malformations with hypermyelination of axons. Currently, status marmoratus is regarded as a pattern of glial
scarring in which astrocytic processes become ensheathed by
myelin lamellae. Status marmoratus has often been described
as a sequela of anoxia.

9. (A) The cellular band on the surface of the cerebellar folia
is the external granular layer of Obersteiner. The presence of

this layer reflects the age of the patient. In a normal, full-
term infant, the layer is approximately 6 cells thick. It undergoes involution with increasing age.

10. (D) The remnants of the external granular layer have
largely disappeared by the ninth postnatal month.

REFERENCES

1. Banker BQ and Larroche JC: Periventricular leukomalacia
    of infancy. A form of neonatal anoxic encephalopathy.
    Arch Neurol 7:386-410, 1962.

2. Borit A and Herndon RM: The fine structure of plaques
    fibromyeliniques in ulegyria and status marmoratus.
    Acta Neuropath 14:304-311, 1970.

3. DeReuck J, et al.: Pathogenesis and evolution of peri-
    ventricular leukomalacia in infancy. Arch Neurol 27:
    229-336, 1972.

4. Leech RW and Alvord EC Jr.: Morphologic variations in
    periventricular leukomalacia. Amer J Path 74:591-600,
    1974.

5. Shaw CM and Alvord EC Jr.: Subependymal germinolysis.
    Arch Neurol 31:374-381, 1974.

6. Towbin A: Cerebral intraventricular hemorrhage and sub-
    ependymal matrix infarction in the fetus and premature
    newborn. Amer J Path 52:121-139, 1968.

7. Towbin A: Cerebral hypoxic damage in fetus and newborn.
    Basic patterns and their clinical significance. Arch
    Neurol 20:35-43, 1969.

: :

CASE 17: An Immature, Acidotic and Anoxic Infant with Foci
          of Intracerebral Discoloration

CLINICAL DATA

This 1060 g female infant was born after a 29-week gestation,
complicated by vaginal bleeding 4 days prior to delivery. The
infant was delivered as a footling breech after spontaneous
rupture of the membranes. Apgar scores were 1 and 3 at 1
and 5 minutes, respectively. The infant's tone and activity
were decreased, sucking and grasp were weak and rooting was
absent. Initial hematological studies disclosed a hemoglobin
of 14.5 g/dl, a hematocrit of 44%, a platelet count of 40,000/
cmm, a prothrombin time of 25.3 sec and a partial thromboplastin time of 103 sec. On 50% oxygen, the pO_2 was 148 mm
Hg, the pCO_2 was 45 mm Hg and the pH was 7.14.

The infant was maintained on a ventilator and an exchange transfusion was performed because of disseminated intravascular
coagulation. Ampicillin and gentamicin were initiated. Subsequently, the acidosis improved but oliguria developed. Two
days later the infant suffered an apneic episode with bradycardia,
and acidosis recurred (pH 6.9). The child developed tonic extensor posturing and the fontanelle was noted to be full. A
lumbar puncture yielded grossly bloodly cerebrospinal fluid and
blood was aspirated from the nasotracheal tube. Another exchange transfusion was performed for disseminated intravascular coagulation. Oliguria and mild acidosis (pH 7.2)
persisted. On the fourth day, rigidity, mottled skin with
petechiae and brawny edema were noted. The infant died
later that day.

At autopsy, a small amount of blood was present in the subarachnoid space over the convexities of the cerebral hemispheres and a larger quantity of blood was present at the base
of the brain and about the foramina of Luschka and Magendie.
Coronal sections of the cerebral hemispheres revealed blood
in the lateral ventricles and beneath the ependyma of the lateral
ventricles. In addition, there were multiple foci of yellow to
orange discoloration maximal in the putamena, pallida, subthalamic nuclei and inferior olives (Fig. 17.1).

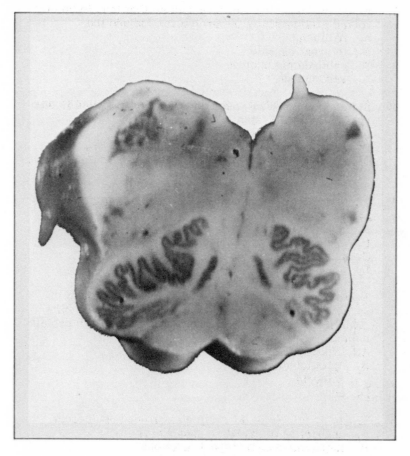

FIG. 17. 1: Transverse section of the infant's brain stem showing yellow to orange discoloration, maximal in the
inferior olives.

QUESTIONS

1. The gross neuropathological diagnoses in this case should
    include
    A. subependymal matrix hemorrhages with intraventricu-
        lar and subarachnoid extension
    B. periventricular leukomalacia
    C. kernicterus
    D. status marmoratus

2. Areas of the central nervous system that tend to be involved preferentially in kernicterus include the
    A. pallidum
    B. internal capsule
    C. subthalamic nucleus
    D. red nucleus

3. In the affected infants, the unconjugated bilirubin is derived principally from
    A. hemoglobin
    B. non-hemoglobin heme compounds
    C. enteric bilirubin glucuronide
    D. maternal bilirubin

4. Factors affecting the conjugation of bilirubin in the neonatal liver include
    A. maternal blood group
    B. "immaturity" of the neonatal liver
    C. maternal administration of certain drugs
    D. genetic defects

5. Factors reported to predispose to the development of kernicterus with low bilirubin levels (the highest bilirubin level recorded in the present case was 5.9 mg/dl) include
    A. hypoalbuminemia
    B. hypoglobulinemia
    C. acidosis
    D. anoxia

6. The toxic effects of bilirubin on neurons result from
    A. uncoupling of oxidative phosphorylation
    B. impairment of transport functions
    C. impairment of protein synthesis
    D. mechanisms that are currently unknown

7. Brains from individuals who survive kernicterus show loss of neurons and gliosis in the
    A. subthalamic nuclei
    B. pallida
    C. hippocampi
    D. superior temporal convolutions

ANSWERS AND DISCUSSION

1. (A, C) The gross neuropathological diagnoses in this premature infant's brain should include subependymal matrix

hemorrhages with intraventricular and subarachnoid extension
and kernicterus (bilirubin encephalopathy). Kernicterus is the
selective staining of various grey matter structures by unconjugated bilirubin.

2.   (A, C) Areas of the central nervous system that tend to be
involved preferentially by kernicterus include the subthalamic
nuclei, pallida, hippocampi, putamena, cranial nerve nuclei,
inferior olives, dentate nuclei, cerebellar flocculi and the grey
matter of the spinal cord.   The cerebral cortex and white
matter tend to be spared, unless they harbor focal destructive
lesions.

It is commonly stated that the abnormal pigmentation fades
rapidly upon storage in formalin. We have encountered no difficulty in detecting kernicterus when the intact brain is fixed in
formalin for the usual 10-14 days.   However, after sectioning
the brain, the yellow to orange discoloration disappears very
rapidly.

3.   (A) The unconjugated bilirubin is derived principally from
the degradation of hemoglobin; therefore, conditions that pro-
mote hemolysis, e.g., Rh incompatibility, ABO incompatibility,
glucose-6-phosphate dehydrogenase deficiency, etc., elevate
the bilirubin level beyond that expected in a normal newborn of
comparable age.

An additional source of bilirubin is from non-hemoglobin heme
compounds.   It has been suggested that the turnover of certain
hepatic heme compounds contribute to neonatal hyperbilirubinemia.

4.   (B, C, D) A major factor affecting the conjugation of bilirubin in the neonate is the "immaturity" of the neonatal liver.
The "immature" liver has markedly reduced uridine diphosphate
glucuronyltransferase (UDP-glucuronyltransferase) activity
and possibly reduced capacity for extracting the bilirubin from
the blood stream.   Normally, full "maturation" requires several weeks but can be hastened by administration of phenobarbital to the mother prior to delivery, or to the newborn
infant.

In rare cases, unconjugated hyperbilirubinemia is due to a
genetic absence or deficiency of UDP-glucuronyltransferase
activity (Crigler-Najjar syndrome), or to a genetic impairment
in the uptake of bilirubin from the blood stream (Gilbert's syndrome).

5. (A, C, D) In the blood, each mole of albumin tightly binds 2 moles of unconjugated bilirubin and prevents it from crossing the blood brain barrier. However, newborn and particularly premature infants have low albumin levels. Furthermore, the binding is reduced by acidosis or drugs (such as the sulfonamides) that compete with bilirubin for the binding sites on the albumin. Anoxia not only produces acidosis but also produces brain damage and increases the permeability of the blood brain barrier in the damaged areas. Thus, kernicterus can develop in certain anoxic and acidotic infants who have relatively low bilirubin levels.

6. (D) The exact mechanism by which the unconjugated bilirubin damages neurons must be regarded currently as unknown. It has been suggested that the bilirubin may uncouple oxidative phosphorylation, interfere with membrane transport systems and impair protein synthesis.

7. (A, B, C) Patients who survive kernicterus commonly show mental retardation and movement disorders. Neuronal loss and gliosis are most pronounced in the subthalamic nuclei, pallida and hippocampi.

REFERENCES

1. Blaw ME: Bilirubin Encephalopathy. In: Handbook of Clinical Neurology. Vinken PJ and Bruyn GW (Eds.). North-Holland, Amsterdam, 1976, Vol. 27, pp. 415-428.

2. Diamond I: Bilirubin Encephalopathy (Kernicterus). In: Scientific Approaches to Clinical Neurology. Goldensohn ES and Appel SH (Eds.). Lea and Febiger, Philadelphia, 1977, pp. 1212-1233.

3. Schmid R: Bilirubin metabolism in man. N Eng J Med 287:703-709, 1972.

: :

CASE 18: A 61-Year-Old Man Who Died 12 Days After a Fall

CLINICAL DATA

This 61-year-old man had a history of multiple disorders including alcoholism, gout, psoriasis, cholelithiasis, hiatal hernia, benign prostatic hypertrophy, chronic obstructive pulmonary disease, congestive heart failure, and hypertension.
Among the medications that he was receiving was a ganglionic
blocking agent. His present illness began with a transient loss
of consciousness attributed to orthostatic hypotension from the
ganglionic blocking agent. He fell backward and struck his
head against a wash basin. He regained consciousness in a
few minutes and had no neurological deficits when seen in the
emergency room. Skull x-rays were normal. The ganglionic
blocking agent was discontinued and the patient was sent home.

Four days later, the patient was brought back to the hospital
complaining of severe headaches and vomiting. On admission,
his blood pressure was 180/110 and his pulse was 64/minute.
He was lethargic and had an unsteady gait. Cranial nerves II
through XII were intact and his deep tendon reflexes were
symmetrical. While in the emergency room, his level of consciousness deteriorated rapidly and he became comatose. He
than displayed a left hemiplegia and a right third nerve palsy.
A right carotid arteriogram showed 2.5 cm of cortical shift
and evidence of uncal herniation. A right temporal craniotomy
was performed and 150 ml of clotted subdural blood was evacu-
ated from over the right temporal and parietal lobes. Postoperatively, the patient exhibited decerebrate posturing. He
died from pneumonia 8 days later.

Fig. 18.1 illustrates the right lateral surface of the brain and
Fig. 18.2 illustrates a coronal section from the parietal level.

QUESTIONS

1.   Subdural hematomas are usually due to
     A. trauma
     B. blood dyscrasias
     C. ruptured aneurysms
     D. hypertension

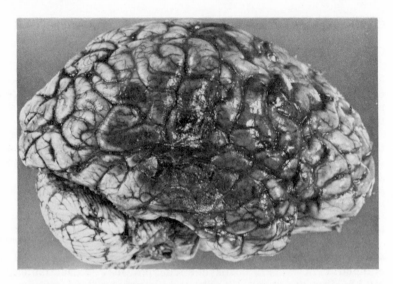

FIG. 18.1: Photograph of the brain showing deformation of the
            right hemisphere resulting from the overlying sub-
            dural hematoma.

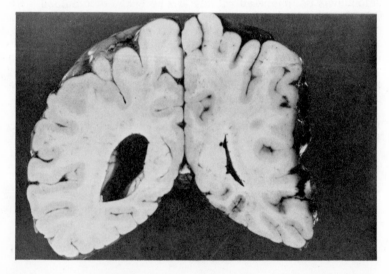

FIG. 18.2: Photograph of a coronal section of the brain showing
            the deformation resulting from the overlying sub-
            dural hematoma.

2. Subdural hematomas are most often located in the
   A. posterior fossa
   B. interhemispheric fissure
   C. posterior frontal-temporal-parietal region
   D. orbitofrontal region

3. Subdural hematomas are especially common in individuals who have a history of
   A. alcoholism
   B. seizures
   C. dementia
   D. hypertension

4. An acute subdural hematoma is generally accompanied by
   A. a fractured temporal bone
   B. intraventricular hemorrhage
   C. subarachnoid hemorrhage
   D. cerebral contusions and lacerations

5. Subdural hematomas become encapsulated as the result of proliferation of
   A. fibroblasts along the dural surface and margins of the hematoma
   B. fibroblasts along the arachnoidal surface and margins of the hematoma
   C. arachnoid cells on the dural and arachnoidal surfaces
   D. fibroblasts on the dural surface and arachnoid cells on the arachnoidal surface

6. Enlargement of a subdural hematoma is due to
   A. increased osmolarity of the sac contents due to blood breakdown products
   B. increased osmolarity due to leakage of protein from the subarachnoid space
   C. episodes of re-bleeding
   D. calcification

7. The inner membrane, as compared with the outer membrane, forms more
   A. rapidly and is thinner
   B. rapidly and is thicker
   C. slowly and is thinner
   D. slowly and is thicker

8. The right oculomotor palsy that the patient developed was due to
   A. irritation of the third nerve by the subdural blood
   B. pressure on the third nerve nucleus in the mesen-cephalon
   C. herniation of the right uncus with displacement and compression of the third nerve
   D. stretching of the third nerve

9. The decerebrate posturing that this patient developed indicates destruction of the
   A. frontal lobe
   B. internal capsule and rostral cerebral peduncle
   C. brain stem rostral to the middle of the pons
   D. medulla

10. The lesion producing the brain stem destruction is a
   A. secondary brain stem hemorrhage
   B. Duret hemorrhage
   C. primary brain stem hemorrhage that occurred when the patient fell
   D. hypertensive hemorrhage

ANSWERS AND DISCUSSION

1. (A) The vast majority of subdural hematomas are due to trauma. The prevalence of subdural hematomas varies among studies reflecting in part the nature of the population under investigation. Figures in the range of 10-15% are usually reported in clinical studies on closed head trauma. Much higher frequencies are reported among fatal cases. Subdural hematomas may result from relatively minor head trauma or falls that are easily and often forgotten. Rarely, subdural hematomas may result from non-traumatic disorders. These include ruptured aneurysms, hemorrhages from metastases and blood dyscrasias.

2. (C) Chronic subdural hematomas usually result from tears in the bridging veins that pass through the subdural space on their way from the surface of the brain to the dural sinuses. In acute subdural hematomas, those developing in a few days, the bleeding is usually from torn vessels immediately overlying a cerebral contusion or laceration. Most subdural hematomas are situated over the lateral surface of the hemisphere, especially over the posterior frontal-temporal-parietal region. About 15% of the subdural hematomas are bilateral. Occasionally, the hematoma is located primarily in the interhemispheric

fissure. Some subdural hematomas are located primarily under
the ventral surface of the temporal lobe. These probably arise
from tears in bridging veins that emerge from the temporal
poles. Posterior fossa hematomas are relatively rare.

3. (A, B, C) Since subdural hematomas usually result from
trauma, they are somewhat more common in men than women,
and are especially common among individuals who sustain frequent head trauma. These include alcoholic, epileptic, demented and psychotic individuals. Demented patients with
marked cerebral atrophy are especially prone to develop subdural hematomas.

4. (C, D) Acute subdural hematomas usually result from contusions or lacerations of the cerebral cortex. They are almost
invariably accompanied by some degree of subarachnoid bleeding. By contrast, the brain under a chronic subdural hematoma
is deformed but usually shows no traumatic lesions.

5. (A) With the passage of time, the subdural hematomas become encapsulated. This is the result of proliferation of fibroblasts along the dural surface and margins of the hematoma.
The arachnoid plays little if any role in the capsule formation.
The encapsulated hematoma can be separated readily from the
arachnoid except when the arachnoid has been torn. The membrane is always adherent to the dura.

6. (C) Enlargement of a subdural hematoma is primarily due
to episodes of re-bleeding. Older concepts regarding the subdural membrane as a semipermeable membrane are probably
not valid. After many years, the membranes of a chronic subdural hematoma may become calcified but this does not contribute to further enlargement.

7. (C) The membrane is formed by proliferation of fibroblasts on the inner surface of the dura and about the margins
of the hematoma. The arachnoid does not contribute to the
membrane. Therefore, the inner membrane is slower to form
and is thinner since these fibroblasts must migrate from the
margins of the hematoma.

8. (C) The ipsilateral oculomotor nerve palsy was due to a
lateral transtentorial hernia (uncal hernia) that caused the third
nerve to be compressed at the incisura of the tentorium by
structures at the base such as the petroclinoid ligament and the
posterior cerebral artery.

9. (C) Lesions that destroy the frontal lobes, internal capsules or rostral cerebral peduncles produce decorticate rigidity. This consists of adduction of the upper extremities with flexion of the wrists and arms and extension, internal rotation and plantar flexion of the lower extremities. Destruction of the brain stem rostral to the midpons results in decerebrate rigidity. This consists of opisthotonos, extension, adduction, and pronation of the arms and extension of the legs.

10. (A, B) The lesion responsible for the brain stem destruction was a secondary brain stem hemorrhage (Fig. 18.3). These are also known as Duret hemorrhages. They are a complication of caudal herniation of the brain stem. The exact pathogenesis has been debated and arterial, venous, and combined arterial and venous origins have been proposed. Most likely the caudal displacement of the brain stem stretches the paramedian arterioles to the lower mesencephalon and pons. This results in foci of ischemia that subsequently become hemorrhagic. These lesions are the immediate cause of death from expanding supratentorial lesions.

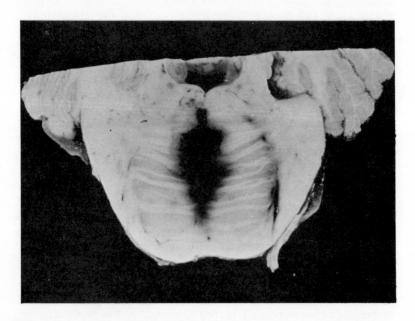

FIG. 18.3: Transverse section of the rostral pons showing a hemorrhagic lesion.

REFERENCES

1. Adams H and Graham DI: The Pathology of Blunt Head
    Injuries. In: Scientific Foundations of Neurology.
    Critchley M, et al. (Eds.). F. A. Davis Co., Philadelphia,
    1972, pp. 478-491.

2. Hassler O: Arterial pattern of human brain stem. Nor-
    mal appearance and deformation in expanding supraten-
    torial conditions. Neurology 17:368-376, 1967.

3. Lindenberg R: Trauma of Meninges and Brain. In:
    Pathology of the Nervous System. Minckler J (Ed.).
    McGraw-Hill Book Co., New York, 1971, Vol. 2, pp.
    1705-1765.

4. Plum F and Posner JB: Diagnosis of Stupor and Coma.
    F. A. Davis Co., Philadelphia, 1972.

: :

CASE 19: A Young Man Who Fell from the Back of a Moving
          Truck

CLINICAL DATA

This 23-year-old man fell from the back of a moving pickup
truck. He was rendered unconscious immediately. He was
taken to a local hospital where he was noted to be responsive
to pain and to have no gross motor deficits or pathological reflexes. Within 45 minutes of his arrival he had regained consciousness and was talking. An occipital scalp laceration was
sutured.

Four hours after his initial hospitalization, he was transferred
to another hospital where he was noted to be somnolent, confused, and complaining of a severe headache. There were no
focal neurological deficits. X-rays of the skull revealed a non-
depressed linear fracture involving the midline of the occipital
bone.

The patient's neurological status improved slightly over the
next three days but he died on the fourth hospital day from
aspiration pneumonia.

QUESTIONS

1. On the basis of the lesions illustrated in Figs. 19.1 and
    19.2, one would conclude that the
    A. patient fell, striking the vertex of his head
    B. patient fell, landing on his buttocks
    C. patient fell, striking his occiput
    D. history is probably erroneous; the patient was prob-
        ably struck on his occiput with a blunt object

2. Given a history of the unsupported head being struck with
    a relatively heavy object, one would expect to find
    A. a depressed or linear skull fracture at the site of the
        impact
    B. a large coup lesion, i.e., contusion at the site of
        impact
    C. minor or no contrecoup lesions
    D. herniation contusions in the cerebellar tonsils and
        medulla

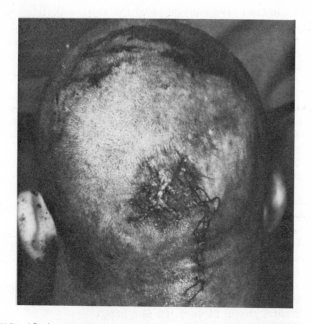

FIG. 19. 1: Photograph of the patient's head showing
the location of the sutured scalp laceration.

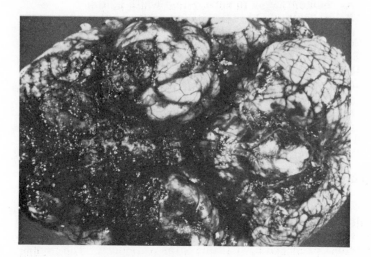

FIG. 19. 2: Photograph of the base of the brain showing
the location of the contrecoup lesion.

3. In the unusual circumstances of the well-supported head being struck, one would expect to find
   A. extensive coup contusions
   B. extensive contrecoup lesions
   C. skull fractures
   D. cerebral lacerations

4. If the patient described in the clinical data had survived, his neurological sequelae may have included
   A. anosmia
   B. personality and behavioral abnormalities
   C. cerebellar ataxia
   D. hemiballismus

5. The histological characteristics of acute contusions include
   A. wedge-shaped areas of necrosis involving especially the crests of gyri
   B. wedge-shaped areas of necrosis involving especially the depths of sulci
   C. linear hemorrhages that are perpendicular to the cortical surface
   D. phagocytosis of corpora amylacea

6. Traumatic cerebral lesions in very young infants differ from those in older individuals and are characterized by
   A. hemorrhages in subcortical white matter
   B. grossly visible tears in the white matter
   C. hemorrhages in the cortex
   D. necrosis in the depths of sulci

7. Histological changes encountered in the brains of individuals who remain comatose for a number of months after severe head injury include
   A. degeneration of white matter
   B. reactive axons
   C. "microglial stars"
   D. neurofibrillary tangles

ANSWERS AND DISCUSSION

1. (C) Injuries sustained in vehicular accidents are often difficult to interpret because of the lack of accurate information regarding the exact sequence of events and because of the complications produced by multiple sites of impact. The findings in the present case are typical of those resulting from a fall with impact on occiput. The brain injuries resulting from the

sudden deceleration of the moving head are characterized by
relatively minor coup lesions beneath the site of impact and
severe contrecoup lesions especially on the ventral surfaces
of the frontal and temporal lobes. The precise mechanism for
the production of the contrecoup lesions has been the subject
of debate and investigation for over 200 years and still has not
been resolved completely. The predilection for the ventral
surfaces of the frontal and temporal lobes appear to be determined in part by the rough floor of the anterior and middle
fossae. The laceration of the scalp and underlying skull fracture are important indicators of the site of impact.   The subjacent cerebral cortex at the coup site may show few or no contusions. The skull fracture itself may produce small contusions on either side of the fracture line remote from the impact
site as the bone strikes against the cortex. These lesions are
called fracture contusions. Lesions within the interior of the
brain, along a line between the coup and contrecoup lesions are
termed intermediary coup lesions. These lesions are relatively
uncommon when the site of impact is on the occiput. They are
especially common in falls on the forehead or convexity of the
head above the level of the corpus callosum.

Contrecoup lesions on the ventral surface of the frontal and
temporal lobes could have been due to impact on the vertex.
In that event, the lacerations and skull fractures would have
been located on the vertex of the head. With impact on the vertex, intermediary coup lesions are often present in the corpus
callosum.   These result from stretching of this commissure
as the brain is deformed. Lesions also may be present in the
unci and about the mammillary bodies as the brain tissue is
momentarily forced ventrally and through the tentorium at the
time of impact.   Still other lesions may be found in the midbrain.   Especially characteristic of this type of impact are
lesions in the brachia conjunctiva.

2.   (A, B, C, D) The pattern of injury resulting from a blow
to the unsupported head by a heavy object is usually quite different from that resulting from a fall.   In the case of a blow
to the stationary but movable head, there is sudden acceleration
of the head at the time of impact.   The majority of these patients have skull fractures, often depressed, at the site of impact.   The underlying brain is usually severely contused, i.e.,
there is an extensive coup lesion. Contrecoup lesions, i.e.,
contusions on the contralateral surface of the brain, are minor
or even absent in the majority of these cases. Herniation contusions resulting from sudden but transient displacement of the
brain at the time of impact may be found in the cerebellar tonsils and dorsal medulla.

3. (C, D) The resulting lesions are quite different from those
produced by falls or blows to the movable head. The differences
are due in part to the lack of acceleration or deceleration of the
head and to the absorption of the force by both the skull and
supporting surface. The skull is often very severely fractured;
nevertheless, coup and contrecoup contusions are generally absent. Extensive laceration of the brain may be produced from
bone fragments about the skull fractures. Despite the severe
skull injuries, the patient may not be unconscious.

4. (A, B) If the patient described in the clinical data had survived, his neurological sequelae may have included a frontal
lobe syndrome as a result of the severe contrecoup injury to
the orbital surfaces of the frontal lobes. This type of frontal
lobe syndrome is characterized by personality and behavioral
abnormalities including social disinhibition. Frontal lobe syndromes resulting from injury predominantly to the convexities
of the frontal lobes are characterized by intellectual deficits.
The patient also may have had anosmia as the result of destruction of the olfactory bulbs and tracts by the contrecoup lesions.
Impairment of hearing and vestibular function can be demonstrated in many patients who have sustained head injury, including relatively mild injury. This results from either bleeding
into the middle ear or injury to the eighth nerve. Visual impairment can result from compression of branches of the anterior
choroidal artery with necrosis in the optic tracts (Fig. 19.3) or
from compression of the posterior cerebral artery at the incisura with necrosis of the calcarine cortex (Fig. 19.4).

5. (A, C) Contusions are characterized by wedge-shaped areas
of necrosis that involve maximally the crests of gyri with relative preservation of the cortex in the sulci. Even when the contusion is large and involves several gyri, the overall lesion has
a roughly wedge-shaped configuration. The preferential involvement of the gyral crests is in contrast to vascular lesions which
maximally involve the depths of sulci. In old vascular lesions
a glial membrane derived from the molecular layer persists
over the gyral crests. Hemorrhages result from damage to
vessels at the moment of impact. These include subarachnoid
hemorrhages from the meninges and hemorrhages in the neural
parenchyma. The latter may appear as punctate hemorrhages
or as linear hemorrhages that are oriented perpendicular to the
cortical surface. The hemorrhages may enlarge during the
first few hours after the injury. With the passage of time, the
contused tissues undergo the same sequence of resorptive changes
as seen with vascular lesions.

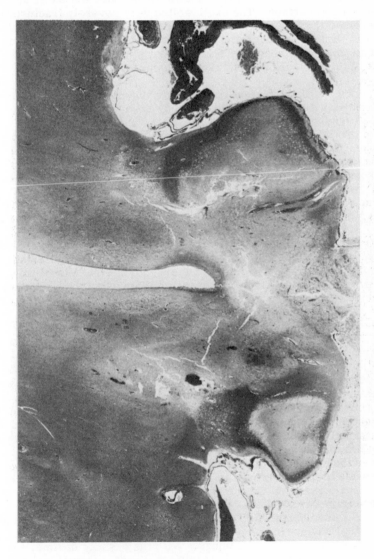

FIG. 19.3: Necrosis of optic tracts due to compression of branches of the anterior choroidal artery.

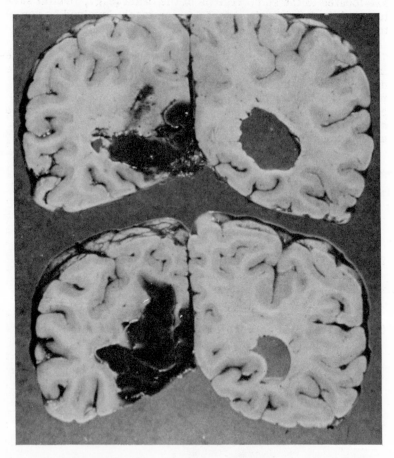

FIG. 19. 4: Necrosis of calcarine cortex due to compression of
the posterior cerebral artery.

6. (B) Traumatic lesions in the immature, poorly myelinated brains of young infants rarely show the same features as contusions in older individuals. The characteristic traumatic lesions in the very young consist of tears in the white matter that are accompanied by relatively little hemorrhage. Even microscopically, necrosis and hemorrhage are minimal. The tears are located in the same regions of the brain (e.g., orbital surfaces of the frontal lobes) that are commonly involved by contusions in older patients.

7. (A, B, C) Patients who sustain severe head injuries and remain comatose for a number of months generally show extensive degeneration of the white matter. This is probably due to the mechanical tearing of nerve fibers and is reflected by the presence of reactive axons, scattered small clusters of macrophages called "microglial stars," and myelin breakdown products that are best demonstrated with Sudan or Marchi stains.

REFERENCES

1. Adams H and Graham DI: The Pathology of Blunt Head Injuries. In: Scientific Foundations of Neurology. Critchley M, et al. (Eds.).   F.A. Davis Co., Philadelphia, 1972, pp. 478-491.

2. Lindenberg R: Trauma of Meninges and Brain. In: Pathology of the Nervous System. Minckler J, et al. (Eds.). McGraw-Hill Book Co., New York, 1971, Vol. 2, pp. 1705-1765.

3. Lindenberg R and Freytag E: The mechanism of cerebral contusions. Arch Path 69:440-469, 1960.

4. Lindenberg R and Freytag E: Morphology of brain lesions from blunt trauma in early infancy. Arch Path 87:298-305, 1969.

: :

CASE 20: A 51-Year-Old Man Who Died After a Gunshot Wound

CLINICAL DATA

This 51-year-old man was brought to the emergency room after
being found with a gunshot wound of his head. An entrance wound
was present in the left supraorbital area; no exit wound was evident.

The patient could be roused only with noxious stimuli. His right
eye displayed a full range of movement and his right pupil was
reactive to light.   His left eye was exophthalmic with marked
hyphemia and vitreous hemorrhage.   The patient had a right
hemiparesis with decerebrate rigidity and bilateral extensor
plantar responses.   Skull x-rays revealed the entrance wound
in the left supraorbital ridge and a large metal fragment to the
left of the midline just above the inion.

A frontotemporal craniotomy was performed for debridement of
the left frontal lobe. The defect in the orbital roof was closed with
a graft and the skin over the left supraorbital ridge was repaired.

Postoperatively the patient continued to have hemiplegia and
decerebrate rigidity on the right. He did not regain consciousness and died three days after the gunshot wound.

QUESTIONS

1.   Features that characterize an entrance wound include
     A.   an abrasion ring
     B.   "tattoos" from unburned or partially burned powder
     C.   outline of gun muzzle
     D.   stretch marks

2.   When present, the exit wound is often
     A.   smaller than the entrance wound
     B.   larger than the entrance wound
     C.   more irregular than the entrance wound
     D.   surrounded by an abrasion ring

3.   Fig. 20.1 shows the entrance wound in the brain and
     Fig. 20.2 shows the exit wound in the brain. The injury
     can be described as a
     A.   penetrating wound of the head
     B.   perforating wound of the head
     C.   penetrating wound of the brain
     D.   perforating wound of the brain

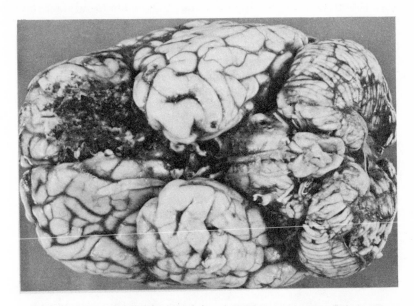

FIG. 20.1: Photograph showing entrance wound in the brain.

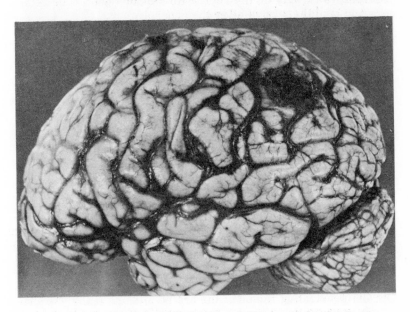

FIG. 20.2: Photograph showing exit wound in the brain.

4. The diameter of the track through the brain is influenced most by
   A. tumbling of the bullet
   B. yaw
   C. the mass of the missile
   D. the velocity of the missile

5. The exit wound in the brain (see Fig. 20.2) is several centimeters dorsal to the site where the bullet was found at the time of autopsy. This was due to
   A. displacement during removal of the brain
   B. internal ricochet
   C. break-up of the missile
   D. cerebral edema

6. The pathologist should determine and be prepared to testify as to the caliber of the bullet on the basis of
   A. the size of the entrance wound
   B. the weight and size of the bullet fragments
   C. the extent of tissue destruction
   D. none of the above

7. Lesions commonly associated with gunshot wounds of the head other than the wound track itself include
   A. orbital roof fractures
   B. uncal contusions
   C. tonsillar contusions
   D. tears of the corpus callosum

8. Among the late or delayed sequelae encountered in patients who survive gunshot wounds to the head are
   A. lead intoxication
   B. low pressure hydrocephalus
   C. epilepsy
   D. abscesses

ANSWERS AND DISCUSSION

1. (A, B, C) The appearance of an entrance wound is influenced by the distance between the skin and the gun muzzle. When the distance is greater than a few feet, the entrance wound is usually smaller than the bullet and the wound is surrounded by an abrasion ring. When the gun muzzle is only a few inches from the skin, the wound is surrounded by "tattoos" produced by the partially burned or unburned powder that accompanies the missile. Obviously, much of the tattooing can be missing if the entrance site is covered by clothing. If the muzzle of the gun is in loose

contact with the skin, the gases that accompany the missile into
the tissues can produce a stellate tear about the entrance wound.
If the gun muzzle is firmly pressed against the skin, the out-
line of the muzzle may be reflected by bruises and the missile
tract will show considerable burning. When the skull is involved, the entrance wound is characterized by a relatively small
defect in the outer table and a larger, crateriform defect in the
inner table.

2.   (B, C) Ordinarily, the exit wound is larger and more irregular than the entrance wound.   There may be several exit
wounds from a single bullet due to fragmentation of the bullet
and the formation of secondary missiles, e.g., fragments of
bone. When the skull is involved, the exit wound is characterized by a relatively small defect in the inner table and a larger
crateriform defect in the outer table.

3.   (A, D) The term "penetrating" is used to indicate that a
specific anatomic structure has an entrance wound but no exit
wound.   The term "perforating" is used to indicate that a specific anatomic structure has both entrance and exit wounds.
In the present case, there is a penetrating wound of the head
but a perforating wound of the brain.

4.   (D) The diameter of the wound track (Fig. 20.3) is influenced by a number of factors including tumbling, yaw, mass
and velocity.   Of these, the velocity is the most important.
Doubling the mass of the bullet doubles the energy that can be
transmitted but doubling the velocity produces a fourfold increase in the amount of energy available.   For this reason,
low velocity civilian weapons usually produce small wound
tracks while high velocity military weapons, even with equal
sized bullets, produce much more massive destruction of
neural parenchyma.

5.   (B) The path of a bullet within the cranium can be deflected
one or more times by contact with the falx, tentorium or the
skull.   This phenomenon is known as internal ricochet.   The
bullet may produce multiple tracks through the neural parenchyma
or, as in the present case, may slide along the inner surface
of the dura. Breakup of the missile and formation of secondary
missiles of bone fragments can also make more complicated
wounds.   For these reasons, it is highly desirable to review
clinical x-rays before performing the autopsy and to x-ray the
brain specimen before dissecting it.

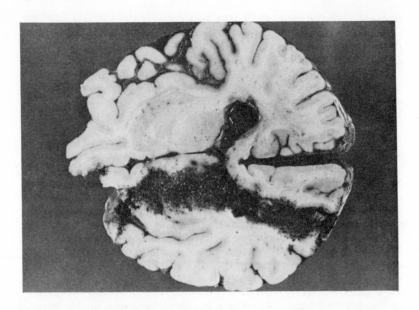

FIG. 20. 3: Photograph showing the wound track. Note the brain
has been sectioned obliquely along a probe gently
passed through the track.

6.   (D) The pathologist should weigh, measure, photograph,
and properly label any bullets or bullet fragments that are obtained at the time of surgery or autopsy. However, determination of the caliber of the bullet and testimony regarding the
caliber of the bullet should be left to ballistics experts.

7.   (A, B, C) As a result of the sudden increase in intracranial
pressure, transient herniation of the unci and cerebellar tonsils
occur and are commonly reflected as herniation contusions. In
addition, the orbital roofs are commonly fractured regardless
of the location and direction of the gunshot. These fractures
can produce exophthalmos secondary to intraorbital hemorrhages.

8.   (C, D) Epilepsy is a common sequela in patients who have
sustained penetrating head wounds and is probably associated
with the hypersensitivity of the cortex surrounding glial-menin-
geal cicatrices. Abscesses may result from wound contamination by clothing, hair, surface dirt, etc., rather than the
missile per se. These abscesses may not become manifested
clinically until months or years after the wound.

REFERENCES

1. Freytag E: Autopsy findings in head injuries from firearms. Arch Path 76:215-225, 1963.

2. Lindenberg R: Trauma of Meninges and Brain. In:
   Pathology of the Nervous System. Minckler J (Ed.).
   McGraw-Hill Book Co., New York, 1971, pp. 1705-1765.

3. Petty CS: Firearms injury research. Amer J Clin Path
   52:277-288, 1969.

4. Rose EF: Forensic Pathology. In: Laboratory Medicine.
   Race GJ (Ed.). Harper and Row, Hagerstown, 1973,
   Vol. 3, pp. 3-36.

: :

CASE 21: A Woman with Chronic Alcoholism and Ascites

CLINICAL DATA

This was the 34th hospitalization for this 56-year-old white woman with chronic alcoholism. She entered the hospital with increasing abdominal girth and peripheral edema. She had gained 20 kg during the 2-1/2 months since her last hospitalization for Laennec's cirrhosis, portal hypertension and Korsakoff's psychosis. She denied hematemesis or melena. She was oriented only to person and place and displayed confabulation.   There were spider nevi on her chest, back and face. She had slight scleral icterus, her pupils were equal and reactive and her extraocular movements were full without nystagmus. The fundi were normal. The neurological examination was essentially normal. She had massive ascites with fluid waves and shifting dullness. The liver was percussed approximately 8 cm below the right costal margin. Rectal examination was normal. She had severe pitting edema of her legs. Laboratory studies revealed a hemoglobin of 10.5 g/dl, hematocrit of 30% and a white cell count of 4,900. The blood urea nitrogen was 25 mg/dl, sodium 134 mEq/l, potassium 4 mEq/l, chloride 111 mEq/l, glucose 118 mg/dl, albumin 1.5 gm/dl, SGPT 20U, SGOT 30U, alkaline phosphatase 14.5 BU and ammonia 80 μg/dl. She died a few days later and at autopsy was found to have marked cirrhosis, pulmonary congestion and 13,500 ml of abdominal ascites.

QUESTIONS

1.   Neuropathological lesions that have an increased prevalence in patients with chronic alcoholism include
     A.   cerebral contusions and subdural hematomas
     B.   peripheral neuropathy
     C.   pneumococcal meningitis
     D.   Wernicke's encephalopathy

2.   Histopathological changes that may be seen in the mammillary bodies from patients with Wernicke's encephalopathy include
     A.   loss of neurons
     B.   accumulation of macrophages
     C.   neurofibrillary tangles
     D.   astrocytosis

3. Wernicke's encephalopathy is generally regarded to be the result of vitamin
   A. A deficiency
   B. B_1 deficiency
   C. B_6 deficiency
   D. B_{12} deficiency

4. The cerebellar degeneration associated with chronic alcoholism is characterized by
   A. atrophy of the superior vermis
   B. atrophy of the inferior vermis
   C. loss of Purkinje cells, granule cells and neurons of the molecular layer
   D. proliferation of Bergmann glia

5. Central pontine myelinolysis is characterized by
   A. loss of neurons from the pons
   B. preservation of neurons in the pons
   C. demyelination in the pons
   D. petechial hemorrhages in the pons

6. Marchiafava-Bignami disease is characterized by degeneration of the
   A. posterior columns of the spinal cord
   B. lateral columns of the spinal cord
   C. corpus callosum
   D. anterior commissure

7. Leigh's disease or subacute necrotizing encephalomyelopathy is characterized by
   A. primarily affecting infants and children
   B. incomplete necrosis in brain stem tegmentum and basal ganglia
   C. demyelination of optic nerves and tracts
   D. necrosis of the mammillary bodies

8. Patients with alcoholic cirrhosis or other hepatic disease occasionally develop hepatic encephalopathy. The changes in the brains of these patients include
   A. proliferation of Alzheimer's type 2 astrocytes
   B. kernicterus
   C. icteric discoloration of the entire brain
   D. icteric discoloration of the dura, choroid plexi and infundibulum

ANSWERS AND DISCUSSION

1.   (A, B, C, D) Traumatic lesions, including contusions and subdural hematomas, are especially common in patients with alcoholism. The high incidence of trauma further complicated by coagulation defects associated with alcoholism accounts for the prevalence of subdural hematomas.

Pneumococcal meningitis is a common form of meningitis in adults and is especially common following trauma and in patients with alcoholism. The higher frequency in alcoholics may be due to the impaired phagocytosis that accompanies alcoholism.

Alcoholic polyneuropathy is encountered most commonly in men during the fifth and sixth decades. The symptoms progress slowly over a period of weeks and tend to be more severe in the legs than the arms. The manifestations include pain, paresthesias and weakness. The morphological lesions are rarely studied at autopsy but consist predominantly of segmental demyelination with relative preservation of the axons.

Wernicke's encephalopathy is found predominantly in alcoholic patients with associated nutritional deficiencies. Fig. 21.1 compares the mammillary bodies from the present case (left) with the mammillary bodies from a non-alcoholic control patient (right). The mammillary bodies from the present case show atrophy and brownish discoloration, changes that are consistent with old Wernicke's encephalopathy. Grossly discernible changes are found in the mammillary bodies from about 75% of patients with Wernicke's encephalopathy. Depending upon the severity and acuteness, the gross changes range from confluent petechial hemorrhages to atrophy and discoloration. Other sites of involvement in descending order of frequency include the walls of the third ventricle, the floor of the fourth ventricle, and the periaqueductal grey matter. In all locations, grossly discernible hemorrhages are relatively uncommon.

2.   (A, B, D) The mammillary bodies invariably show histopathological changes in patients with Wernicke's encephalopathy. However, the spectrum of alterations varies with the severity and acuteness of the disorder. In the acute cases, the mammillary bodies show edema, prominent blood vessels, demyelination, abundant macrophages and swollen astrocytes. Hemorrhages may be present but are unusual. In the older cases, the mammillary bodies show loss of neurons, loss of myelin, scattered perivascular macrophages and increased numbers of astrocytes. In all cases, the loss of myelin appears to be more severe than the loss of axis cylinders.

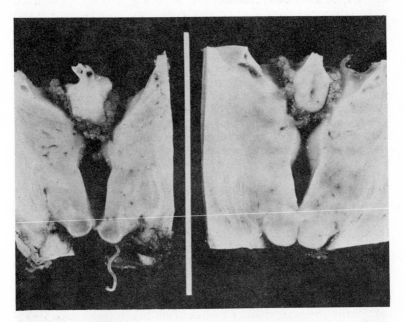

FIG. 21.1: Mammillary bodies from the present case (left)
compared with mammillary bodies from a non-
alcoholic control patient (right).

Neurofibrillary tangles are not a feature of Wernicke's encephalopathy but may be found in the mammillary bodies in patients with
Alzheimer's disease.

3. (B) The metabolic basis of Wernicke's encephalopathy is
now generally regarded to be vitamin B_1 or thiamine deficiency.
The active form of the vitamin, thiamine pyrophosphate, is a
coenzyme in the decarboxylation of alpha-ketoacids such as
pyruvic acid. It is also involved in the pentose phosphate shunt
as a cofactor to transketolase. The transketolase activity is
apparently even more susceptible to thiamine deficiency than
the pyruvate decarboxylase activity. Determinations of blood
pyruvate or assays of transketolase activity can be used in the
clinical diagnosis of Wernicke's encephalopathy. However,
some authors feel that neither of these enzyme deficiencies is
directly responsible for the morphologically demonstrable
lesions.

4.   (A, C, D) Cerebellar degeneration is commonly encountered
in patients with severe chronic alcoholism. The lesion consists
of folial atrophy that is largely restricted to the superior portion
of the vermis.   The changes are best demonstrated grossly by
a sagittal section through the cerebellar vermis (Fig. 21.2).
Histologically, the atrophied folia show extensive loss of neurons including Purkinje cells, granule cells and neurons from
the molecular layer. In addition, there is proliferation of the
Bergmann glia, the astrocytes that are found adjacent to the
Purkinje cells. In some patients, there are also changes in
the inferior olivary nuclei consisting of loss of neurons from
the dorsal laminae.

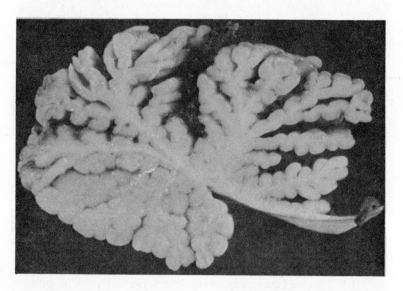

FIG. 21.2: Sagittal section of the cerebellar vermis from a
           patient with severe chronic alcoholism.

Although this type of cerebellar degeneration is found predominantly in patients with chronic alcoholism, the lesions are probably due to associated nutritional deficiencies. Somewhat similar morphological changes may be encountered in patients with
diphenylhydantoin intoxication.

5.   (B, C) Central pontine myelinolysis is an uncommon disorder that has been encountered most often in patients with
chronic alcoholism or other disorders that produce severe

nutritional deficiencies. Central pontine myelinolysis is rarely diagnosed clinically; most cases have been recognized only at the time of autopsy.   The lesion consists typically of a single diamond-shaped area of demyelination in the center of the basis pontis (Fig. 21.3). Within the lesion, myelin sheaths and oligo-dendrocytes are largely destroyed while neurons and axis cylinders are preserved.

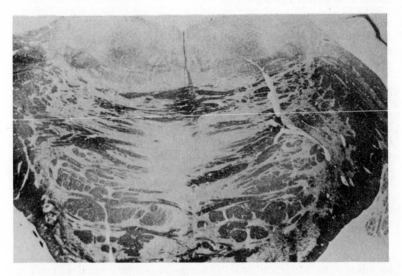

FIG. 21. 3: Transverse section of a pon showing central pon-
          tine myelinolysis.

6.   (C, D) Marchiafava-Bignami disease is an extremely rare disorder found predominantly, but not exclusively, in middle-aged Italian men who are addicted to red wine. Pathologically, the lesions consist of demyelination or partial necrosis of the corpus callosum with lesser degrees of involvement of the anterior commissure, posterior commissure and centrum semiovale. Within the corpus callosum the midportion is most severely affected with relative sparing of the dorsal and ven-tral surfaces.   Clinically, the disorder is characterized by mental symptoms, convulsions, tremors, and motor disabilities.

7.   (A, B, C) Leigh's disease is a rare metabolic disorder that has been described primarily in infants and children.   It is characterized by multiple, often bilaterally symmetrical areas of incomplete necrosis that are encountered most often

in the tegmentum of the brain stem, the spinal cord, and the basal ganglia. In the destructive foci, there is relative sparing of the neurons and striking hyperplasia of the capillaries. The optic nerves and tracts often show demyelination. The disorder is occasionally designated erroneously as "infantile Wernicke's encephalopathy." The mammillary bodies are rarely involved in Leigh's disease whereas they are always affected in Wernicke's encephalopathy.

The presence of an inhibitor of adenosine triphosphate-thiamine pyrophosphate phosphotransferase, the enzyme responsible for forming thiamine triphosphate, has been proposed to be the biochemical basis of Leigh's disease.

8. (A, D) Brains from patients with hepatic encephalopathy may show bile staining but only in areas where the blood-brain-barrier is incompetent. The dura, choroid plexi and infundibulum are the most obviously icteric structures. Focal destructive lesions such as infarcts and metastases also become discolored. Microscopically, the most consistent alteration is a proliferation of distinctive astrocytes, the so-called Alzheimer's type 2 glia. These cells usually have vesicular, often multilobed nuclei and inconspicuous cytoplasm. Many of the nuclei contain acidophilic inclusions thought to be glycogen. These changes are due at least in part to the elevated ammonia levels.

REFERENCES

1. Brion S: Marchiafava-Bignami Syndrome. In: Handbook of Clinical Neurology. Vinken PJ and Bruyn GW (Eds.). North-Holland, Amsterdam, 1976, Vol. 28, pp. 317-329.

2. David RB, et al.: Necrotizing Encephalomyelopathy (Leigh). In: Handbook of Clinical Neurology. Vinken PJ and Bruyn GW (Eds.). North-Holland, Amsterdam, 1976, Vol. 28, pp. 349-363.

3. Goebel HH and Herman-Ben Zur P: Central Pontine Myelinolysis. In: Handbook of Clinical Neurology. Vinken PJ and Bruyn GW (Eds.). North-Holland, Amsterdam, 1976, Vol. 28, pp. 285-316.

4. Valsamis MP and Mancall E: Toxic cerebellar degeneration. Human Path 4:513-520, 1973.

5. Victor M, et al.: The Wernicke-Korsakoff Syndrome. F. A. Davis Co., Philadelphia, 1971.

: :

CASE 22: A Young Man who Died 10 Days After Attempting
Suicide with Automobile Exhaust

CLINICAL DATA

This 24-year-old man attempted suicide by carbon monoxide inhalation. He had connected the end of a hose to the exhaust pipe
of his automobile and passed the other end through the car win-
dow. He was taken to a local hospital where he was found to be
comatose and in an opisthotonic posture. Only a trace of corneal reflex and no gag reflex were obtainable. The deep tendon
reflexes were hyperactive. He was treated with oxygen and
given supportive care. The next day he was transferred to the
university hospital.

Physical examination upon admission to the university hospital
revealed a blood pressure of 150/80 mm Hg, pulse of 100/min
and a temperature of 39°C. The patient was still comatose and
assumed a decerebrate posture upon stimulation. His pupils
were dilated but reacted to light. Eye movements upon caloric
stimulation and doll's head maneuver were normal. The carboxyhemoglobin saturation was 9.8%. Despite treatment with
oxygen, ventilatory support and antibiotics, the patient remained comatose and died ten days later.

QUESTIONS

1. The toxicity of carbon monoxide is due to
   A. its non-reversible combination with hemoglobin
   B. the greater affinity of hemoglobin for carbon
      monoxide than for oxygen
   C. its combination with myoglobin
   D. its combination with cytochrome oxidase

2. Patients who die acutely from carbon monoxide intoxication
   often show
   A. cherry-red colored skin, mucous membranes and blood
   B. petechiae
   C. elevated levels of carbon monoxide in the blood
   D. pallidal necrosis

3. Patients with carbon monoxide intoxication who suffer "de-
   layed deaths" often show
   A. elevated levels of carbon monoxide in the blood
   B. coma
   C. hypertonia
   D. hyperglycemia

4. Fig. 22.1 illustrates the neuropathological lesions that are
    typically encountered in delayed deaths from carbon
    monoxide intoxication. These include
    A. cortical "border zone" infarcts
    B. pallidal necrosis
    C. scattered foci of demyelination or necrosis in the white
        matter
    D. putamenal necrosis

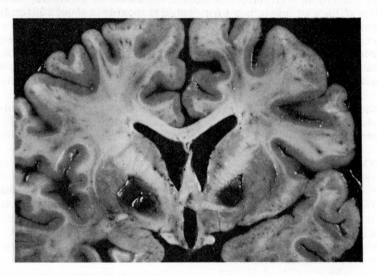

FIG. 22.1: Coronal section of the cerebral hemispheres
           showing necrosis of the globi pallidi and scat-
           tered foci of demyelinization in the white matter.

5. Other conditions in which this combination of neuropatho-
    logical lesions has occasionally been reported include
    A. cardiac arrest
    B. cyanide poisoning
    C. morphine poisoning
    D. strangulation

6. Visceral lesions that have been described in carbon
    monoxide intoxication include
    A. hemorrhagic pancreatitis
    B. centrolobular hepatic necrosis
    C. necrosis of cardiac muscle
    D. toxic megacolon

7. A blue-green discoloration of the fresh brain suggests in-
    toxication by
    A. cyanides
    B. hydrogen sulfide
    C. carbon tetrachloride
    D. methanol

ANSWERS AND DISCUSSION

1. (B) The toxic effect of carbon monoxide is asphyxia, since
the affinity of hemoglobin for carbon monoxide is about 250 times
greater than for oxygen.   Thus, carbon monoxide combines
rapidly with hemoglobin, forming carboxyhemoglobin and re-
duces the blood's oxygen carrying capacity. Furthermore, the
binding sites on the remaining hemoglobin are altered in such
a manner that oxygen is released to the tissues less readily
than normal. Death ensues when approximately two-thirds of
the hemoglobin is converted to carboxyhemoglobin. Convulsions, syncope, dizziness, etc. occur with lesser degrees
of saturation.

The reaction between the carbon monoxide and hemoglobin is
reversible. A normal man breathing air eliminates one-half of
his blood carbon monoxide in four hours and virtually all within
18 hours. Oxygen therapy speeds up the elimination of carbon
monoxide fourfold to sixfold. Carbon monoxide also combines
with myoglobin and cytochrome oxidase. The significance of
these reactions in producing carbon monoxide intoxication has
not been established.

2. (A, B, C) Patients who die acutely from carbon monoxide
intoxication often have cherry-red colored skin, mucous membranes, viscera and blood. This color is not pathognomonic
since a similar red color can be seen in individuals who die from
cyanide poisoning or freezing. Bullae and petechiae may be
present, but these too may be seen with other intoxicants. In
acute deaths, there are no characteristic neuropathological
findings. The nature of the intoxication can be established by
determination of blood or tissue carbon monoxide levels. Prolonged exposure of a cadaver to carbon monoxide will not
spuriously elevate the level of carbon monoxide in heart blood
and the determinations can even be made on putrefied tissue.

3. (B, C, D) Patients who suffer delayed deaths from carbon
monoxide intoxication are generally in profound coma with diminished to absent corneal, gag and pupillary reflexes. Hypertonia
is common and is often accompanied by trismus. Decerebration

may occur and is often accompanied by respiratory and vaso-
motor disturbances. Laboratory studies may reveal hyperglycemia, respiratory alkalosis or metabolic acidosis and
azotemia. Unless performed immediately, blood carbon
monoxide levels are of little value since the carbon monoxide
is eliminated rather rapidly.

4. (B, C) Neuropathological lesions typically encountered in
delayed deaths due to carbon monoxide intoxication include
necrosis of the globus pallidus and scattered foci of demyelination or necrosis in the white matter.

Pallidal necrosis in carbon monoxide poisoning has long been
recognized and was probably first described by von Recklinghausen.
The presumed selective necrosis of the globus pallidus by carbon monoxide was one of the lesions on which C. and O. Vogt
based their famous theory of "Pathoclisis," a concept of selective vulnerability of certain "topistic" constituents of the central
nervous system. In a review of the cerebral lesions in 22 fatal
cases of carbon monoxide poisoning, Lapresle and Fardeau
found necrosis of the pallidum in 16 of their 22 cases. The extent of necrosis was variable. The necrotic foci were often
small and confined to the anterior superior portion of the internal nucleus of the globus pallidus. The necrosis was commonly
bilateral but often asymmetrical, appearing on only one side in
a given coronal section. Many authors now regard pallidal
necrosis as a lesion common to many forms of severe anoxia
with the necrosis resulting from impaired perfusion in branches
of the anterior choroidal artery. Brucher, in particular, has
emphasized the incomplete involvement of the pallidum and the
encroachment of the necrosis into the adjacent internal capsule
as evidence of a vascular process rather than selective vulnerability of the pallidum to carbon monoxide.

Lesions of the white matter also have long been recognized in
carbon monoxide poisoning. Lapresle and Fardeau found lesions of the cerebral white matter in 16 of their 22 fatal cases.
They classified the lesions into four groups that differed only
in severity ranging from demyelinization to necrosis. The
mechanism for production of these lesions is controversial. A
specific histotoxic effect of carbon monoxide, the combined
effect of anoxia and acidosis and the effect of circulatory insufficiency secondary to cardiac damage have all been proposed.

Lapresle and Fardeau encountered necrotic lesions of the isocortex in 12 of their 22 cases and injury to Ammon's horn in 10
of 20 cases. Cerebellar lesions were present in many of the

cases and consisted of foci of necrosis, pallor of white matter and lysis of the granule cells with relative preservation of the Purkinje cells.

5. (A, B, C, D) While carbon monoxide intoxication is the most common cause of pallidal necrosis, other agents and events have been reported to cause the same lesion. These include anoxia due to pulmonary disturbances, strangulation, sequela of nitrous oxide anesthesia, post-hemorrhagic anemia, cyanide poisoning, barbiturate poisoning, morphine poisoning, cardiac arrest, trauma and hypoglycemia. Similarly, the white matter lesions have been described with anesthetic accidents, closed head injuries, cardiac arrest, postoperative shock, cyanide poisoning, carbon disulfide poisoning, morphine poisoning, sodium nitrate poisoning, strangulation and hypoglycemia. Thus, the combination of pallidal necrosis and scattered white matter lesions are typical but not pathognomonic of carbon monoxide intoxication and have been reported occasionally in other conditions.

6. (C) Necrosis of cardiac muscle, especially the papillary muscles has been described in association with carbon monoxide intoxication.

7. (B) There are several reports of a peculiar blue-green discoloration of the fresh brain from individuals who have died acutely from inhalation of very high concentrations of hydrogen sulfide. The discoloration rapidly disappears during formalin fixation. The chemical composition of the colored material is unknown although it is assumed to result from a reaction between the hydrogen sulfide and hemoglobin. The material is apparently not sulfhemoglobin or sulfmethemoglobin.

REFERENCES

1. Adelson L and Sunshine I: Fatal hydrogen sulfide intoxication. Arch Path 81:375-380, 1966.

2. Bour H, et al.: The central nervous system and carbon monoxide poisoning. I. Clinical data with reference to 20 fatal cases. Prog Brain Res 24:1-30, 1967.

3. Brucher JM: Neuropathological problems posed by carbon monoxide poisoning and anoxia. Prog Brain Res 24:75-100, 1967.

4.   Finck PA: Exposure to carbon monoxide: Review of the
     literature and 567 autopsies. Mil Med 131:1513-1539,
     1966.

5.   Gonzales TA, et al.: Legal Medicine: Pathology and
     Toxicology, 2nd Edition. Appleton-Century-Crofts,
     New York, 1954.

6.   Lapresle J and Fardeau M: The central nervous system
     and carbon monoxide poisoning. II. Anatomical study
     of brain lesions following intoxication with carbon
     monoxide (22 cases). Prog Brain Res 24:31-74, 1967.

: :

CASE 23: An Elderly Man who Committed Suicide with a
          Heating Compound

CLINICAL DATA

This 62-year-old man attempted suicide by ingesting an eight-
ounce can of a commercial heating compound that contained
85% methanol. One hour after the ingestion, he was hospitalized
and given intravenous fluids and bicarbonate. He remained
alert throughout the day but complained of abdominal pain and
nausea and vomited twice. The next day he was transferred to
the university hospital because of lethargy and respiratory
distress.

Physical examination on admission to the university hospital
revealed a lethargic, disoriented man with hyperventilation.
His blood pressure was 130/80 mm Hg, his pulse was 120/mm
and his temperature was 37.2°C. Skin turgor was poor. His
vision was impaired but he could count fingers. His pupils
were dilated and responded poorly to light. Funduscopic examination revealed edema of the nerve head and segmental
narrowing of the retinal arterioles. Corneal and gag reflexes
were decreased. Muscle tone was normal but he was areflexic.
The blood pH was 7.30 on admission. He was treated with
ethanol infusion, bicarbonates, steroids and antibiotics. The
patient eventually died 7 days after the methanol ingestion.

QUESTIONS

1. The usual lethal dose of ingested methanol is
    A. 5-50 ml
    B. 50-100 ml
    C. 200-300 ml
    D. highly variable

2. Intoxication from methanol is due to
    A. cerebral depression from the methanol per se
    B. hypocalcemia due to formation of calcium oxalate
    C. metabolic acidosis due to formation of formic and
        other organic acids
    D. toxic effects of formaldehyde

3. Prominent clinical manifestations in methanol intoxication
    include
    A. visual impairment
    B. abdominal pain
    C. headache
    D. respiratory distress

4. Other exogenous poisons that cause severe metabolic
    acidosis include
    A. ethylene glycol
    B. paraldehyde
    C. barbiturates
    D. glutethimide

5. The visual disturbances are due to
    A. selective injury to the visual cortex in the occipital
        lobes
    B. selective injury to the neurons of the lateral geniculate
        bodies
    C. selective injury to the retinal ganglion cells
    D. retinal edema

6. Fig. 23.1 illustrates the neuropathological changes typically
    found in delayed deaths from methanol intoxication. These
    include
    A. cerebral edema
    B. necrosis of the globus pallidus
    C. necrosis of the lateral portion of the putamen
    D. laminar necrosis of the cerebral cortex

7. Visceral changes that have been described in methanol in-
    toxication include
    A. pulmonary congestion
    B. intranuclear inclusion in renal tubular cells
    C. pancreatic necrosis
    D. perivascular eosinophil infiltrates

8. Morphological findings in the nervous system of patients
    who have ingested ethylene glycol include
    A. cerebral edema
    B. perivascular mononuclear cell infiltrates
    C. perivascular deposits of birefringent crystals
    D. perivascular eosinophil infiltrates

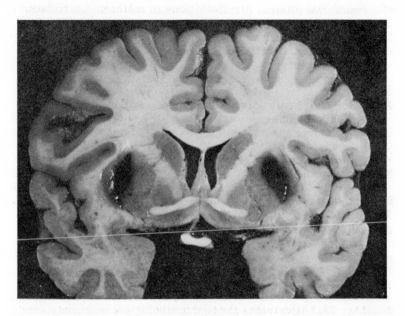

FIG. 23.1: Coronal section of the cerebral hemispheres show-
       ing bilateral hemorrhagic necrosis of the putamena.

ANSWERS AND DISCUSSION

1. (B, D) There is marked variation in individual susceptibility
to ingested methanol. Blindness has followed the ingestion of
as little as 4 ml and death has resulted from the consumption
of only 15 ml of 40% methanol. The usual lethal dose is 70 to
100 ml. However, at least one person survived after consuming 500 ml of 40% methanol. Severe intoxication can also result from inhalation of methanol vapors.

2. (A, C, D) Methanol produces toxic effects in at least three
different ways. Methanol itself can produce a moderate degree
of central nervous system depression. However, the serious
sequelae result from its catabolism. Methanol is oxidized primarily by hepatic alcohol dehydrogenase but only about one-
seventh as rapidly as ethanol. Some is excreted in the urine
and a considerable quantity is eliminated in the expired air.
Methanol is oxidized to formaldehyde which is at least 30 times
as toxic as the original methanol. It is also oxidized to formic
acid which contributes to the resulting severe metabolic acidosis.

The exact mechanism for the development of the metabolic acidosis is not clear. It is more severe than can be accounted for on the basis of formic acid production alone. Some of the acidosis results from the reaction of the formaldehyde with amino compounds.

3. (A, B, C, D) In the series of 323 patients reported by Bennett, et al., following ingestion of whiskey containing 35-40% methanol, visual disturbances were a universal complaint. Central nervous system symptoms ranged from those of a "hangover" to convulsions and coma. Headache was described by more than one-half of the patients. Two-thirds complained of severe upper abdominal pain. Only one-fourth of the patients mentioned respiratory distress, however, a "peculiar cessation of respiration" was the prime cause of death in their series. They emphasized that dyspnea was a poor indicator of the degree of acidosis resulting from the methanol intoxication.

4. (A, B) Other exogenous poisons that produce profound metabolic acidosis include ethylene glycol and partially decomposed paraldehyde. Ethylene glycol, which is found in certain antifreezes, is oxidized to oxalic acid. This produces profound acidosis and leads to the precipitation of calcium oxalate crystals in the proximal tubules of the kidneys and about blood vessels in the brain and meninges. Paraldehyde, when partially decomposed, is metabolized to acetic acid and produces acidosis.

5. (C, D) The visual disturbances are due to pathological changes within the eyes. Ophthalmoscopic examination reveals retinal edema and hyperemia of the optic disc. Bennett, et al., found these funduscopic changes to correlate more closely with the degree of acidosis than any of the other clinical manifestations. Histopathological studies on fatal cases of methanol intoxication have demonstrated degeneration of the retinal ganglion cells with lesser degrees of injury to the rods and cones. The optic nerves and tracts are relatively well preserved, though edematous.

6. (A, C) The neuropathological changes in patients with delayed death from methanol intoxication include cerebral edema and a distinctive, often hemorrhagic necrosis of the lateral aspect of the putamen. Orthner observed this pattern of necrosis in 41 of 124 fatal cases of methanol intoxication. The claustrum and external capsule often showed ischemic necrosis while the caudate and globus pallidus were uniformly spared. In one patient who survived for 17 days, there were also large areas of hemorrhagic necrosis in the white matter of the cerebrum and cerebellum. The exact pathogenesis of these lesions in unclear.

7.   (A, C) General autopsy findings in patients with methanol
intoxication usually include pulmonary congestion, gastritis,
and mild fatty degeneration of the liver. Of particular interest
is pancreatic necrosis. This was reported in 13 of 17 cases
necropsied by Bennett, et al. It probably accounts for the abdominal pain and elevated serum amylase levels noted clinically.

8.   (A, B, C) Ethylene glycol is metabolized to oxalic acid
which in turn forms insoluble calcium oxalate. Birefringent
crystals of calcium oxalate are found in the perivascular spaces
and in the walls of vessels within the nervous system. They are
accompanied by mild mononuclear inflammatory cell infiltrates
and cerebral edema.

REFERENCES

1.   Bennett IL Jr, et al.: Acute methyl alcohol poisoning:
     A review based on experiences in an outbreak of 323
     cases. Medicine 32:431-463, 1953.

2.   Orthner H: Methylalkoholvergiftung mit besonders
     schweren Hirnveranderungen. Virchows Archiv 323:
     442-464, 1953.

3.   Parry MF and Wallach D: Ethylene glycol poisoning.
     Amer J Med 57:143-150, 1974.

: :

CASE 24: Rapidly Progressive Encephalopathy in a 4-Month-
        Old Girl

CLINICAL DATA

This 4-month-old girl had a "cold" for about a week. She then
began vomiting and became febrile. The next day, she was
taken to a local hospital comatose, hyperventilating and febrile
(103°F). She had scattered rales but no skin lesions. A blood
glucose was 9 mg/dl. Intravenous glucose, fluids and antibiotics were given. A lumbar puncture was performed and
yielded clear cerebrospinal fluid with no cells, a protein of 45
mg/dl and a glucose of 11 mg/dl. Later the same day, she
developed seizures and vomited guaiac-positive material.

She was transferred to the university hospital. On admission,
her blood pressure was 70 mm Hg systolic, pulse 160/min and
temperature 103°F. She was unresponsive and had fixed dilated
pupils. Her fontanelle was tense and there was no response
upon caloric stimulation. The liver was firm and extended
4 cm below the costal margin. Laboratory studies disclosed a
hemoglobin of 10 g/dl, a hematocrit of 31%, a white blood cell
count of 16,500 (42% neutrophils), a serum glutamic oxaloacetic
transaminase (SGOT) of 1697 units, a blood ammonia of 653
μg/dl and a prothrombin time of 30.5 sec. The infant died a
few hours after admission.

QUESTIONS

1. The clinical data are most consistent with
    A. viral encephalitis
    B. infectious hepatitis
    C. Reye's syndrome
    D. drug intoxication

2. The antecedent illnesses in patients who develop Reye's
    syndrome are most commonly due to
    A. influenza B
    B. parainfluenza
    C. poliovirus
    D. varicella

3. Characteristic clinical laboratory findings in patients with
    Reye's syndrome include
    A. elevated serum glutamic oxaloacetic transaminase
    B. elevated serum bilirubin

C. prolonged prothrombin time
D. elevated blood ammonia

4. Characteristic morphological changes in the livers of
    patients with Reye's syndrome include
    A. fatty degeneration
    B. glycogen depletion
    C. Mallory's bodies
    D. acidophilic intranuclear inclusion bodies in hepatocytes

5. Characteristic morphological changes in the brains of
    patients with Reye's syndrome include
    A. diffuse cerebral edema
    B. perivascular lymphocytic infiltrates
    C. microglial nodules
    D. acidophilic intranuclear inclusion bodies in neurons
        and oligodendrocytes

6. The encephalopathy in Reye's syndrome has been
    attributed to
    A. hyperammonemia
    B. circulating short chain fatty acids
    C. generalized mitochondrial injury
    D. hypoglycemia

ANSWERS AND DISCUSSION

1. (C) The clinical data, as presented, are most consistent
with a diagnosis of Reye's syndrome. This is an acute encephalopathy that usually develops within a few days of an antecedent
viral illness. The initial manifestation of the syndrome is generally vomiting. This is quickly followed by alterations in the
state of consciousness, convulsions, hyperventilation and coma.
Fever may be present. As the coma deepens, fixed dilated
pupils and decerebrate rigidity may develop; this may then be
replaced by flaccidity. Although the intracranial pressure is
elevated, papilledema is often not evident. The encephalopathy
is accompanied by enlargement of the liver in 50-70% of the
patients.

2. (A, D) Reye's syndrome has followed a wide variety of
viral infections; however, the most common antecedent illnesses
are due to influenza B or varicella. In Thailand, large numbers of children have an identical or at least similar disease
that is precipitated by food contaminated with aflatoxin, a myco-
toxin produced by Aspergillus flavus. Other nonviral agents and
diseases may also precipitate some cases of Reye's syndrome.

3. (A, C, D) Abnormalities of hepatic function are reflected by elevation of various enzymes (SGOT, SGPT, LDH, etc.) and prolongation of the prothrombin time; however, the bilirubin generally remains normal. Hypoglycemia, encountered in over 50% of the patients, is also a manifestation of liver involvement.

The cerebrospinal fluid is acellular and the protein usually remains normal. The spinal fluid glucose may be depressed, reflecting the blood glucose level.

Of particular interest, with regard to pathogenesis of the encephalopathy, are elevations in blood ammonia and short chain fatty acids.

4. (A, B) Patients with Reye's syndrome commonly have enlarged pale tan to yellow livers. Histologically, the most conspicuous alteration is the presence of numerous lipid droplets in the cytoplasm of the hepatocytes. The droplets tend to be very small (microvesicular steatosis) and are more abundant in the hepatocytes toward the periphery of the liver lobules (Fig. 24.1). Glycogen depletion is a more variable feature. The hepatocyte nuclei may be enlarged and vesicular but do not harbor intranuclear inclusion bodies. Small foci of necrosis and sparse periportal inflammatory cell infiltrates may be encountered in some cases.

Electron microscopy discloses marked enlargement of the hepatocyte mitochondria. The cristae may be deranged and flocculent dense material may be present in the matrix compartment. Mitochondrial dense bodies are generally absent.

Small droplets of fat may also accumulate in the myocardium and the renal tubular epithelium.

5. (A) The brain characteristically shows severe cerebral edema. There are no perivascular inflammatory cell infiltrates, microglial nodules, intranuclear inclusion bodies or other morphological evidence of viral encephalitis. Recently, cytoplasmic inclusion bodies have been described in the cerebellum; their significance remains to be determined.

Varying degree of ischemic necrosis of neurons may be seen but are undoubtedly secondary to impaired perfusion from the increased intracranial pressure.

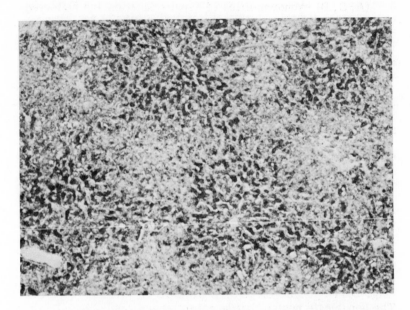

FIG. 24.1: Microscopic section of liver, stained with oil-red-O, from a patient with Reye's syndrome. Note the numerous fat droplets in the hepatocytes, especially at the periphery of the lobules.

6. (A, B, C, D) The pathogenesis of the encephalopathy is still controversial. Some authors attribute the encephalopathy to hyperammonemia. This in turn, has been attributed to inherited or acquired deficiencies in the activities of ornithine transcarbamylase and/or carbamyl phosphate synthetase. These are mitochondrial enzymes involved in the urea cycle. Arguments against hyperammonemia being the cause of the cerebral dysfunction include the lack of cerebral edema with other forms of liver failure and the lack of correlation between the ammonia levels and the clinical status of the patient.

Short chain fatty acids have been implicated by some authors. The blood levels of these compounds have been shown to be elevated in many patients with Reye's syndrome. Furthermore, infusion of these compounds simulate many of the features of Reye's syndrome in laboratory animals.

Some authors attribute the encephalopathy of Reye's syndrome to a generalized mitochondrial injury that affects all tissues including the brain. Nevertheless, the exact nature of the mitochondrial injury and its evolution from the antecedent viral illness remain unclear.

REFERENCES

1. Bove KE, et al.: The hepatic lesion in Reye's syndrome. Gastroenterology 69:685-697, 1975.

2. Brown T, et al.: Transiently reduced activity of carbamyl phosphate synthetase and ornithine transcarbamylase in liver of children with Reye's syndrome. N Eng J Med 294:861-868, 1976.

3. DeVico DC: Reye syndrome: A metabolic response to an acute mitochondrial insult? Neurology 28:105-108, 1978.

4. Huttenlocher PR and Trauner DA: Reye's Syndrome. In: Handbook of Clinical Neurology. Vinken PJ and Bruyn GW (Eds.). North-Holland, Amsterdam, 1977, Vol. 29, pp. 331-334.

5. Partin JC: Mitochondrial ultrastructure in Reye's syndrome (encephalopathy and fatty degeneration of the viscera). N Eng J Med 285:1339-1343, 1971.

6. Snodgrass PJ and DeLong GR: Urea-cycle enzyme deficiencies and an increased nitrogen load producing hyperammonemia in Reye's syndrome. N Eng J Med 294:855-860, 1974.

7. Trauner DA, et al.: Biochemical correlates of illness and recovery in Reye's syndrome. Ann Neurol 2:238-241, 1977.

: :

CASE 25: A Moribund 11-Day-Old with a Tense Fontanelle

CLINICAL DATA

This 11-day-old male infant was delivered by a cesarean section after a full term pregnancy. He did well for ten days.   The night before hospitalization he was excessively irritable and did not feed well. The next morning he was brought to the emergency room in a moribund condition.   His anterior fontanelle was tense and the sutures were spread. His pupils were "pinpoint" in size and did not respond to light.   The child was unresponsive to pain and had decreased tendon reflexes.   His extremities were cold and his mucous membranes were cyanotic. No petechiae were evident.

A lumbar puncture yielded cerebrospinal fluid under increased pressure containing 25 neutrophils/cmm, 496 mg/dl of protein and no glucose.   A smear of the cerebrospinal fluid sediment disclosed gram-positive cocci in chains. The peripheral white blood cell count was 67,000 with 15% mature neutrophils and 30% immature neutrophils.

Despite vigorous therapy with antibiotics, intravenous fluids and oxygen, the child died on the day of admission. The results of the cerebrospinal fluid cultures were not available until after the child's death.

QUESTIONS

1. The clinical data are most consistent with a diagnosis of
    A. Escherichia coli meningitis
    B. pneumococcal meningitis
    C. Group B streptococcal meningitis
    D. staphylococcal meningitis

2. The bacteria that most commonly cause meningitis during the neonatal period are
    A. Listeria monocytogenes
    B. Escherichia coli
    C. Group B streptococci
    D. Hemophilus influenzae

3. Group B streptococcal infections in neonates commonly produce
    A. brain abscesses
    B. subdural empyema
    C. a syndrome of early-onset sepsis
    D. a syndrome of delayed-onset sepsis and meningitis

4. Fig. 25.1 illustrates the appearance of the brain from the present case. Morphological features of neonatal meningitis include
   A. congestion of leptomeningeal vessels
   B. exudate in the subarachnoid space
   C. arteritis and phlebitis
   D. cerebral edema

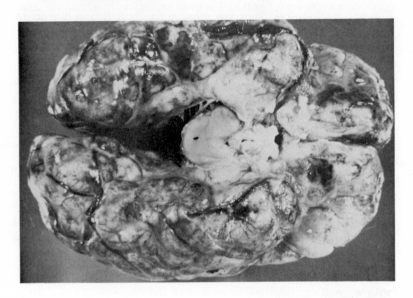

FIG. 25.1: Photograph of the base of the brain with the cerebellum removed. Note the exudate in the subarachnoid space.

5. Factors predisposing to neonatal meningitis include
   A. meningomyeloceles
   B. prolonged rupture of membranes
   C. neonatal sepsis
   D. advanced maternal age

6. Neonatal meningitis has a high mortality rate and many of the survivors have serious sequelae. Among the sequelae are
   A. subependymal matrix cysts
   B. mineralization in the globus pallidus
   C. subdural hygroma
   D. hydrocephalus

7. Listeria monocytogenes
    A. is a gram-negative coccus
    B. is a recognized cause of neonatal meningitis
    C. can be transmitted transplacentally
    D. may produce abortions

ANSWERS AND DISCUSSION

1. (C) The clinical data are most consistent with a diagnosis
of Group B streptococcal meningitis. During the neonatal period, bacterial meningitis poses special diagnostic problems.
The neonate with meningitis is often excessively irritable or
lethargic, feeds poorly, vomits and has seizures but lacks the
characteristic meningeal signs such as neck stiffness, Kernig's
sign and Brudzinski's sign. Fever may or may not be present;
premature infants are often hypothermic. A bulging fontanelle
may not develop until the infection is well established. Cerebrospinal fluid examination is essential to make the diagnosis
and should be performed whenever meningitis or sepsis is suspected. The cellular response consists predominantly of neutrophils but varies greatly in number. The glucose is generally
between zero and 15 mg/dl but is influenced by a number of factors. The precise mechanism for the reduction in the glucose
level has been debated for many years and is variously attributed
to consumption by the organisms, consumption by the leukocytes
or increased utilization by the neural parenchyma. As in the
present case, the protein content of the cerebrospinal fluid in
neonatal meningitis may be quite high and is especially high
with E. coli meningitis. A smear of the cerebrospinal fluid
sediment usually reveals the causative organisms and permits
a tentative specific diagnosis. In the present case, the chains
of gram-positive cocci, i.e., streptococci, were strongly suggestive of Group B streptococcal meningitis.

2. (B, C) Escherichia coli is the most common cause of meningitis during the neonatal period and accounts for 40-50% of
such cases. It has a high mortality rate and the survivors
usually have serious sequelae. In recent years, Group B, beta-
hemolytic streptococci have emerged as the second most common cause and in some areas, the leading cause of neonatal
meningitis. Cultures of the spinal fluid from the present case
yielded Group B streptococci. Serotyping was not performed.
Other enteric bacteria such as Klebsiella and Pseudomonas,
staphylococci and Listeria monocytogenes are responsible for
some cases of neonatal meningitis. Hemophilus influenzae is
the most common cause of meningitis between the ages of 6
months and 3 years but is uncommon during the neonatal period.

3.   (C, D) Group B streptococcal infections in neonates can be
divided into two syndromes or patterns of illness according
to the age at onset. The early-onset (or acute) syndrome occurs in neonates less than five days old and is characterized by
sepsis with respiratory distress and pneumonia. Some of these
patients may also have meningitis. The early-onset (or acute)
syndrome can be caused by any of the five Group B streptococcus serotypes. The delayed-onset or late-onset syndrome
occurs in neonates older than 10 days of age and is characterized by sepsis and meningitis. Almost all of the cases of de-
layed- or late-onset disease are caused by the type III Group
B streptococcus serotype. The type III serotype is also responsible for many of the early-onset or acute cases with meningitis. These observations have been interpreted as suggesting that the type III serotype has invasive properties and a special predilection for the meninges. The early-onset or acute
syndrome is generally regarded as resulting from intrapartum
infection from the maternal vaginal flora. The mechanism for
development of the delayed-onset or late-onset syndrome is
currently unknown.

4.   (A, B, C, D) The gross pathological features of bacterial
meningitis in the neonate are basically the same as in older individuals. The leptomeningeal blood vessels are usually intensely congested. Depending more upon the stage of the disease than on the nature of the causative agent, a variable
quantity of exudate is present in the subarachnoid space. The
exudate is more abundant in the sulci than over the gyri and is
especially copious in the various cisterns. Many types of meningitis, especially in the very young, are accompanied by
arteritis and phlebitis. The associated infarcts produce many
of the serious sequelae. Meningitis is commonly accompanied
by ventriculitis and choroid plexitis. The brain itself is usually
severely swollen or edematous.

5.   (A, B, C) There are many factors that predispose to neonatal meningitis. Premature infants are generally more susceptible than full term infants and males are often more affected
than females. Prolonged rupture of maternal membranes and
traumatic delivery are important intrapartum factors. Congenital malformations such as meningomyeloceles and dermal
sinuses are important portals of infection. Acquired respiratory, intestinal or umbilical infections can lead to septicemia
and subsequently meningitis.

6.   (C, D) Hydrocephalus is one of the most common serious
sequela of neonatal meningitis. It may be due to occlusion of

the aqueduct from the associated ventriculitis, from obstruction of the outlet foramina of the fourth ventricle or from blockage of subarachnoid cerebrospinal fluid pathways by exudate or meningeal fibrosis. Seizures and various neurological deficits may be attributable to the parenchymal destruction resulting from the associated arteritis and phlebitis. Subdural hygromas or effusions are less common but potentially serious sequelae. Their formation has been attributed to altered permeability of the arachnoid permitting passage of fluid from the subarachnoid space into the subdural space.

7. (B, C, D) Listeria monocytogenes is a motile, gram-positive bacillus that has long been known to produce infections in man and animals. The organism can be transmitted transplacentally from an asymptomatic or minimally ill mother to her child. This may result in a generalized infection leading to abortion, stillbirth or prematurity. The organism has a predilection for the nervous system and produces meningitis especially in neonates and elderly individuals. Other cases of listeriosis occur in individuals with malignancies.

REFERENCES

1. Baker CJ and Barrett FF: Group B streptococcal infections in infants. JAMA 230:1158-1160, 1974.

2. Baker CJ and Kasper DL: Correlation of maternal antibody deficiency with susceptibility to neonatal group B streptococcal infection. N Eng J Med 294:753-756, 1976.

3. Bell WE and McCormick WF: Neurologic Infections in Children. W.B. Saunders Co., Philadelphia, 1975, pp. 3-41.

4. Friede RL: Developmental Neuropathology. Springer-Verlag, New York, 1975, pp. 166-178.

5. Lavette A, et al.: Meningitis due to Listeria monocytogenes. A review of 25 cases. N Eng J Med 285:598-603, 1971.

: :

CASE 26: A 62-Year-Old Man with Chronic Alcoholism,
          Headache and Stiff Neck

CLINICAL DATA

This 62-year-old man with a long history of chronic alcoholism
was admitted to the hospital because of headache and swelling
of his feet and abdomen.

On physical examination he was noted to be poorly responsive
to verbal commands, in moderate respiratory distress, icteric,
and to have severe pitting edema of both lower limbs and abdominal swelling. His temperature was 102°F, pulse was 130/
min and respiratory rate was 36/min. Vascular "spiders"
were present on his chest and abdomen. His neck was stiff and
there were positive Kernig and Brudzinski signs.

Shortly after admission the patient had a grand mal seizure. A
lumbar puncture yielded cerebrospinal fluid under increased
pressure containing 300 white blood cells/cmm, 6 mg/dl of
glucose and 360 mg/dl of protein. Gram-positive diplococci
were noted in a smear of the cerebrospinal fluid sediment.

The patient expired shortly after hospitalization. The results
of the cultures of the cerebrospinal fluid were not available until
after the patient's death.

QUESTIONS

1. The clinical data are most consistent with a diagnosis of
    A. Group B streptococcal meningitis
    B. Hemophilus influenzae meningitis
    C. meningococcal meningitis
    D. pneumococcal meningitis

2. Special circumstances that particularly predispose to the
    development of pneumococcal meningitis include
    A. alcoholism
    B. head trauma
    C. splenectomy in childhood
    D. splenectomy in adulthood

3. Fig. 26.1 illustrates the brain from the patient described
    in the clinical data. A gross diagnosis specifically of
    pneumococcal meningitis is suggested by
    A. the quantity of exudate in the subarachnoid space
    B. the greenish-yellow color of the exudate

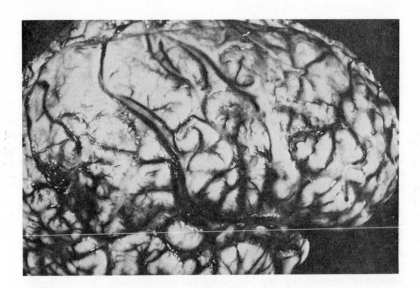

FIG. 26.1: Photograph of the patient's brain showing the quantity and distribution of the exudate.

    C. the distribution of the exudate
    D. none of these features

4. Meningococcal meningitis may be accompanied by
    A. the Waterhouse-Friderichsen syndrome
    B. petechial skin lesions
    C. myocarditis
    D. Babes' nodes

5. Histological characteristics of pyogenic leptomeningitis
    include
    A. inflammatory cell exudate in the subarachnoid space
    B. inflammation of the neural parenchyma
    C. extension of inflammatory cell exudates along the
        Virchow-Robin spaces
    D. inflammation of the ependyma and choroid plexi

6. Pachymeningitis hemorrhagica is due to
    A. Treponema pallidum
    B. Nocardia asteroides
    C. Actinomyces israelii
    D. trauma

ANSWERS AND DISCUSSION

1.   (D) The clinical data are strongly indicative of pneumococcal meningitis. Diplococcus pneumoniae or Streptococcus pneumoniae as it has been designated more recently, is one of the
most common causes of meningitis. Pneumococcal meningitis
is especially prevalent in the elderly and in young children beyond the neonatal period. It is often associated with pulmonary
infections, otitis or sinusitis. Modern therapy has greatly reduced the mortality from pneumococcal meningitis but it is still
fatal in over half of the elderly cases. The characteristic gram-
positive diplococci can usually be recognized in the spinal fluid
sediment. Other gram-positive cocci usually occur in special
situations or different age groups.

Group B streptococcal meningitis, while common in the neonatal
period, is quite uncommon in older patients. Staphylococcal
meningitis is relatively uncommon in adults and in most instances is associated with open penetrating injuries or surgical
procedures in the skull. The bacteria causing Hemophilus influenzae meningitis are pleomorphic gram-negative bacilli but
because of uneven staining, may be misinterpreted as gram-
positive cocci.   Hemophilus influenzae is the most common
cause of meningitis between the ages of 6 months and 3 years
but rarely causes meningitis in persons over 5 years of age.
Meningococcal meningitis is most common in children and young
adults and is caused by a gram-negative diplococcus.

2.   (A, B, C) There are a number of special circumstances
that predispose individuals to the development of pneumococcal
meningitis. Of these, alcoholism is the most common.   The
increased prevalence of pneumococcal meningitis among these
individuals has been attributed to an alcohol-induced defect in
chemotaxis or impaired phagocytosis. Similarly, the age-de-
pendent decline in the competence of the immune system may
account for the general increased prevalence of meningitis in
the elderly.

Head trauma with basal skull fractures predisposes to pneumococcal meningitis by providing access to the subarachnoid space
from the nasal cavities, paranasal sinuses, ears and mastoids.
Many of these occur in individuals who were thought initially to
have sustained closed head injuries. Persistent dural defects
may result in recurrent infection. Sickle cell disease and
splenectomy during childhood are associated with an increased
prevalence of pneumococcal meningitis. Splenectomy in the
adult, however, does not carry the same associated risk.

3. (D) Attempts to correlate the etiologic agent with the color, quantity and distribution of the exudate have been largely unsuccessful in patients with pyogenic meningitis. The quantity of exudate corresponds more closely with the stage of the disease than causative agent. Over the convexities of the cerebral hemispheres, exudate tends to be most conspicuous along the vessels and in the sulci. The exudate is generally most abundant at the base of the brain and in the cisterns. The dorsal surface of the spinal cord is generally more thickly covered by exudate than the ventral surface of the cord. This is related to the patient's position and cerebrospinal fluid circulation. The typical "meningeal signs" of meningitis are largely related to inflammation of pain-sensitive spinal nerves and roots.

In some cases of Hemophilus influenzae meningitis, the causative agent can be suspected grossly because of the extensive cortical necrosis that is often encountered in this condition. Tuberculous and other forms of granulomatous meningitis can usually be distinguished from pyogenic meningitis by the presence of miliary and confluent granulomas. However, grossly, the various types of granulomatous meningitis are virtually indistinguishable from one another.

4. (A, B, C) Meningococcal meningitis occurs most often in children and young adults, especially in crowded conditions where the nasopharyngeal carriers can come into contact with susceptible individuals. The underlying meningococcemia produces vascular damage that is responsible for the skin petechiae and the adrenal hemorrhages of the Waterhouse-Friderichsen syndrome. Myocarditis is an important aspect of the disease and may be responsible for many of the deaths in adults. Although meningococcal meningitis is generally thought of as a fulminating illness, a chronic form has been described.

Babes' nodes have no relation to meningococcal meningitis. This is an eponym used to designate the focal microglial infiltrates that are seen in rabies.

5. (A, C, D) Regardless of the causative organism, the histological changes in purulent meningitis are essentially the same. The subarachnoid space contains polymorphonuclear leukocytes, macrophages, occasional lymphocytes and plasma cells, fibrin and bacteria. The relative proportions change with the passage of time, i.e., the polymorphonuclear leukocytes decrease and the mononuclear cells increase. The walls of the meningeal vessels, both veins and arteries, become surrounded by and

infiltrated with inflammatory cells. The neural parenchyma
shows edema but relatively little inflammation. Inflammatory
cell infiltrates extend along penetrating vessels but the cells
are in extensions of the subarachnoid space, the Virchow-
Robin spaces. Infarction of neural parenchyma occurs as a
complication of the associated vasculitis. The ependyma and
choroid plexi are focally to extensively coated by the inflammatory cell exudate.

6. (D) Pachymeningitis hemorrhagica was the term applied to
the hemorrhagic dural lesions found in patients with general
paresis. Although once regarded as a specific manifestation
of syphilis, this lesion is now regarded as a resorbing and
organizing subdural hematoma.

REFERENCES

1. Artenstein M: Meningococcal Meningitis. In: Handbook
   of Clinical Neurology. Vinken PJ and Bruyn GW (Eds.).
   North-Holland, Amsterdam, 1978, Vol. 33, 21-33.

2. Bell WE and McCormick WF: Neurologic Infections in
   Children. W. B. Saunders Co., Philadelphia, 1975,
   pp. 43-71.

3. Harris AA, et al.: Pneumococcal Meningitis. In: Handbook of Clinical Neurology. Vinken PJ and Bruyn GW
   (Eds.). North-Holland, Amsterdam, 1978, Vol. 33,
   pp. 35-52.

4. Mathies AW Jr.: Influenza Meningitis. In: Handbook of
   Clinical Neurology. Vinken PJ and Bruyn GW (Eds.).
   North-Holland, Amsterdam, 1978, Vol. 33, pp. 53-59.

: :

CASE 27: A 3-Year-Old with Headaches, Fever and Lethargy

CLINICAL DATA

This 3-year-old girl was in good health until two weeks before
hospitalization, when her parents noted the onset of headaches,
malaise, anorexia, and occasional emesis. Ten days before
admission, she was given tetracycline for a four day period.
Five days prior to hospitalization, she was noted to have repetitive movements of her left ankle and was waking at night because of headaches.

On admission, the child was lethargic and had a temperature of
100.6°F. There was mild nuchal rigidity. The right pupil was
1 mm larger than the left but otherwise the cranial nerves were
intact. The patient was able to move all extremities but the
deep tendon reflexes were hyperactive with a Babinski sign on
the left. Sensory examination revealed no deficits. General
physical examination was normal except for rales in the right
lower lobe.

The white blood cell count was 18,600 with 72% neutrophils and
28% lymphocytes. A lumbar puncture yielded cerebrospinal
fluid under increased pressure that contained 1 lymphocyte/
cmm, 92 mg/dl of protein and 85 mg/dl of glucose.

The next day the child rapidly became more lethargic. Her left
pupil was dilated and unreactive to light. An angiogram revealed
a deep right fronto-parietal lesion. Burr holes were made and
purulent material was aspirated from an abscess. Aspiration
of the left ventricle yielded cloudy ventricular fluid containing
27,000 cells/cmm. Smears revealed gram-positive cocci.

Postoperatively, the child continued to deteriorate and developed
Cheyne-Stokes respiration followed by respiratory arrest.

QUESTIONS

1. Clinical features that supported the diagnosis of an abscess
    included
    A. rapid evolution of the illness
    B. evidence of infection
    C. evidence of increased intracranial pressure
    D. evidence of focal neurological dysfunction

2. Lumbar puncture in a patient with a brain abscess usually reveals
    A. increased cerebrospinal fluid pressure
    B. elevated cerebrospinal fluid protein content
    C. a marked pleocytosis
    D. a markedly diminished glucose content

3. Conditions that predispose to brain abscesses include (Fig. 27.1)
    A. pulmonary infections
    B. congenital heart disease
    C. hypertensive cardiovascular disease
    D. ear and paranasal sinus infections

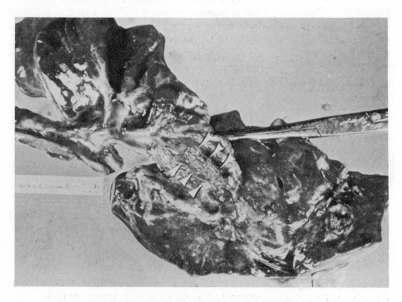

FIG. 27. 1: Right lung with aspirated spikelet of timothy (arrows) in lower lobe bronchus.

4. The major pathogens in brain abscess are
    A. staphylococci
    B. gram-negative bacilli
    C. Bacteroides
    D. anaerobic streptococci

5.   Fig. 27.2 illustrates the abscess from the present case.
     The abscess is
     A.   located in the fronto-parietal white matter
     B.   completely encapsulated by a uniformly thick
          fibrous wall
     C.   surrounded by a hyperemic border
     D.   surrounded by edematous neural parenchyma

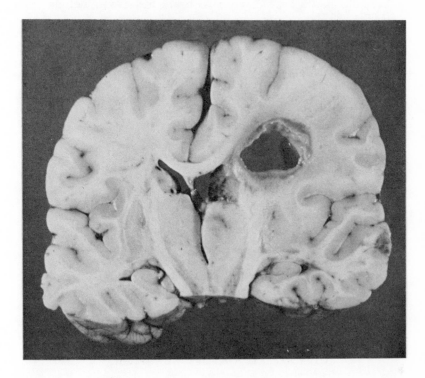

FIG. 27.2: Coronal section of cerebral hemispheres showing
            an abscess involving the right frontal and parietal
            lobes.

6.   Deaths from brain abscesses are due to
     A.   destruction of vital centers
     B.   rupture
     C.   herniation
     D.   hydrocephalus

7. Fig. 27.3 illustrates the histological appearance of the
    abscess from the present case. Which of the following are
    the characteristic features?
    A. Central focus of suppurative material
    B. Layer of granulation tissue
    C. Collagenous capsule
    D. Edematous gliotic neural parenchyma

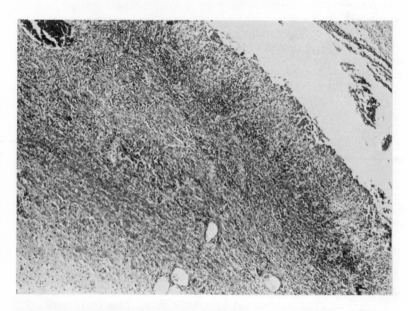

FIG. 27. 3: Microscopic section of the wall of the abscess. Sup-
             purative material has fallen out of the center of the
             abscess (upper right). Edematous gliotic neural
             parenchyma is seen in the lower left.

ANSWERS AND DISCUSSION

1. (A, B, C, D) The predominant clinical manifestations of a
brain abscess are those of an expanding mass lesion.   Headache is the most common initial symptom and is accompanied
by or followed by other signs of increased intracranial pressure such as nausea and vomiting, alteration in the level of consciousness and in about one-half the cases, papilledema. The
constellation of focal neurological dysfunctions depends on the
location of the abscess, e.g., seizures and hemiparesis with
frontal lobe abscess, visual field defects with temporal lobe

abscess and ataxia with cerebellar abscess. The illness tends to evolve rather rapidly except in those rare instances when the abscess results from a retained foreign body. Thus, the development of additional signs and symptoms from an abscess is usually more rapid than from a neoplasm. Many of the patients show evidence of infection with mild temperature elevation and leukocytosis and occasionally an extracerebral suppurative focus can be demonstrated or is known historically.

2. (A, B) The cerebrospinal fluid pressure in a patient with a brain abscess is usually moderately to markedly elevated. The protein content of the cerebrospinal fluid is generally elevated, often to over 100 mg/dl. The cell count generally ranges from normal to only moderately elevated unless the abscess is at the surface of the brain or is accompanied by ventriculitis or meningitis. Rupture of an abscess will cause the cell count to rise precipitously. The glucose level is usually normal unless the meninges have been invaded by the bacteria.

3. (A, B, D) Brain abscesses generally develop secondary to an extracerebral focus of suppuration. Otitis, mastoiditis, and sinusitis are major sources of infection accounting for 20 to 60% of brain abscesses. With the decline in mastoiditis, paranasal sinus infections have become a relatively more important source. Blood-borne infections from distant sites are responsible for 15 to 50% of brain abscesses. Among the distant sites, lung and pleura are the most important. In the present case, the general autopsy disclosed an aspirated spikelet of timothy grass in the right lower lobe bronchus (Fig. 27.1) with a surrounding suppurative focus. Congenital heart disease, especially cyanotic congenital heart disease is now one of the most important lesions predisposing children to brain abscesses. The relative importance of venous blood unfiltered by passage through the lungs, reduced oxygen tension and marantic heart lesions is not clear. Most of the children with congenital heart disease and brain abscesses do not have bacterial endocarditis; however, brain abscesses may be found in patients with either subacute or acute bacterial endocarditis. Open injuries and complications of surgery are responsible for a few brain abscesses. Retained foreign bodies with delayed development of brain abscesses are relatively rare in most civilian series but may follow combat injuries.

4. (A, B, C, D) Over the years many different organisms have been regarded as the major pathogens in brain abscesses. Current evidence seems to indicate that anaerobic streptococci, including peptostreptococci, and anaerobic bacilli, such as

Bacteroides, are frequent agents. The previous failure to
recognize the importance of anaerobes can be attributed to
improper specimen handling and culture techniques. Aerobic
organisms that are implicated frequently include staphylococci
and gram-negative bacilli, especially Proteus mirabilis.
Occasionally, abscesses have mixed flora. Reports of sterile
abscesses usually result from previous antibiotic therapy or
improper techniques. Smears will often demonstrate bacteria
in these cases. Some large, often multiloculated abscesses
are due to nocardia species. Abscesses that develop as complications of surgery or open wounds are often due to staphylococci.

5. (A, C, D) Abscesses typically arise in the white matter
and are most often found in the frontal and parietal lobes. The
relative decline in the frequency of temporal lobe involvement
reflects the decrease in mastoiditis. The brain stem is an uncommon site for brain abscesses. Multiple abscesses are found
in nearly 50% of the patients at autopsy but are diagnosed clinically in only 15-20% of all patients.

The abscess begins as a poorly localized area of cerebritis that
undergoes suppuration and gradually becomes surrounded by
granulation tissue derived from proliferation of blood vessels
and their adventitial cells. When the granulation tissue becomes
organized, the resulting collagenous capsule is rarely of uniform thickness, and is often thinner along the deeper surfaces.
In the past, anaerobes were thought to produce less complete
encapsulation than aerobes but this distinction appears to be
completely invalid. The average thickness of the capsule
correlates best with the duration of the process.

The hyperemic border surrounding an abscess is a very characteristic gross morphologic feature and serves to distinguish
an abscess from a largely necrotic metastatic neoplasm. The
neural parenchyma surrounding an abscess is usually markedly
edematous. The edema is due to the increased permeability of
the proliferating capillaries in the abscess wall and gradually
subsides in the more chronic cases.

6. (B, C) Deaths from brain abscesses are due to herniation
in about two-thirds of the fatal cases. Rupture with ventriculitis
and meningitis is catastrophic but not invariably fatal. Without
treatment, brain abscesses are almost uniformly fatal. Even
with currently optimal therapy, the mortality is high, over 30%
of cases.

7. (A, B, C, D) The center of an abscess is composed of suppurative material, i.e., necrotic tissue and inflammatory cells. This is surrounded by granulation tissue that is composed of proliferating capillaries, fibroblasts and inflammatory cells. If the abscess has been present sufficiently long, the granulation tissue undergoes organization and the abscess is partially surrounded by a collagenous capsule. The surrounding neural parenchyma is severely edematous and gliotic. As a result of the edema, adjacent myelin shows pallor of staining. The astrocytes are enlarged, have abundant visible cytoplasm and may be multinucleated. The blood vessels are often heavily encircled by chronic inflammatory cells.

REFERENCES

1. Bell WE and McCormick WF: Neurologic Infections in Children. W.B. Saunders Co., Philadelphia, 1975, pp. 90-101.

2. Bellar AJ, et al.: Brain abscess. J Neurol Neurosurg Psychiat 36:757-768, 1973.

3. Garfield J: Brain Abscesses and Focal Suppurative Infections. In: Handbook of Clinical Neurology. Vinken PJ and Bruyn GW (Eds.). North-Holland, Amsterdam, 1978, Vol. 33, pp. 107-147.

4. Morgan H, et al.: Experience with 88 consecutive cases of brain abscess. J Neurosurg 38:698-704, 1973.

5. Samson DS and Clark K: A current review of brain abscess. Am J Med 54:201-210, 1973.

6. Shaw MDM and Russell JA: Cerebellar abscess. J Neuro Neurosurg Psychiat 38:429-435, 1975.

: :

CASE 28: A 45-Year-Old Man with Headaches, Fever and
          Night Sweats

CLINICAL DATA

This 45-year-old man was admitted to the hospital complaining
of headaches, fever and night sweats for three days' duration.
He denied cough, weight loss or tuberculosis contacts. On admission, his blood pressure was 148/100, pulse 100 and temperature 103ºF. He was confused and disoriented. His neck
was supple and examination of heart, lungs, abdomen and nervous system showed no abnormalities. However, a chest x-
ray revealed multiple pulmonary calcifications and pleural
thickening. A white cell count revealed 5,500 leukocytes with
65% neutrophils, 21% lymphocytes, and 13% monocytes.

Two days later he became comatose and was noted to have nuchal rigidity. A lumbar puncture revealed 169 leukocytes with
90% lymphocytes, a protein of 655 mg/dl and a glucose of 81
mg/dl. Brain scan and arteriograms were reported as normal.
Cultures of the cerebrospinal fluid for the usual aerobic and
anaerobic bacteria and for fungi were negative. Eventually,
acid-fast bacilli were cultured from the cerebrospinal fluid.

Despite continued antituberculous therapy, the patient fluctuated
between moderate disorientation and coma and eventually developed akinetic mutism. His serum sodium was low and remained so despite fluid restriction and supplemental sodium
chloride. The patient continued to deteriorate and died six
weeks after admission.

QUESTIONS

1. Cerebrospinal fluid findings characteristic of tuberculous
    meningitis include
    A. elevated protein
    B. lymphocytosis
    C. decreased glucose
    D. elevated glucose

2. Tuberculous meningitis is
    A. more common in men than in women
    B. more common in parts of Asia, Africa, and South
        America than the United States
    C. commonly encountered in children
    D. usually secondary to pulmonary tuberculosis

3. Processes involved in the development of tuberculous
    meningitis include
    A. hematogenous dissemination
    B. establishment of a superficial cortical tuberculoma
        prior to the involvement of the subarachnoid space
    C. establishment of a tuberculoma in the choroid plexus
        prior to involvement of the subarachnoid space
    D. establishment of vasculitis prior to involvement of the
        subarachnoid space

4. Grossly discernible features of tuberculous meningitis in-
    clude
    A. abundant exudate especially at the base of the brain
    B. multiple miliary granulomas
    C. occlusive vasculitis
    D. obstructive hydrocephalus

5. Major complications of tuberculous meningitis include
    A. hydrocephalus
    B. secondary fungal meningitis
    C. encephalomalacia secondary to the obliterative
        arteritis
    D. myelomalacia

6. Histological characteristics of tuberculous meningitis
    include
    A. caseation necrosis
    B. giant cells
    C. obliterative arteritis
    D. acid-fast bacilli

7. Tuberculomas are
    A. common space occupying intracranial lesions in
        countries where tuberculosis is still rampant
    B. commonly infratentorial in children
    C. occasionally calcified
    D. usually cystic

8. Sarcoidosis of the central nervous system is characterized
    by
    A. granulomatous involvement of the leptomeninges and
        hypothalamus
    B. caseation necrosis
    C. small numbers of weakly acid-fast bacilli
    D. cranial nerve palsies

ANSWERS AND DISCUSSION

1. (A, B, C) The diagnosis of tuberculous meningitis can be established with certainty only by demonstration of acid-fast organisms in smears of the cerebrospinal fluid sediment or by isolation of the organism in culture. This may be difficult to achieve. Nevertheless, other cerebrospinal fluid findings can be quite characteristic and provide the usual basis for initiating antituberculous therapy. The typical changes include a moderate elevation of the cerebrospinal fluid pressure, an opalescent appearance, a moderate pleocytosis usually less than 500 cells/cmm with a predominance of lymphocytes, an elevated protein content that may be as high as 200 mg/dl even without spinal block, and a moderate reduction in the glucose. The chloride level is no longer considered a useful determination since it is often not reduced early in the course of the infection. Additional supportive data include a non-reactive test for syphilis, negative india ink preparation for cryptococci and negative cultures for the usual bacteria and fungi.

2. (B, C, D) Tuberculous meningitis affects the sexes in approximately equal proportions. The general decline in the prevalence of tuberculosis in the United States since about 1940 has been accompanied by a marked decline in the prevalence of tuberculous meningitis. Tuberculosis still persists as a very common disease in many parts of Asia, Africa, and South America, and in such areas tuberculous meningitis is more common than in the United States. In countries with a high prevalence of tuberculosis, tuberculous meningitis is very commonly encountered under the age of 5 years and often comprises the major cause of childhood meningitis. Owing to modern diagnosis and therapy, there has been a tendency to encounter tuberculous meningitis in progressively older age groups. Almost all cases are now due to the human rather than bovine strains.

3. (A, B) It is generally agreed that tuberculous meningitis develops as the result of hematogenous dissemination from some other site, usually the lungs. The precise mechanism by which the meninges and subarachnoid space become infected secondary to the hematogenous dissemination has been debated over the years. Because of the prominent vasculitis in association with tuberculous meningitis, Hektoen had suggested that the meningeal infection was secondary to infection of small vessels. Because of the prevalence of granulomas in the choroid plexi, Kment suggested that the ventriculitis and meningitis were

secondary to these foci. Most workers now agree with Rich and
McCordock, who proposed that tuberculous meningitis results
from extension of the infection from small tuberculomas on the
surface of the cortex or in the meninges. However, once the
meningitis becomes extensive, it is difficult to determine
whether a small cortical focus caused or resulted from the
meningitis.

4.   (A, B, C, D) As seen in Fig. 28.1, tuberculous meningitis
is characterized by a thick exudate that is generally most abundant at the base of the brain. Depending upon the duration of
the disease and whether treated or not, the exudate may be soft
and gelatinous or firm and fibrous. The cranial nerves and
blood vessels are commonly obscured. Multiple small miliary
granulomas (arrows in Fig. 28.2) can be seen on the convexities
of the cerebral hemispheres and are most conspicuous along
the cortical veins. The granulomas may occur singly or in
small clusters. Where the exudate densely encases arteries,
the vessels respond with an obliterative arteritis. This process may be evident grossly as thick-walled vessels with very
small lumens (Fig. 28.3). Accumulation of exudate and thickening of the meninges about the foramina of Luschka and
Magendie may result in obstructive hydrocephalus. Less often
obstructive hydrocephalus may result from partial or total
occlusion of the aqueduct. Hydrocephalus also may result from
obliteration of the subarachnoid space or interference with absorption at the Pacchionian granulations.

5.   (A, C, D) Hydrocephalus and obliterative arteritis are two
of the most important complications of tuberculous meningitis.
The vasculitis is manifested predominantly by intimal proliferation with relatively little necrosis of the vessel wall. The process closely resembles both histologically and angiographically
Heubner's syphilitic arteritis. As a result of the obliterative
arteritis, the brains and spinal cords from patients with tuberculous meningitis often contain foci of encephalomalacia and
myelomalacia. These secondary vascular lesions probably
account for many of the deaths and many of the permanent sequelae from tuberculous meningitis. Hemorrhagic infarction
is considerably less common than ischemic necrosis but may
occur. Dastur has also described an allergic tuberculous encephalopathy in the absence of overt infarction, hydrocephalus,
or tuberculomas. The significance of this process remains
to be determined.

6.   (A, B, C, D) The histological characteristics of tuberculous meningitis (Fig. 28.4) are similar to those encountered in tuberculous lesions in other parts of the body.

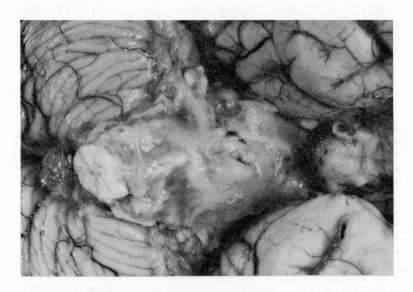

FIG. 28. 1: Photograph of the base of the brain showing the thick exudate obscuring the vessels and nerves.

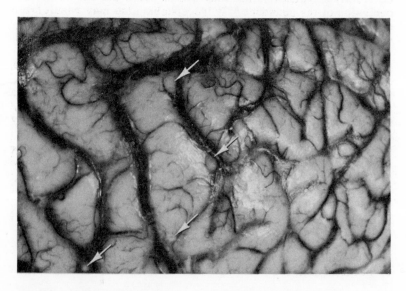

FIG. 28. 2: Photograph of the convex surface of the cerebral hemisphere showing the miliary granulomas (arrows).

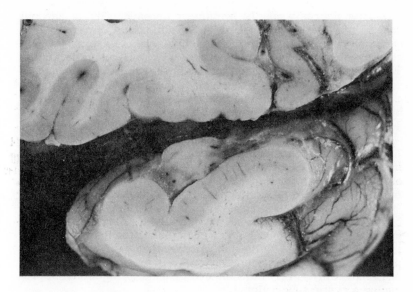

FIG. 28. 3: Photograph showing exudate surrounding arteries and producing an obliterative arteritis.

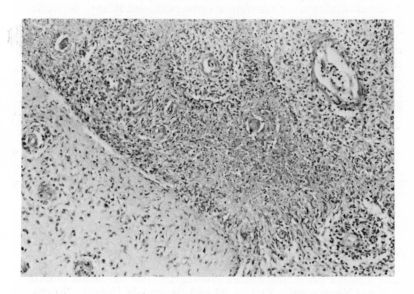

FIG. 28. 4: Microscopic section showing the histological characteristic of the exudate in the subarachnoid space.

Caseation necrosis may be prominent or especially in chronic
cases, may be overshadowed by an admixture of chronic inflammatory cells and fibroblasts.   Plasma cells may be encountered among the inflammatory cells.   Giant cells with
multiple nuclei are found especially in the vicinity of the cas-
eous foci.   As previously mentioned, obliterative arteritis is
a prominent feature.   Acid-fast bacilli can be demonstrated
best in regions of caseation but may be very difficult or im-
possible to demonstrate in partially treated patients.

7.   (A, B, C) Tuberculomas are common space occupying lesions
in countries where tuberculosis is still rampant.   In a series
of 1,000 intracranial space occupying lesions reported from
India, 22.6% were tuberculomas.   Two-thirds of these were
supratentorial lesions, however, among children, two-thirds
of the tuberculomas were infratentorial. Histologically, tuberculomas of the nervous system show caseation necrosis, epithelioid cells, giant cells and lymphocytes with occasional
plasma cells.   Some become extensively or even totally mineralized.   Only rarely does the center undergo liquefaction producing a cystic tuberculoma.

8.   (A, D) Sarcoidosis is a systemic granulomatous disease of
unknown etiology.   Some workers have regarded it as a variant
of tuberculosis whereas others have regarded it as a peculiar
allergic or immune response to a variety of different agents.
The central nervous system is involved in 2-7% of patients with
sarcoidosis.   The disease in the central nervous system is
manifested predominantly as a non-caseating granulomatous
meningitis with a predilection for the base of the brain and hypothalamus.   Clinical manifestations include cranial nerve
palsies, blindness, anosmia, and diabetes insipidus.   Acid-fast
organisms cannot be demonstrated morphologically or by cultures.

REFERENCES

1.   Dastur DK: Neurotuberculosis. In: Pathology of the Ner-
     vous System. Minckler J (Ed.). McGraw-Hill Book Co.,
     New York, 1972, Vol. 3, pp. 2412-2422.

2.   Dastur DK and Lalitha VS: The Many Facets of Neuro-
     tuberculosis: An Epitome of Neuropathology. In: Progress
     in Neuropathology. Zimmerman H (Ed.). Grune and
     Stratton, New York, 1973, Vol. II, pp. 351-408.

3.   Tandon PN: Tuberculous Meningitis. In: Handbook of Clini-
     cal Neurology. Vinken PJ and Bruyn GW (Eds.). North-
     Holland, Amsterdam, 1978, Vol. 33, pp. 195-262.

: :

CASE 29: An Elderly Woman with Chronic Lymphocytic
Leukemia who Developed Hemiplegia

CLINICAL DATA

This 73-year-old woman had been found to have a white blood
cell count of 60,000 but refused further evaluation. Three
years later, she was admitted to the hospital with a one-month
history of weakness and fever. Physical examination revealed
hepatosplenomegaly and lymphadenopathy. A white blood cell
count was 200,000 cells/cmm and the cells consisted predominantly of lymphocytes. A bone marrow aspiration confirmed
the diagnosis of chronic lymphocytic leukemia. She did reasonably well without therapy for another five months before
treatment with prednisone, chlorambucil, and allopurinol was
instituted. One month later, she was readmitted to the hospital with a weight loss of ten pounds, increasing weakness,
cough and night sweats. On physical examination she was found
to be febrile and to have rales. Except for generalized weakness, her neurological examination was within normal limits.
Chest x-rays showed a right lower lobe infiltrate. Her chemotherapy was discontinued and antibiotics were instituted with
favorable results. Eight days later, the fever and the right
lower lobe infiltrate recurred. Despite additional antibiotics,
the patient remained febrile and developed a stiff neck. A lumbar puncture yielded cerebrospinal fluid containing 60 cells/
cmm, 75 mg/dl of protein and 75 mg/dl of glucose. Neurological examination the next day disclosed an absent left corneal reflex, a left central facial weakness, left hemiplegia and
questionable sensory deficits. Choriform movements of the
right hand developed later in the day. The patient died on the
following day.

QUESTIONS

1. Fig. 29.1 illustrates a coronal section from this patient's
   brain. There was no grossly discernible exudate or hemorrhage in the subarachnoid space and no major arterial or
   venous thromboses. The most appropriate gross diagnosis
   is
   A. progressive multifocal leukoencephalopathy
   B. leukemic infiltration
   C. disseminated necrotizing leukoencephalopathy
   D. opportunistic mycotic infection

2. Fig. 29.2 illustrates the fungus in the brain of this patient
    as seen with a Grocott methenamine silver stain.   From
    this appearance, one should make a diagnosis of
    A. Aspergillus fumigatus
    B. Aspergillus species
    C. invasive septate fungus morphologically consistent
        with an Aspergillus species
    D. invasive non-septate fungus morphologically consistent
        with an Aspergillus species

3. Cerebral aspergillosis is generally a component of dis-
    seminated aspergillosis.   Other sites that are commonly
    involved include the
    A. lungs
    B. heart
    C. gastrointestinal tract
    D. eye

4. Other fungi with septate hyphae that have been reported
    to involve the brain include
    A. Penicillium
    B. Cladosporium
    C. Sporotrichum
    D. Rhizopus

5. Conditions that predispose to disseminated and cerebral
    candidiasis include
    A. prolonged antibiotic therapy
    B. intravenous catheters
    C. abdominal operations
    D. onychomycosis

6. Morphological characteristics of Candida in tissue include
    the presence of
    A. septate hyphae
    B. ovoid yeasts
    C. gram-positive pseudohyphae
    D. gram-negative pseudohyphae

7. Clinical features that are commonly associated with cere-
    bral phycomycosis are
    A. poorly controlled diabetes
    B. history of injury from rose thorns
    C. history of residence in San Joaquin Valley or Arizona
    D. rapidly progressive periorbital swelling and proptosis

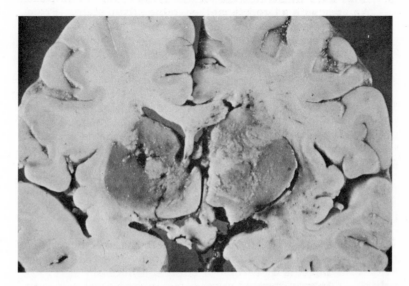

FIG. 29.1: Coronal section of the cerebral hemispheres showing bilateral, focally hemorrhagic encephalomalacia.

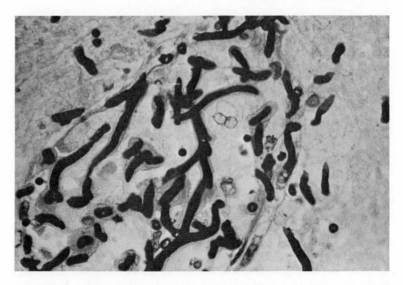

FIG. 29.2: Microscopic section showing the morphology of the
fungus.

8. In tissue, the Phycomycetes appear as
    A. narrow septate hyphae
    B. broad septate hyphae
    C. broad non-septate hyphae
    D. broad pseudohyphae

ANSWERS AND DISCUSSION

1. (D) The bilateral, focally hemorrhagic areas of encephalomalacia in this immunosuppressed patient without major arterial
or venous thromboses are strongly suggestive of an opportunistic mycotic infection. Aspergillosis is the most common fungal infection encountered under these circumstances. The
organism has a marked propensity to invade and occlude small
blood vessels, thus accounting for the usual gross appearance
as an area of focally hemorrhagic encephalomalacia. The infection can also result in frank abscesses or granulomas.

The clinical setting, i.e., an immunosuppressed patient, is
more suggestive of the diagnosis than any of the neurological
signs or symptoms or results of clinical laboratory determinations. Aspergillosis is more common among patients with
leukemia than lymphoma and is especially prevalent in renal
transplant recipients. In man, aspergillosis is most often due
to Aspergillus fumigatus.

Toxoplasmosis in the immunosuppressed individual can produce
cerebral lesions that are grossly indistinguishable from aspergillosis. However, opportunistic toxoplasmosis is far less
common than opportunistic mycotic infections.

Progressive multifocal leukoencephalopathy usually occurs in
immunosuppressed individuals, most of whom have leukemia or
lymphoma. Grossly, the lesions are destructive and demyeli-
native but involve predominantly the white matter.

Disseminated necrotizing leukencephalopathy is characterized
by multiple discrete or confluent necrotic lesions in the white
matter. This recently described entity has been found in the
brains of children who have received intrathecal chemotherapy
and irradiation for their leukemia.

2. (C) The identification of the genus and species of a fungus
can be done only by culturing the organism and observing such
features as colony shape, color, spore color, shape of fruiting
heads, number and arrangement of sterigmata, etc. A presumptive diagnosis of Aspergillus in tissue is based on the

presence of dichotomously branching septate hyphae with a
relatively uniform diameter of 3 to 6 microns. The fungi are
generally poorly stained by hematoxylin-eosin and can be demonstrated to better advantage with a periodic acid-Schiff or methenamine silver stain. Occasionally, as in the present specimen,
the hyphae are surrounded by a homogeneous eosinophilic material that is thought to result from an antigen-antibody reaction,
the so-called Hoeppli-Splendore phenomenon.

When the Aspergillus grows in cavities exposed to air, fruiting
heads will develop. These facilitate the diagnosis of the genus
Aspergillus in tissue. We have not seen these structures in
brain tissue.

3.   (A, B, C) The lungs are usually the portal of entry for Aspergillus and are thus the organs most commonly involved in
disseminated aspergillosis. In the immunocompetent individual,
the fungus may be present as a mass, an aspergilloma, in pre-
existing bronchiectatic or tuberculous cavities. An allergic
form of bronchopulmonary aspergillosis has also been described.
The heart is commonly involved in disseminated aspergillosis.
Aspergillus endocarditis is an important complication following
implantation of prosthetic heart valves. The brain is the third
most commonly involved organ in patients with hematogenously
disseminated aspergillosis. In addition, a few cases with cerebral involvement arise as the result of extension from the ears
or paranasal sinus. Involvement of the gastrointestinal tract
is common in disseminated aspergillosis and is manifested by
mucosal ulcerations. Superficial aspergillosis of the eye, i.e.,
keratomycosis, is considered common but endogenous involvement as part of disseminated aspergillosis is generally considered rare. This has not been thoroughly investigated by
autopsy studies.

4.   (A, B) Although very rare, a number of other fungi with
septate hyphae have been reported to involve the brain. These
include Penicillium, Hormodendrum and Cladosporium. While
there are suggestive morphological features such as the paucity
of septa in the hyphae of Penicillium and the brown color of Hormodendrum and Cladosporium, the final diagnosis depends on
cultural characteristics.

In tissue, Sporotrichum usually appears as small ovoids; hyphae
are very rare. Rhizopus forms prominent broad hyphae in tissue
but they are non-septate.

5. (A, B, C) Although once considered rare, candidiasis is
now the most common mycotic infection of the nervous system
encountered at autopsy. This reflects the increasing prevalence of disseminated candidiasis and other opportunistic infections in the compromised host. Factors that appear to be
especially important in predisposing the patient to candidiasis
include long-term, broad spectrum antibiotic therapy, prolonged
use of intravenous catheters and abdominal operations. Within the brain, candidiasis may be manifested as abscesses,
multiple foci of cerebritis or miliary microabscesses.

6. (B, C) In tissue, Candida appears as a mixture of ovoid
yeasts and thin pseudohyphae. The organisms are often detectable with hematoxylin-eosin and are gram-positive but are best
demonstrated with the periodic acid-Schiff or methenamine silver stains. The tissue reaction elicited by the Candida ranges
from suppurative to granulomatous. Positive identification, as
with other fungi, depends on isolation and cultural characteristics. Disseminated candidiasis is often diagnosed antemortem
by blood cultures.

7. (A, D) Phycomycosis occurs most frequently in individuals
with poorly controlled diabetes or other conditions with keto-
acidosis. It has also been observed in immunosuppressed patients and rarely in the absence of recognized predisposing conditions. Cerebral phycomycosis usually results from direct
extension of the mycotic infection from the nose or paranasal
sinuses often by way of the orbit. This produces periorbital
swelling, external ophthalmoplegia, proptosis and loss of vision.
Rarely, the organism appears to reach the brain by hematogenous spread from an extracranial site. The hyphae have a marked
propensity for vascular invasion and produce extensive cerebral infarction.

A history of injury from rose thorns is classically associated
with sporotrichosis, and a history of residence in the San Joaquin Valley or Arizona is suggestive of coccidioidomycosis.

8. (C) In tissue, the Phycomycetes appear as broad, irregularly branched, non-septate hyphae. Only if proven by culture,
should the more specific terms mucor, mucormycosis or
Rhizopus be used.

REFERENCES

1. Bell WE and McCormick WF: Neurologic Infections in
    Children. W.B. Saunders Co., Philadelphia, 1975,
    pp. 301-350.

2. Fetter BF, et al.: Mycoses of the Central Nervous System. Williams and Wilkins Co., Baltimore, 1967.

3. Meyer RD, et al.: Aspergillosis complicating neoplastic disease. Am J Med 54:6-15, 1973.

4. Pena CE: Aspergillosis. In: Human Infection with Fungi, Actinomycetes and Algae. Baker RD (Ed.). Springer-Verlag, New York, 1971, pp. 762-831.

5. Price DL, et al.: Intracranial phycomycosis: A clinicopathological and radiological study. J Neurol Sci 14:359-375, 1971.

6. Rosen PP: Opportunistic Fungal Infections in Patients with Neoplastic Diseases. In: Pathology Annual. Sommers S (Ed.). Appleton-Century-Crofts, New York, 1976, pp. 255-315.

: :

CASE 30:   A 51-Year-Old Man with Systemic Lupus, Fever
           and Obtundation

CLINICAL DATA

This 51-year-old farmer had been diagnosed as having systemic
lupus erythematosus with Raynaud's phenomenon, polyserositis,
hemolytic anemia and positive "LE preps."   He was being
treated with corticosteroids. When he developed fever, more
severe anemia and bizarre behavior, these changes were attributed to progression of his collagen-vascular disease.   His
steroids were increased and Cytoxan was added to his regimen.
Within a month, he developed an intermittent spiking fever.
Cultures of urine, blood and sputum failed to reveal any pathogens. Despite the addition of antibiotics and still further increases in his steroids, the fever persisted, he became
obtunded and died.

QUESTIONS

1. Grossly the brain showed mildly opacified leptomeninges
    and parenchymal lesions, as illustrated in Fig. 30.1.
    These were maximal in the basal ganglia. The most
    appropriate gross diagnosis is
    A. lupus encephalopathy
    B. thrombotic thrombocytopenic purpura
    C. cryptococcosis
    D. aspergillosis

2. Morphological characteristics of cryptococci in tissue in
    clude
    A. variable-sized spheres
    B. budding with narrow site of attachment
    C. thick refractile cell walls
    D. endospores

3. Central nervous system cryptococcosis usually results
    from
    A. direct extension from nose and paranasal sinuses
    B. direct extension from cutaneous infection involving
        scalp
    C. hematogenous dissemination from cutaneous infection
    D. hematogenous dissemination from pulmonary infection

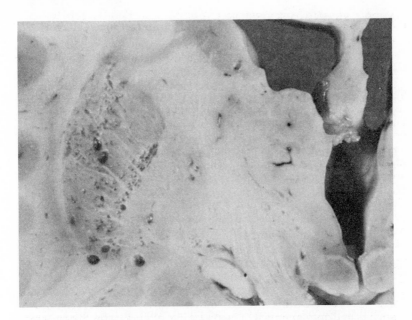

FIG. 30.1: Coronal section of the cerebral hemispheres showing small cystic lesions in the putamen.

4. Central nervous system blastomycosis may be manifested
   as
   A. hemorrhagic infarction
   B. pachymeningitis
   C. leptomeningitis
   D. abscesses

5. A fungus infection characteristically associated with the
   San Joaquin Valley and Arizona is
   A. histoplasmosis
   B. coccidioidomycosis
   C. blastomycosis
   D. paracoccidioidomycosis

6. Nocardiosis of the central nervous system
   A. is manifested as meningitis or abscesses
   B. is usually manifested as calcified miliary granulomas
   C. usually results from hematogenous dissemination from
      a pulmonary focus
   D. usually results from direct extension from a sinus
      infection

ANSWERS AND DISCUSSION

1.   (C) The most appropriate gross diagnosis is cryptococcosis.
This is one of the common mycotic infections of the central nervous system but is now less commonly encountered at autopsy
than opportunistic aspergillosis or candidiasis. Even with cryptococcosis, about one-half of the cases occur in association with
malignancies, long-term corticosteroid therapy or other immunosuppressive conditions.

Cryptococcosis commonly produces meningitis. The gross alterations in the meninges range from mild opacification of the
leptomeninges to distension of the subarachnoid space by gelatinous exudate. Occasionally, small granulomas are found along
the cortical veins.

Within the brain there may be small intraparenchymal cysts.
These are often most numerous in deep grey matter. In the
present case, the putamen and the substantia nigra were the
most severely affected structures. Similar appearing cysts
may be found in the cortex. Regardless of location, the cysts
are derived primarily from distension of the perivascular
spaces and displacement of neural parenchyma by the organisms
and their mucopolysaccharide capsules. There is relatively
little tissue destruction. The ventricular system is often enlarged, the ependymal surfaces may be studded by ependymal
granulations and the choroid plexi may harbor the organisms.
Occasionally, Cryptococci will produce solitary or multiple
granulomas called "torulomas."

The usual neuropathological changes attributable directly to systemic lupus erythematosus are small infarcts that may be visible
grossly. Rarely, hemorrhages, petechial or larger, also may
occur.

Thrombotic thrombocytopenic purpura is a syndrome characterized by a triad of hemolytic anemia, thrombocytopenia and
bizarre neurological disturbances. The lesions in the central
nervous system appear grossly as small infarcts and hemorrhages. Microscopically ectatic small vessels are partially or
completely filled with eosinophilic granular material. The
eosinophilic material often becomes covered by endothelial
cells.

2.   (A, B) In tissue, Cryptococci appear as variable sized
spheres that range from 2 to 15 microns in diameter (Fig. 30.2).
The organisms form buds that characteristically have a narrow

site of attachment. Occasionally, the buds elongate and form
short pseudohyphae. The organisms are surrounded by a variable quantity of mucopolysaccharide capsular material. Although the capsular material is highly characteristic of Cryptococci, it may be quite sparse in tissues. The fungi can be seen
with hematoxylin-eosin but are better demonstrated with the
periodic acid-Schiff or methenamine silver stains. The capsules are seen as "halos" in India ink preparations of the spinal
fluid or tissue smears. The capsules can be stained by mucopolysaccharide stains, such as alcian blue and colloidal iron.
The tissue reaction to the Cryptococci is highly variable, ranging from almost no cellular infiltrate to a frankly granulomatous response.

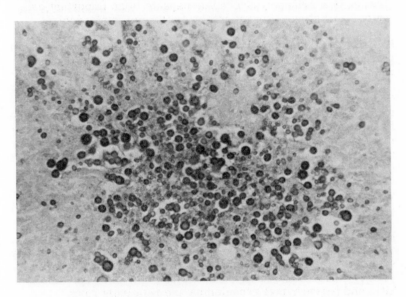

FIG. 30.2: Microscopic section showing the organisms stained
with the alcian blue stain.

3. (D) Cryptococcosis of the central nervous system usually
results from hematogenous dissemination from a pulmonary infection. The pulmonary lesions are usually located in the lower
lobes, may be quite small and rarely calcify or cavitate. The
central nervous system manifestations are often the initial or only
clinical manifestations. The central nervous system is estimated
to be involved in 90-100% of the cases of disseminated cryptococcosis. Only rarely is the skin the site of primary infection.

4. (B, C, D) Central nervous system involvement by blastomycosis is relatively uncommon, and usually results from
hematogenous dissemination from a primary pulmonary infection. The central nervous system involvement may be in the
form of leptomeningitis, intraparenchymal abscesses or granulomas, or pachymeningitis when the adjacent bone and epidural
tissues are involved. The organisms elicit both suppurative and
granulomatous tissue reactions.

The fungi appear as thick-walled yeasts that range from 8 to 12
microns in diameter. The thick cell wall is highly refractile
and poorly stained while the cytoplasm is deeply stained. The
yeasts form single buds that have broad attachment sites. The
absence of a mucopolysaccharide capsule is an important criterion for distinguishing Blastomyces from Cryptococci.

5. (B) Coccidioidomycosis is encountered in the southwestern
portion of the United States and is especially prevalent in the
San Joaquin Valley and parts of Arizona. The infection primarily
involves the lungs and becomes disseminated in only a very few
instances. Involvement of the central nervous system is the
most serious complication of dissemination and is usually in the
form of meningitis. Less commonly, there are intraparenchymal granulomas. In tissue, the fungi form distinctive large
sporangia that measure up to 60-70 microns in diameter. These
become filled with endospores. When the sporangia rupture,
the endospores are released. When this occurs, the tissue reaction becomes purulent in addition to the general granulomatous reaction.

Histoplasmosis is especially associated with the Ohio and Mis-
sissippi River Valleys. The involvement of the central nervous
system is relatively uncommon and usually minimal. During
primary dissemination vascular lesions may develop. Meningitis and parenchymal granulomas are relatively rare.

Paracoccidioidomycosis is endemic in Mexico, Central and
South America and is especially prevalent in Brazil. Involvement of the central nervous system is relatively uncommon.

6. (A, C) Nocardia and Actinomyces are commonly discussed
with fungi but are now classified among the bacteria. Nocardiosis of the central nervous system is almost always produced by
Nocardia asteroides and may appear as meningitis, cerebritis
or abscesses. The organisms reach the nervous system by
hematogenous dissemination from a pulmonary focus. In tissue,
the organisms appear as thin branched filaments that are best

demonstrated with the methenamine silver or Gram stains. The tissue reaction is predominantly suppurative.

REFERENCES

1. Brown JR: Human actinomycosis: A study of 181 subjects. Hum Pathol 4:319-330, 1973.

2. Fetter BF, et al.: Mycoses of the Central Nervous System. Williams and Wilkins Co., Baltimore, 1967.

3. Littman ML and Zimmerman LE: Cryptococcosis, Torulosis or European Blastomycosis. Grune and Stratton, New York, 1956.

4. Selby RC and Lopez NM: Torulomas (cryptococcal granulomata) of the central nervous system. J Neurosurg 38:40-46, 1973.

: :

CASE 31:   A Female Infant with Rapidly Developing Hydro-
            cephalus and an Elevated Cerebrospinal Fluid
            Protein

CLINICAL DATA

This female infant was the product of an uncomplicated full-
term pregnancy and a normal delivery. At birth, the child
weighed 7 lbs, 4-3/4 oz and her head measured 13-1/4 in in
circumference. When seen at two weeks of age, her head circumference had increased to 16 in. She was referred to the
university hospital for evaluation.

Physical examination revealed a grossly enlarged head, measuring 40 cm in circumference, with widely spread sutures and
a full anterior fontanelle. The left eye was smaller than the
right and both were deviated downward and medially. The liver
was palpable 1-2 cm below the right costal margin and the tip
of the spleen was palpable. There was questionable decerebrate posturing.

X-rays of the skull confirmed the hydrocephalus but showed no
intracranial calcification. The cerebrospinal fluid contained
1,000 cells/cmm of which most were neutrophils, 50 mg/dl of
glucose and 4.2 g/dl of protein. A ventriculogram revealed
massive hydrocephalus with severe loss of neural parenchyma.
Only about 1 cm of cerebral parenchyma was present in the left
frontal region and almost none on the right. The third ventricle
could not be visualized with air or contrast media. "TORCH"
titers were obtained and reported to be negative for cytomegalovirus, rubella and herpes but positive at a dilution of 1:256 for
toxoplasmosis. The child died at the age of six weeks. General autopsy findings included moderate hepatomegaly and
splenomegaly.

QUESTIONS

1. The clinical data are most consistent with a diagnosis of
    A. congenital toxoplasmosis
    B. congenital cytomegalovirus infection
    C. perinatal herpes simplex infection
    D. congenital rubella

2. Laboratory studies that can be employed to establish a
    diagnosis of congenital toxoplasmosis include
    A. Sabin-Feldman dye test

B. determination of IgM toxoplasma antibodies in blood
C. demonstration of organisms in ventricular fluid
D. fluorescent antibody test

3. Figs. 31.1 and 31.2 show this infant's brain. The gross
    pathological changes of congenital toxoplasmosis include
    A. hydrocephalus
    B. scattered foci of necrosis
    C. scattered foci of mineralization
    D. enlarged perivascular spaces containing gelatinous
        exudate

4. The histological features of toxoplasmosis include
    A. necrosis
    B. free toxoplasma trophozoites
    C. toxoplasma cysts
    D. glial and inflammatory cell infiltrates

5. Ophthalmic manifestations of toxoplasmosis include
    A. microphthalmia
    B. chorioretinitis
    C. intraglobal masses of cartilage
    D. glaucoma

6. Severe congenital toxoplasmosis usually results from
    maternal infections
    A. before pregnancy
    B. during the first trimester
    C. during the second trimester
    D. during the third trimester

7. Acquired toxoplasmosis in the immunocompetent adult
    most commonly results in
    A. fatal encephalitis
    B. lymphadenopathy
    C. pneumonitis
    D. myocarditis

8. Toxoplasmosis in the immunosuppressed adult with a
    malignant neoplasm is
    A. usually a recently acquired infection
    B. probably reactivation of a dormant infection
    C. the cause of the neoplasm
    D. usually manifested as encephalitis

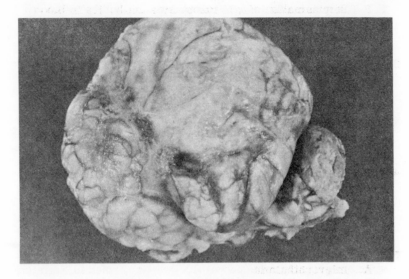

FIG. 31.1: Photograph of the brain showing extensive destruction of the cerebral hemispheres.

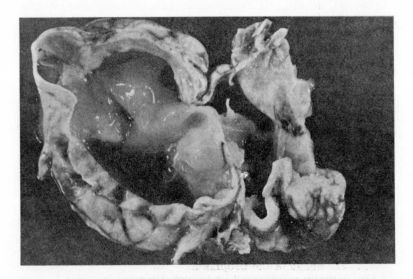

FIG. 31.2: Coronal section of the cerebral hemispheres showing the extensive destruction of neural parenchyma,
hydrocephalus and the precipitated protein from the
ventricular fluid.

9. Toxoplasmosis is acquired by
    A. sexual intercourse
    B. transplacental passage
    C. eating undercooked meat
    D. contamination with cat feces

ANSWERS AND DISCUSSION

1.   (A) The clinical data are clearly indicative of a diagnosis
of congenital toxoplasmosis. In its most severe form, the disease may cause abortion or death shortly after birth.   Prematurity is common.   Often the infected newborn infant initially
appears to be normal but develops clinical manifestations of
the disease within a few days to a few weeks after delivery.
Convulsions, intracerebral calcifications, hydrocephalus or
microcephalus, chorioretinitis and microphthalmia are among
the more typical manifestations and reflect the predilection of
the organisms for the central nervous system and eye.   Associated evidence of systemic involvement include hepatomegaly,
splenomegaly, lymphadenopathy, jaundice, anemia, pneumonitis and myocarditis.   These various signs and symptoms
are largely indistinguishable from those produced by other members of the so-called "TORCH complex" (T, toxoplasmosis; O,
other; R, rubella; C, cytomegalovirus; H, herpesvirus) and
specific diagnosis depends upon laboratory criteria. In this
case, the specific diagnosis was established by the 1:256 titer
for toxoplasmosis and negative titers for the other agents.

It must be noted that severe disease as in the present case is
the exception rather than the rule with congenital toxoplasmosis. Among 59 non-aborted cases of congenital toxoplasmosis
reported by Desmonts and Couvreur, two died, seven had
severe disease, 11 had mild disease and 39 had subclinical illness.

2.   (A, B, C, D) The Sabin-Feldman dye test has long been
used for the serological diagnosis of toxoplasmosis. This test
is based on the fact that Toxoplasma from mouse peritoneal
exudate swell and stain with methylene blue after being incu-
bated with normal human serum. By contrast, Toxoplasma exposed to antibody-containing serum remain thin and do not stain.
This procedure is being replaced by direct fluorescent antibody
tests that are technically simpler.   In suspected congenital
toxoplasmosis, these tests must be repeated in order to rule
out passive transfer of maternal antibodies. A fluorescent anti-
IgM antibody test is now available for use on cord blood.

Examination of the ventricular fluid can be highly informative
or even diagnostic. The protein content is extraordinarily high
in patients with severe congenital disease, e.g., 4.2 grams/dl in
the present case. Antibody titers may be far higher than in
blood, e.g., 1:1024 in the present case. Occasionally, the organisms can be seen in smears of the ventricular fluid; more often
they can be recovered by inoculation in Toxoplasma-free mice.

3. (A, B, C) In congenital toxoplasmosis there is a variable
degree of destruction of the central nervous system. The lesions are predominantly necrotic and may be small and multifocal or extensive and confluent. The necrotic foci are initially
soft, yellow-grey and shrunken. Later these undergo partial
mineralization. The necrotic lesions involve cortex, white
matter and deep ganglionic grey matter. The ventricular surfaces are directly involved by the necrosis of periventricular
structures and by extensive development of ependymal granulations. Frenkel has suggested that seepage of highly antigenic
ventricular fluid through ependymal defects leads to vasculitis
and promotes further necrosis of the periventricular tissue.
The aqueduct commonly becomes occluded from necrosis of
periaqueductal structures, from the ependymal granulations or
merely from the necrotic debris in the ventricular system. As
a result, the brains are often hydrocephalic. The brain stem
and cerebellum are somewhat less severely affected than the
cerebral hemispheres. The leptomeninges may harbor foci of
necrosis and the subarachnoid space often contains abundant
grey-white exudate.

Enlargement of perivascular spaces producing grossly visible
intraparenchymal cysts containing gelatinous exudate is a characteristic of cryptococcosis, not toxoplasmosis.

4. (A, B, C, D) The lesions of toxoplasmosis are determined
by the rate of proliferation and virulence of the Toxoplasma
and by the immune response of the host. In congenital toxoplasmosis, the interplay of these factors leads to a variety of
histopathological changes that vary in severity from area to area.
The neural parenchyma shows mild to intense inflammation.
Free trophozoites produce a mixed inflammatory cell response
that includes the presence of plasma cells. Cysts, on the other
hand, are accompanied by little or no inflammation (Fig. 31.3).
Diffusion of antigen from the ventricular system elicits an im-
mune-mediated vasculitis and tissue destruction remote from
sites of actual parasitic infection. Furthermore, proliferation
of trophozoites in vessel walls can lead to thrombosis of small
vessels and infarction distally. With the passage of time, there
is increasing gliosis and deposition of mineral about the foci of
necrosis. The free trophozoites may be sparse and difficult to
distinguish from the smaller granules of mineral.

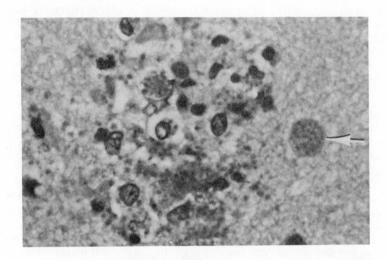

FIG. 31.3: Microscopic section showing Toxoplasma trophozoites and cysts (arrow).

5. (A, B) Ocular damage is a common complication of congenital toxoplasmosis. A few of the patients have microphthalmia
(Fig. 31.4) and many of the patients have chorioretinitis (Fig.
31.5). In contrast to rubella, cataracts and glaucoma are uncommon. The role of acquired toxoplasmosis in producing
uveitis in the immunocompetent adult remains controversial.

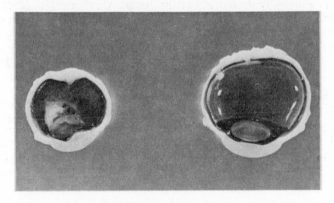

FIG. 31.4: Photograph comparing the severely dis-
organized microphthalmic left eye with
the more nearly normal right eye.

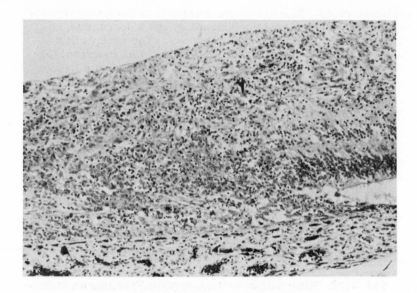

FIG. 31.5:   Microscopic section showing the severe chorioretinitis.

6.   (B, C) The time at which maternal infection is acquired
appears to be of great significance in determining the risk to
the fetus.   Maternal infections acquired before or very soon
after conception, i.e., earlier than the first month of pregnancy, generally do not affect the fetus. Conversely, subclinical infantile infections commonly result from maternal infection
during the third trimester.   Desmonts and Couvreur have con-
cluded that fetal death or severe congenital toxoplasmosis results only from maternal infections during the second to sixth
months of gestation.

7.   (B) Acquired toxoplasmosis in the immunocompetent adult
is usually subclinical or manifested by lymphadenopathy involving especially cervical, suboccipital, supraclavicular and
axillary lymph nodes.   Clinically, these enlarged nodes may be
mistaken for lymphoma.   Myocarditis and pneumonitis have
been reported on rare occasions in apparently immunocompetent
adults.

8.   (B, D) Immunosuppressed individuals have an increased
prevalence of severe toxoplasmosis.   Most of these patients
have malignant neoplasms, usually lymphomas, and are taking

corticosteroids. The symptoms referable to the toxoplasmosis are central nervous system dysfunction and a necrotizing encephalomyelitis may be found at autopsy. The encephalitis is thought to result from reactivation of a dormant infection. The necrotic brain lesion may be grossly indistinguishable from that produced by an opportunistic mycotic infection.

9. (B, C, D) Congenital toxoplasmosis is transmitted from the mother to the fetus by transplacental passage of the parasites. Infection in the older individual is acquired by consumption of undercooked meat containing Toxoplasma cysts or by contamination from cat feces. It has been shown that the parasites complete their life cycle in the cat and infectious oocysts are present in cat feces.

REFERENCES

1. Carey RM, et al.: Toxoplasmosis. Am J Med 54:30-38, 1973.

2. Desmonts G and Couvreur J: Congenital toxoplasmosis. N Eng J Med 290:1110-1116, 1974.

3. Frenkel JK: Toxoplasmosis. In: Pathology of the Nervous System. Minckler J (Ed.). McGraw-Hill Book Co., New York, 1972, Vol. 3, pp. 2521-2538.

4. Townsend JJ, et al.: Acquired toxoplasmosis. Arch Neurol 32:335-343, 1975.

: :

CASE 32: A Mexican-American Woman with Hydrocephalus and an Intraventricular Cystic Lesion

CLINICAL DATA

This 21-year-old, pregnant, Mexican-American woman had nearly constant headaches accompanied by nausea and vomiting for the past eight months. During the past three months, she noted progressive decrease in her visual acuity. She had had no seizures or syncopal episodes.

Physical examination on admission revealed a lethargic woman who was approximately eight months pregnant. Her visual acuity was markedly reduced. Her pupils were equal and reacted sluggishly to light. Her fundi showed papilledema. There was no nystagmus. The remainder of her cranial nerves appeared to be intact. There was mild generalized weakness and spasticity in both legs. The deep tendon reflexes were increased in the lower limbs and a Babinski sign was present on the left. The sensory examination was normal.

A ventriculogram demonstrated hydrocephalus and apparent upward displacement of the fourth ventricle. A ventriculo-atrial shunt was inserted to relieve the intracranial pressure. One month later, after the patient delivered, an angiogram and a pneumoencephalogram were performed. These studies demonstrated a midline, fourth ventricular mass. A posterior fossa exploration was performed and a cyst was removed from the fourth ventricle. The patient did well postoperatively.

QUESTIONS

1. The surgical specimen consisted of a partially collapsed grey-white cyst that measured approximately 3 cm in diameter. The microscopic appearance is shown in Fig. 32.1. The most appropriate diagnosis is
    A. colloid cyst of the fourth ventricle
    B. Cysticercus
    C. Coenurus cerebralis
    D. hydatid cyst

2. Cysticercus cellulosae is the larval form of
    A. Taenia saginata
    B. Taenia solium
    C. Multiceps multiceps
    D. Echinococcus granulosus

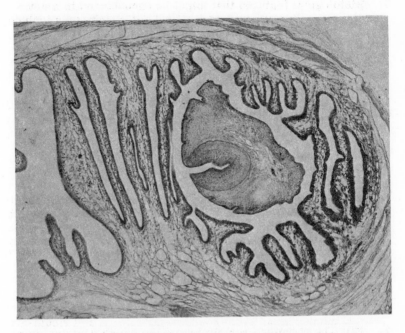

FIG. 32. 1: Microscopic section showing the structure of the cyst
removed from the fourth ventricle.

3. In neural parenchyma, living cysticerci usually elicit
    A. an intense suppurative reaction
    B. an intense granulomatous reaction
    C. intense gliosis
    D. minimal tissue reaction

4. In trichinosis, the ingested larvae
    A. mature in the gastrointestinal tract and new larval
        progeny invade and encyst in skeletal muscle
    B. are freed from their cysts in the stomach and migrate
        to skeletal muscles without further maturation
    C. are freed from their cysts in the stomach and migrate
        to the heart without further maturation
    D. mature in the gastrointestinal tract and new larval
        progeny invade and encyst in skeletal and cardiac
        muscle

5. Histological features that might be encountered in a muscle biopsy specimen from a patient with trichinosis include
    A. enlarged basophilic myofibers
    B. encysted larvae
    C. interstitial and perivascular inflammatory cell reaction containing eosinophils
    D. target fibers

6. Eosinophilic meningitis is caused by the larvae of
    A. Trichinella spiralis
    B. Toxocara canis
    C. Angiostrongylus cantonensis
    D. Enteriobius vermicularis

7. A parasitic meningoencephalitis, characteristically contracted by swimming in fresh or brackish water, is caused by
    A. Entamoeba histolytica
    B. Strongyloides stercoralis
    C. Nosema cuniculi
    D. Naegleria fowleri

ANSWERS AND DISCUSSION

1. (B) The structure removed from the fourth ventricle is an encysted parasitic larva. The cyst wall is composed of three layers: an outer cuticular layer, an intermediate cellular layer and an inner fibrillary or reticular layer. The plicated structure within the cyst is the scolex and is characteristic of a cysticercus. A specific diagnosis of Cysticercus cellulosae should be made only after demonstrating that the cyst contains a single invaginated scolex that has four suckers and an anterior circle of hooklets. The detailed structure of the scolex is best determined by examining the opened cyst as a whole mount pressed between two slides. Serial sections are needed to demonstrate the hooklets after the cyst has been embedded in paraffin, such as in the present case. Cysticerci in the ventricles and the subarachnoid space may give rise to large loculated or multivesicular masses that are called racemose cysticerci. These are probably viable but degenerate forms of Cysticercus cellulosae and characteristically lack the invaginated scolex. When cysticerci die, the previously clear vesicle fluid becomes turbid and the scolex undergoes mineralization.

A coenurus differs from a cysticercus by possessing multiple invaginated scolices. A hydatid cyst has a distinctive laminated wall and contains multiple brood capsules and scolices.

2.   (B) Cysticercus cellulosae is the encysted larval stage of
Taenia solium, the pork tape worm. Man is the definitive host
for this parasite and harbors the tape worm in the small intestine.   The adult worm attains a length of two to seven meters
and lives for many years.   Relatively few symptoms are
directly attributable to the intestinal parasitism.   Periodically
gravid proglottids filled with ova are shed from the strobila,
the segmented body of the worm.   When the proglottids or ova
are ingested by an intermediate host, usually a hog, the embryos
or oncospheres invade the intestinal lymphatics and venules.
They are carried throughout the body where they metamorphose
into cysticerci.   Man acquires the adult tape worm by consuming raw or inadequately cooked pork.

Human cysticercosis develops when man acts as the intermediate host. Man usually acquires the ova from fecally contaminated food or water but autoinfection may occur in individuals
who harbor the adult worm.   The frequent development of cysticerci in the nervous system contributes significantly to the
seriousness of cysticercosis.   Although relatively uncommon
in the United States, cysticerci have been reported to comprise
as many as 25% of intracranial space-occupying masses in
some Mexican series.

Man is the definitive host for Taenia saginata, the beef tape-
worm.   The larval form, Cysticercus bovis develops in cattle
and certain other herbivorus animals but not in man.   The dog
and wolf are the usual definitive hosts for Multiceps multiceps
and sheep are the usual intermediate hosts.   Man is involved
occasionally as an intermediate host.   The larval stage is a
coenurus rather than a cysticercus.   The dog is the definitive
host for Echinococcus granulosus with sheep, hogs and a wide
variety of herbivorous wild animals as common intermediate
hosts.   Man is involved occasionally as an intermediate host.
The larvae form hydatid cysts that have distinctive laminated
walls and contain multiple brood capsules and scolices.

3.   (D) Intraparenchymal, living cysticerci evoke almost no
inflammatory reaction and only mild gliosis.   When the parasites die, however, they evoke an intense inflammatory response
with polymorphonuclear leukocytes, lymphocytes, plasma cells,
macrophages, epitheloid cells and foreign body giant cells.
Whether the reaction is toxic, allergic or both is disputed.
When the parasites are in the ventricular system, they may
produce granular ependymitis.   When the parasites die or the
cysts are ruptured in the subarachnoid space, a severe meningitis and vasculitis may result.

4. (A) Man usually develops trichinosis by consuming inadequately cooked pork that contains viable encysted trichina larvae. The larvae are freed from their cysts in the stomach and undergo maturation in the proximal small intestine. Here mature gravid females discharge larvae that penetrate the bowel wall and enter the blood stream. The larvae are carried throughout the body but undergo further development and encyst only in skeletal muscle. The larvae begin to penetrate into the skeletal muscle fibers eight to ten days after the original ingestion. They undergo further maturation and reach their maximal development about a month after entering the myofibers. All skeletal muscles are not affected equally; the diaphragm and tongue are among the most heavily parasitized. The majority of fatalities are due to myocarditis; however, the larvae do not encyst in cardiac muscle.

5. (A, B, C) The parasitized myofibers undergo a series of changes. Initially the parasitized fiber loses its cross-striations, becomes homogeneous, basophilic, and contains multiple central nuclei. Approximately ten days after myofiber penetration, the larvae has a "U"-shaped configuration as it begins to assume its final "corkscrew" form. The myofiber bulges about the parasite and the adjacent endomysial connective tissue proliferates. Eventually a cyst forms. The cyst wall is composed of an amorphous capsule and a basophilic coat derived from the sarcoplasm. The central cavity contains the coiled parasite. The derivation of the capsule is disputed; endomysial connective tissue, sarcoplasm and antigen-antibody complexes have been suggested. The muscle shows an interstitial and perivascular inflammatory cell response that often includes numerous eosinophils. Eventually the cysts undergo mineralization. Target fibers are characteristic of denervation, not trichinosis.

6. (C) Eosinophilic meningitis is a relatively common disease in Southeast Asia and certain Pacific islands. The disease is characterized by severe headaches and the usual signs of meningeal irritation. As suggested by the name, the cerebrospinal fluid contains a variable number of eosinophils. The disease is caused by the larvae of Angiostrongylus cantonensis, the rat lung worm. Histopathological changes include collections of inflammatory cells including plasma cells and eosinophils in the meninges and along tracks in the neural parenchyma. The vessels show arteritis and thrombosis. Granulomas develop about the dead larvae.

7.   (D) A hemorrhagic meningoencephalitis is produced by certain free-living soil amebas. The exact taxonomy of these organisms is currently under debate, but they are often designated as Naegleria fowleri. Infection is characteristically acquired from swimming in fresh or brackish water. Within a week to ten days the infected individuals develop a fulminating meningoencephalitis and most die. Histologically, the meninges and neural parenchyma show intense inflammation and hemorrhage. The amebas are 10-12 microns in diameter and have a single nucleus with a prominent karyosome.   The amebas may infiltrate along blood vessels beyond the inflammatory infiltrates.

REFERENCES

1.   Escobar A and Nieto D: Parasitic Disorders. In: Pathology of the Nervous System. Minckler J (Ed.). McGraw-Hill Book Co., New York, 1972, Vol. 3, pp. 2503-2521.

2.   Marquez-Monter H: Cysticerosis. In: Pathology of Protozoal and Helminthic Diseases. Marcial-Rojas RA (Ed.). Williams and Wilkins Co., Baltimore, 1971, pp. 592-617.

3.   Martinez AJ, et al.: Primary Amebic Meningoencephalitis. In: Pathology Annual. Sommers S and Rosen PP (Eds.). Appleton-Century-Crofts, New York, 1977, Part 2, pp. 225-250.

4.   Nye SW, et al.: Lesions of the brain in eosinophilic meningitis. Arch Path 89:9-19, 1970.

5.   Ribas-Mujal D: Trichinosis. In: Pathology of Protozoal and Helminthic Diseases. Marcial-Rojas RA (Ed.). Williams and Wilkins Co., Baltimore, 1971, pp. 677-710.

: :

CASE 33: A Man with Fever, Headaches, Olfactory Hallucinations and Irrational Behavior

CLINICAL DATA

This 38-year-old midwestern farmer developed fever and headaches on the first of December. The next day he complained of
peculiar odors and intermittent tingling in his left hand. His
behavior became irrational and he was hospitalized on the third
day of his illness.

On admission, the patient seemed oriented but had a short attention span and was restless. His blood pressure was normal,
his pulse rate was increased and his temperature was 104°F.
His neck was somewhat stiff. The remainder of his neurological
examination and his general physical examination were within
normal limits.

His peripheral white blood cell count was 12,300 cells/cmm
and consisted of 80% polymorphonuclear leukocytes. A lumbar
puncture yielded clear, colorless cerebrospinal fluid with an
elevated opening pressure. The cerebrospinal fluid contained
24 cells/cmm, 96 mg/dl of glucose and 56 mg/dl of protein.
A brain scan revealed increased isotope uptake in the left
posterior temporal area. An electroencephalogram showed
slowing over the left hemisphere with delta waves over the left
temporal region.

On the second hospital day, the patient's left pupil appeared
larger than the right but was still reactive to light. A left
carotid angiogram revealed bowing of the posterior temporal
arteries and minimal shift of the anterior cerebral artery.

Despite measures to combat cerebral edema, the patient became
progressively more obtunded. His temperature remained between 104°F and 105°F. A left subtemporal trephination and
temporal lobe biopsy were performed. Two days after surgery,
the patient had a respiratory arrest. After two isoelectric electroencephalograms, the patient was pronounced dead.

QUESTIONS

1. The most appropriate clinical diagnosis is
   A. glioblastoma multiforme
   B. eastern equine encephalitis
   C. herpes simplex encephalitis
   D. mumps encephalitis

2. The cerebrospinal fluid from patients with herpes simplex encephalitis may show
   A. mild to moderate pleocytosis
   B. increased pressure
   C. red cells and xanthochromia
   D. reduced glucose content

3. Herpes simplex encephalitis in older children and adults is caused
   A. predominantly by type-1 herpes simplex virus
   B. predominantly by type-2 herpes simplex virus
   C. predominantly by type-3 herpes simplex virus
   D. equally by types-1 and 2 herpes simplex viruses

4. Gross neuropathological changes typical of herpes simplex encephalitis include
   A. petechial hemorrhages in the mammillary bodies, about the third ventricle and about the aqueduct
   B. hemorrhagic necrosis largely confined to the pons
   C. petechial hemorrhages located predominantly in the corpus callosum and centrum semiovale
   D. hemorrhagic necrosis located predominantly in the medial portion of the temporal lobe and the inferior and medial portions of the frontal lobe

5. Histological changes characteristic of herpes simplex encephalitis include
   A. perivascular inflammatory cell infiltrates
   B. hemorrhagic necrosis
   C. acidophilic intracytoplasmic inclusions
   D. acidophilic intranuclear inclusions

6. Disseminated herpes simplex and herpes simplex encephalitis in the neonate is caused
   A. predominantly by type-1 herpes simplex virus
   B. predominantly by type-2 herpes simplex virus
   C. predominantly by type-3 herpes simplex virus
   D. equally by types-1 and 2 herpes simplex viruses

7. In addition to genital herpes, type-2 herpes simplex virus infection in the adult may produce
   A. aseptic meningitis
   B. dermatitis herpetiformis
   C. herpes zoster
   D. infectious mononucleosis

8. Neurological disorders in which the Epstein-Barr virus has
    been implicated include
    A. Bell's palsy
    B. Guillain-Barre syndrome
    C. transverse myelitis
    D. herpes zoster

9. Herpes simiae (B-virus) generally produces
    A. stomatitis in monkeys
    B. stomatitis in man
    C. fatal encephalitis in monkeys
    D. fatal encephalitis in man

ANSWERS AND DISCUSSION

1. (C) The most appropriate clinical diagnosis is herpes simplex encephalitis.   This is now regarded as the most common
type of severe, often fatal, non-epidemic viral encephalitis.

In general, viral infections of the nervous system are uncommon
but serious complications of systemic infections by common
viruses.   The viruses that are most frequently responsible for
diseases of the nervous system include the echoviruses, Coxsackie viruses, mumps virus, lymphocytic choriomeningitis
virus, arboviruses and herpes viruses.   The polioviruses are
no longer included in this group as a result of the widespread
immunization programs for the control of poliomyelitis.   Many
of these agents produce serious disease or at least more serious
disease only when the central nervous system is involved.

In evaluating patients with viral infections of the nervous system, consideration should be given to the environment and sea-
son.   The echoviruses and coxsackie viruses, the most common causes of viral meningitis, are encountered primarily in
late summer and early fall, especially in crowded urban en-
vironments. Mumps, the most common cause of viral meningitis and mild encephalitis, is encountered primarily in late
winter and early spring.   The arboviruses are transmitted by
various types of mosquitoes and are a serious consideration
only when and where the appropriate mosquitoes are abundant.
By contrast, herpes simplex encephalitis is sporadic and shows
no seasonal variation.

Herpes simplex encephalitis is commonly preceded by one to
several days of a prodromal "flu"-like illness. Bizarre mental changes, olfactory or gustatory hallucinations and memory

loss are common early features of the disease.   Focal neurological signs, seizures, and obtundation progressing to coma
commonly follow.   These clinical manifestations reflect the
usual involvement of the inferior frontal and medial temporal
lobe areas.

The electroencephalogram is almost always abnormal although
not specific for herpes simplex encephalitis.   Brain scan and
contrast studies may be of assistance in localizing the process
and distinguishing the encephalitis from a neoplasm.

2.   (A, B, C, D) The spinal fluid from patients with herpes
simplex encephalitis is under increased pressure.   The cell
count varies with the stage of the disease and ranges from near
normal to 700-800 cells/cmm.   These may be either mononuclear cells or polymorphonuclear leukocytes.   Erythrocytes and
xanthochromia may be present and reflect the hemorrhagic
necrosis produced by this infection.   The protein content ranges
from normal to markedly elevated.   The glucose content may
be normal, mildly reduced or even markedly reduced.   Other
viral infections that occasionally produce hypoglycorrhachia
include mumps meningoencephalitis and lymphocytic choriomeningitis.

3.   (A) Herpes simplex encephalitis in older children and adults
is caused predominantly by type-1 herpes simplex virus (HSV-1).
The precise pathogenesis of the encephalitis is unclear.   Serological surveys have indicated that type-1 herpes simplex virus
antibodies are present in 40 to 90% of adults, depending on their
socioeconomic status.   Furthermore, it has been shown that the
type-1 herpes simplex virus persists in and can be recovered
from nearly one-half of trigeminal ganglia obtained from routine
autopsies.   Reactivation of a latent infection followed by spread
along neural pathways from the ganglia would seem to be the
most likely pathogenesis of herpes simplex encephalitis in the
adult.   The type-1 herpes simplex virus cannot be recovered
from the cerebrospinal fluid or blood with any regularity. The
diagnosis of herpes simplex encephalitis must be confirmed by
cerebral biopsy with demonstration of acidophilic intranuclear
inclusions, isolation of the virus, or identification of the virus
by fluorescent or electron microscopy. Serological tests are
of little diagnostic significance because of the prevalence of
herpes simplex antibodies and the delay in demonstrating a rise
in the titer.   Furthermore, a rise in the antibody titer may result from an exacerbation of a non-cerebral herpes simplex infection during the illness.

4.   (D) Gross neuropathological changes typical of herpes simplex encephalitis include cerebral edema and hemorrhagic
necrosis that is most pronounced in the medial portion of the
temporal lobes (Fig. 33.1) and the inferior and medial portions
of the frontal lobes.

Petechiae in the mammillary bodies, about the third ventricle
and about the aqueduct are characteristic of Wernicke's
encephalopathy.   Petechiae predominantly in the corpus callosum and centrum semiovale are characteristic of fat embolism.

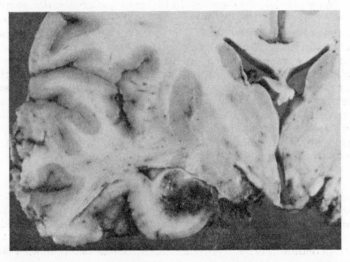

FIG. 33. 1: Coronal section of cerebral hemispheres showing
              the maximal lesions in the medial portion of the
              temporal lobe.

5.   (A, B, D) The light microscope characteristics of herpes
simplex encephalitis include hemorrhagic necrosis of both
grey and white matter.   The blood vessels are surrounded
by inflammatory cell infiltrates that include polymorphonuclear leukocytes.   Inflammatory cells are also scattered
throughout the necrotic neural parenchyma.   The most distinctive findings consist of acidophilic intranuclear inclusions
(Fig. 33.2).   Many of these are typical Cowdry type A inclusions, that is, acidophilic, relatively large and surrounded
by a clear "halo" due to margination of chromatin.   The majority of the inclusion-bearing cells appear to be oligodendrocytes.   By electron microscopy, many more cells and cells
of all types are found to harbor intranuclear virions (Fig. 33.3).

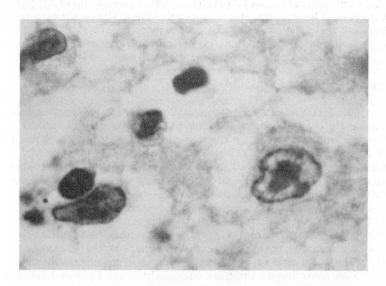

FIG. 33. 2: Microscopic section showing a Cowdry type A
intranuclear inclusion.

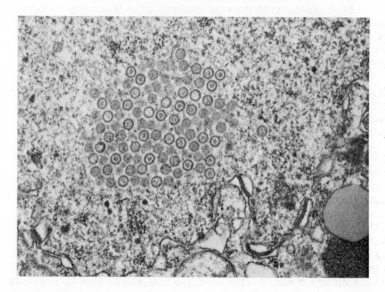

FIG. 33. 3: Electron micrograph showing intranuclear herpes virions.

These virions are characteristic of the entire group of herpes-viruses. The various members cannot be distinguished on the basis of the appearance of the nucleocapsids. Usually, a mixture of immature nucleoids, empty capsids and mature nucleo-capsids are encountered. An envelope is acquired by passage through the nuclear membrane, which is typically thickened and redundant.

6. (B) Disseminated herpes simplex and herpes simplex encephalitis in the neonate are caused predominantly by type-2 herpes simplex virus. In the neonate the infection is acquired during delivery or, rarely, as the result of transplacental transmission. In the adult, type-2 herpes simplex is transmitted venereally and is the cause of genital herpes. Serological surveys show antibodies to type-2 herpes simplex in 10 to 50% of adults, depending upon socioeconomic status. About one-half of the infants born to actively infected women become infected. The type-2 herpes simplex virus is disseminated hematogenously and can be recovered from the cerebrospinal fluid and from the buffy coat of centrifuged blood. A smaller number of neonates have herpes simplex encephalitis due to type-1 herpes simplex virus. Under these circumstances, the type-1 herpes simplex virus can be isolated from the cerebrospinal fluid.

7. (A) In addition to genital lesions, type-2 herpes simplex virus may produce aseptic meningitis in adults. Type-2 herpes simplex virus has been recovered from the sacral ganglia. This may be the source of virus in recurrent genital herpes infections.

Herpes zoster is produced by recrudescence of latent varicella-zoster virus. Infectious mononucleosis has been attributed to infection with another herpesvirus, the Epstein-Barr virus (EBV).

8. (A, B, C) The Epstein-Barr virus has been implicated in certain cases of Bell's palsy, Guillain-Barre syndrome, and transverse myelitis. In some, but not all, of these patients, there has been concurrent heterophil-positive infectious mononucleosis.

9. (A, D) Herpes simiae (B-virus) occurs naturally in monkeys where it produces stomatitis and occasionally, mild meningo-encephalitis. This is the only "non-human" herpesvirus known to infect man. The resulting disease in man is generally a fatal encephalitis. This disorder should always be considered in a patient who develops encephalitis after exposure to monkeys.

REFERENCES

1. Baringer JR: Human Herpes Simplex Virus Infections.
    In: Infectious Diseases of the Central Nervous System.
    Thompson RA and Green JR (Eds.). Raven Press,
    New York, 1974, pp. 41-51.

2. Baringer JR: Herpes simplex virus infection of nervous
    tissue in animals and man. Prog Med Virol 20:1-26, 1975.

3. Grose C, et al.: Primary Epstein-Barr virus infections in
    acute neurologic diseases. N Eng J Med 292:392-395, 1975.

4. Hanshaw JB and Dudgeon JA: Viral Diseases of the Fetus
    and Newborn. W. B. Saunders Co., Philadelphia, 1978,
    pp. 153-181.

5. Johnson RT: Pathophysiology and Epidemiology of Acute
    Viral Infections of the Nervous System. In: Infectious
    Diseases of the Central Nervous System. Thompson RA
    and Green JR (Eds.). Raven Press, 1974, pp. 27-40.

6. Nahmias AJ and Roizman B: Infections with herpes-simplex
    virus 1 and 2. N Eng J Med 289:667-674; 289:719-725;
    289:781-789, 1973.

: :

CASE 34: An Obtunded Infant with Pneumonia and Hepato-
          splenomegaly

CLINICAL DATA

This 10-week-old male infant was the product of a normal pregnancy and delivery. His birth weight was 6 lbs, 11 oz. There
were no perinatal complications and he was sent home on the
fourth postnatal day. At the time of his 6-week examination,
he weighed 9 lbs, 15 oz, appeared well and was given his
initial immunizations.

Sixteen days prior to hospitalization, he developed mild fever,
rhinorrhea and diarrhea. Nine days prior to admission, he
developed a persistent non-productive cough. Two days before
hospitalization, his diarrhea became worse, his temperature
rose to 102°F and his abdomen became distended.

On physical examination, he appeared severely obtunded and in
shock. His chest was markedly congested and x-rays revealed
severe, diffuse pneumonia. His peripheral white cell count
was elevated and showed a shift to the left. Despite intravenous fluids, digitalization, corticosteroids and antibiotics, he
suffered a cardio-respiratory arrest and died on the day of admission. The general autopsy findings included pneumonia,
pulmonary congestion and hepatosplenomegaly.

QUESTIONS

1. The brain was grossly normal with no malformations or
    visible areas of mineralization or necrosis. Microscopi-
    cally, changes, as illustrated in Fig. 34.1, were present
    throughout the brain but were most pronounced in the
    striata and medulla. The most appropriate diagnosis is
    A. subacute sclerosing panencephalitis
    B. disseminated herpes simplex
    C. cytomegalovirus infection
    D. Coxsackie virus infection

2. Transplacental infection of the fetus by cytomegalovirus
    may produce
    A. asymptomatic infection in neonates reflected only by
        viuria
    B. cataracts
    C. microcephaly with intracerebral mineralization
    D. stillbirths

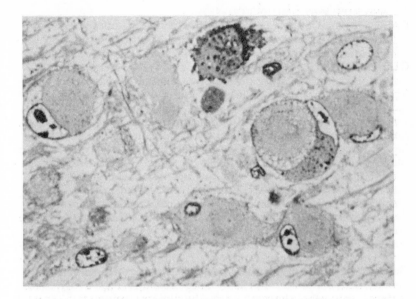

FIG. 34.1: Microscopic section of brain showing the presence of large cells with prominent intranuclear inclusions and abundant granular cytoplasm.

3. Sources of perinatal infections are
    A. blood transfusions
    B. infected maternal saliva
    C. infected breast milk
    D. infected maternal genital tract

4. Active cytomegalovirus infections are prevalent among adults who
    A. are renal transplant recipients
    B. work in primate colonies
    C. have Addison's disease
    D. have had rhinoplasty

5. Hemorrhagic dorsal root ganglia may occur in an infection with
    A. herpes simplex
    B. cytomegalovirus
    C. herpes varicellae
    D. Epstein-Barr virus

ANSWERS AND DISCUSSION

1.   (C) The histological changes in this brain are those of cytomegalovirus infection.   This herpesvirus infection characteristically produces prominent Cowdry type-A intranuclear inclusions in markedly enlarged cells that often have abnormal
granular cytoplasm.   The nuclear inclusions contain myriads
of nucleocapsids that are ultrastructurally indistinguishable
from other herpesviruses. The abnormal granular cytoplasm
contains membrane-bounded aggregates of virions and homogeneous, osmiophilic, dense bodies. All types of cells within
the central nervous system can be affected; however, the distortion produced by the cytomegaly often precludes precise
identification of cell type by light microscopy.   In addition to
the large inclusion-bearing cells, there are inflammatory cell
infiltrates, foci of necrosis and areas of mineralization. These
changes are often most severe in the periventricular regions.
The immature central nervous system is especially susceptible
to damage from the cytomegalovirus infection. Other organs
that are commonly involved in generalized cytomegalovirus infections include the salivary glands, kidneys (Fig. 34.2), lungs,
liver, pancreas, thyroid, adrenals, and gastrointestinal tract.

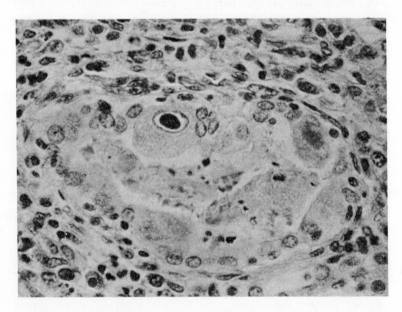

FIG. 34. 2: Microscopic section showing similar cells in a re-
            nal tubule.

2.   (A, C, D) The consequences of transplacental infection of
the fetus by the cytomegalovirus are highly variable.   In the
most severe form, the infection may result in stillbirths.
Classically, but relatively infrequently, the infection results
in microcephaly with intracerebral mineralization, hepatosplenomegaly, thrombocytopenia, purpura, pneumonitis, gastrointestinal disorders, and chorioretinitis.   This spectrum
of manifestations overlaps with the sequelae from the other
"TORCH" agents.   However, microcephaly is more often associated with cytomegalovirus infection or rubella than with toxoplasmosis.   The intracerebral calcification is classically periventricular with cytomegalovirus infection and more widespread
with toxoplasmosis.   Cataracts are especially prominent with
rubella, while chorioretinitis is more typically seen in association with cytomegalovirus infections and toxoplasmosis.

More recently it has been realized that the majority of transplacental cytomegalovirus infections are asymptomatic in the
neonate and can be recognized only by viuria.   Surveys have
indicated that as many as 1 to 2% of all neonates have cyto-
megaloviuria at birth.   Some of these asymptomatic newborns
may develop focal neurological deficits, deafness or mental
retardation later in life.

3.   (A, B, C, D) Serological surveys have demonstrated antibodies to the cytomegalovirus in as many as 80% of the adult
population.   There is considerable evidence that the infection
can be spread among adults during sexual activity.   Maternal
infection at the time of delivery has been found in 3 - 6% as
determined by viuria and 5 - 28% as determined by cervical cultures during the third trimester.   Some infants born to these
infected mothers acquire the infection during parturition.
Other perinatal routes of infection include contact with infected
saliva and breast milk, and from transfusions.   However, in
contrast to the transplacental infections, virtually none of these
infants demonstrate serious neurological damage from their
cytomegalovirus infections.

4.   (A) An increased prevalence of active cytomegalovirus infections has been described in patients with leukemias and
lymphomas and in patients who are receiving immunosuppressive
therapy.   Active cytomegalovirus infections have been especially
frequent among renal transplant recipients.   Many of these patients develop pulmonary cytomegalovirus infections and some
develop encephalitis.   The cerebral lesions consist of scattered
clusters of reactive astrocytes and inflammatory cells with or
without the characteristic cytomegalic cells.

5. (C) Herpes varicellae or varicella-zoster virus is the
agent responsible for causing chickenpox. This very common
exanthematous disorder is only rarely accompanied by neurological complications. When present, these include an acute
cerebellar ataxia of unknown pathogenesis and an encephalomyelitis that is probably due to direct involvement of the nervous system by the virus.

"Shingles" or herpes zoster is caused by the same virus, predominantly in older individuals. It results from reactivation
of a latent herpes varicellae infection that has been harbored
in dorsal root or cranial ganglia. The affected ganglia may
show hemorrhagic necrosis. The virus moves centrifugally
along the nerve through the axons and Schwann cells and produces a vesicular rash in the corresponding dermatomes. The
peripheral nerves may show demyelination. The skin shows
typical viral vesicles or bullae with intranuclear inclusion
bodies in the surrounding epidermal cells.

REFERENCES

1. Bell WE and McCormick WF: Neurologic Infections in
    Children. W. B. Saunders Co., Philadelphia, 1975,
    pp. 215-242.

2. Dorfman LJ: Cytomegalovirus encephalitis in adults.
    Neurology 23:136-144, 1973.

3. Hanshaw JB and Dudgeon JA: Viral Diseases of the Fetus
    and Newborn. W. B. Saunders Co., Philadelphia, 1978,
    pp. 97-152.

4. Reynolds DW, et al.: Maternal cytomegalovirus excretion
    and perinatal infection. N Eng J Med 289:1-5, 1973.

5. Weller TH: The cytomegaloviruses: Ubiquitous agents
    with protean clinical manifestations. N Eng J Med 285:
    203-214; 285:267-274, 1971.

: :

CASE 35: An Infant with a Cataract and a Heart Murmur

CLINICAL DATA

This male infant was the first child born to this 19-year-old woman. The mother's pregnancy had been complicated at about the seventh week by an erythematous rash that began on her face and rapidly spread to the rest of her body. The rash lasted about two days and was accompanied by generalized malaise and lymphadenopathy.

The child's delivery was uncomplicated, his birth weight was 5 lbs, 4 oz, and initially he was thought to be healthy. At six weeks of age he was noted to have a cataract in the left eye, a high arched palate and a heart murmur. Chest x-rays showed an enlarged heart and pulmonary congestion. Cardiac catheterization demonstrated a patent ductus arteriosus. The child was also thought to have decreased hearing since he did not respond to loud noises. Laboratory studies were within normal limits except for a rubella antibody titer that was 1:512.

At age 10 weeks, the patent ductus arteriosus was ligated. Initially, the child did well but he died on the fourth postoperative day.

QUESTIONS

1. Lesions typically associated with the congenital rubella syndrome include
    A. congenital heart defects
    B. hydranencephaly
    C. microcephaly
    D. cataracts

2. Currently, the fetal risk from first trimester maternal rubella is estimated to be about
    A. 100%
    B. 75%
    C. 20-50%
    D. less than 5%

3. The affected offspring
    A. harbor no virus since the damage is due to a toxic byproduct from the mother
    B. harbor virus in the cerebrospinal fluid for many months
    C. shed virus in pharyngeal secretions
    D. have elevated IgM

4.   Ocular lesions are among the most common abnormalities
     and include
     A. cataracts
     B. iridocyclitis
     C. colobomas
     D. intraocular cartilagenous masses

5.   Gross neuropathological changes that are observed con-
     sistently in the brains of children with the congenital
     rubella syndrome are
     A. polymicrogyria and pachygyria
     B. micrencephaly
     C. subependymal matrix cysts
     D. none of the above

6.   The histological changes that are observed most commonly
     in the brains of children with the congenital rubella syn-
     drome include
     A. leptomeningeal inflammatory cell infiltrates
     B. intraparenchymal perivascular inflammatory cell
         infiltrates
     C. mineral deposits in and about vessel walls
     D. intracytoplasmic inclusions

7.   Recently a chronic progressive panencephalitis has been
     described as a late sequela of the congenital rubella syn-
     drome. This condition is characterized by
     A. late onset of new symptoms including seizures, mental
         deterioration and ataxia
     B. elevated cerebrospinal fluid, total protein and gamma
         globulin
     C. perivascular inflammatory cell infiltrates
     D. acidophilic intranuclear inclusions

ANSWERS AND DISCUSSION

1.   (A, C, D) The teratogenic potential of maternal rubella during the first trimester of pregnancy was first appreciated following an epidemic of this disease in Australia during 1940.   Congenital heart defects, cataracts, deafness, microcephaly, and
a low birth weight were soon regarded as typical sequelae of
maternal rubella.   It was also realized that the spectrum of lesions varied according to the time of exposure.   Initially, the
fetal risk from maternal rubella during the first trimester was
overestimated.

Following the 1964 epidemic in this country, additional lesions that had not been emphasized previously were added to the so-called "expanded rubella syndrome." These included hepatosplenomegaly, jaundice, thrombocytopenic purpura, myocarditis, pneumonitis, meningoencephalitis, and skeletal anomalies.

2. (C) The fetal risk from first trimester rubella is difficult to determine. The earliest reports overestimated the risk in part because they were retrospective studies designed to identify the components of the syndrome. More recent studies have cited a wide range of fetal risks but most fall between 20 and 50% for first trimester maternal infection. All are in agreement that the fetal risk is greatest during the first eight weeks of pregnancy and declines thereafter. Although the risk becomes quite small, fetal deaths and serious malformations have resulted even from second trimester maternal infections. Determination of the risk is complicated by the fact that up to 40% of the maternal infections may be subclinical. Pregnant women should not be given the rubella vaccine.

3. (B, C, D) The fetal damage results from transplacental infection during the period of maternal viremia that extends for about a week before and after the appearance of the rash. As a result of the infection, organogenesis is affected by retardation of cell multiplication. This probably accounts for the small size of the affected offspring and some of the specific defects. Other lesions result from persistent infection that continues throughout the pregnancy and into the postnatal period. The affected offspring shed virus in the pharyngeal secretions for a number of months and the virus can be recovered from the cerebrospinal fluid for as long as 18 months. The infection is reflected by elevated levels of IgM in the blood and a lymphocyte pleocytosis in the spinal fluid. The initially elevated cerebrospinal fluid protein decreases with the passage of time.

4. (A, B) A variety of ocular lesions have been encountered in children with the congenital rubella syndrome. Cataracts were emphasized in the initial studies on the complications of maternal rubella. The cataracts may be unilateral or bilateral and may occur in normal-sized or mildly microphthalmic eyes. Clinically, the cataracts appear densely white and fill the area of the undilated pupils. Histologically, these cataracts are different from other types of congenital cataracts and show the most marked alterations centrally. The sclerotic nuclear cataract is sharply demarcated and the component cells contain persistent pycnotic and karyorrhectic nuclei. The surrounding lens cortex shows varying degrees of liquefaction and degeneration.

Zimmerman regards iridocyclitis and its sequelae to be the most constant alterations. This appears as a nongranulomatous inflammation in the iris and ciliary body or as atrophy of the iris. The retina shows depigmentation of the retinal pigment epithelium.

Marked microphthalmia, retinal dysplasia, and colobomas are not features of rubella. Cartilaginous masses within the globes have been regarded as characteristic of the 13-15 trisomy.

5. (D) A wide spectrum of gross neuropathological changes including polymicrogyria, pachygyria, cerebellar malformations, aqueductal stenosis, etc., have been described in the brains from children with the congenital rubella syndrome but none are observed consistently. The heads are very often microcephalic and the brains micrencephalic. More often the brain size is reduced in comparison to normal specimens but is in proportion to the reduced mass of the total body. Subependymal matrix cysts have been reported in a number of cases. Shaw and Alvord have suggested some of the subependymal matrix cysts may result from the lysis of undifferentiated cells in the germinal matrix. Among the agents capable of producing this change are rubella virus and cytomegalovirus. Nevertheless, these cysts are not encountered consistently in patients with the congenital rubella syndrome. More frequently, however, subependymal matrix cysts are the sequelae of subependymal matrix hemorrhages; lesions that are characteristically encountered in premature infants who have suffered anoxic insults.

6. (A, B, C) Hematoxylinophilic deposits of mineral (Fig. 35.1) are commonly encountered in and about the walls of intraparenchymal blood vessels. Similar deposits can also be found in leptomeningeal blood vessels. The deposits stain intensely with the periodic acid-Schiff stain and with stains for iron. The von Kossa stain for "calcium" (actually a stain for phosphate) is usually less intense. The deposits are regarded as iron and calcium containing mineral bound to a mucopolysaccharide-protein substrate. They are interpreted as evidence of vascular damage from the viral infection. Somewhat less common than the mineral deposits are leptomeningeal and perivascular inflammatory cell infiltrates (see Fig. 35.1). These are regarded as morphological evidence of the persistent infection. Inclusion bodies have not been described with rubella.

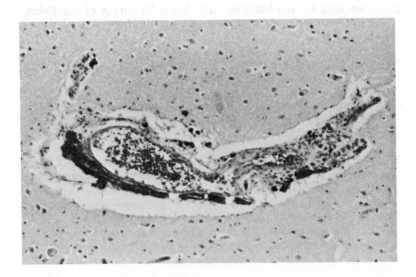

FIG. 35.1: Microscopic section showing vascular mineralization and perivascular inflammatory cell infiltrates.

7. (A, B, C) Recently, chronic progressive encephalitis has
been described by Townsend, et al., and by Weil, et al., as a
late sequela of the congenital rubella syndrome. These children
developed additional neurological symptoms after a latent period
of ten or more years. The new symptoms included further mental deterioration, seizures and ataxia. All had elevated cerebrospinal fluid protein levels and, where assayed, elevated
gamma globulin and rubella antibodies. Two autopsied cases
showed diffuse destruction of white matter while a biopsy specimen from a third case showed uneven staining and pallor of the
white matter. Perivascular inflammatory cell infiltrates containing lymphocytes and plasma cells, microglial nodules and
leptomeningeal inflammatory infiltrates were prominent.
Neuronal loss was maximal in the cerebellum. In contrast to
subacute sclerosing panencephalitis, which this disorder resem-
bled morphologically, no inclusion bodies were present and vascular mineralization characteristic of rubella was present.

REFERENCES

1.   Bell WE and McCormick WF: Neurologic Infections in
     Children. W. B. Saunders Co., Philadelphia, 1975,
     pp. 262-282.

2. Hanshaw JB and Dudgeon JA: Viral Diseases of the Fetus and Newborn. W. B. Saunders Co. , Philadelphia, 1978, pp. 17-96.

3. Shaw CM and Alvord EC Jr.: Subependymal germinolysis. Arch Neurol 31:374-381, 1974.

4. Townsend JJ, et al.: Progressive rubella panencephalitis. Late onset after congenital rubella. N Eng J Med 292: 990-993, 1975.

5. Weil L, et al.: Chronic progressive panencephalitis due to rubella virus simulating subacute sclerosing panencephalitis. N Eng J Med 292:994-998, 1975.

::

CASE 36:   A 9-Year-Old Boy with Deteriorating School
              Performance and Seizures

CLINICAL DATA

This 9-year-old boy had been the product of a normal pregnancy
and an uncomplicated delivery. His neonatal period was normal
and he passed his developmental milestones at appropriate
times.   At the age of eighteen months, he contracted rubeola
from which he recovered without apparent sequelae.

The child had been in good health and did well in the first grade
of school. At the age of seven, he became progressively more
hyperactive, his attention span became shorter and his performance in school deteriorated.   He displayed periods of confusion and recurrent episodes of crying. Approximately nine
months prior to admission, he began to have focal seizures that
progressed to generalized convulsions.

Physical examination revealed a cooperative child whose attention span and comprehension were reduced for his age. Extraocular muscle function and the fundi were normal.   There was
no weakness, sensory deficits or ataxia. Muscle tone and deep
tendon reflexes were normal.   The remainder of the physical
examination was normal.

Skull x-rays and a brain scan were within normal limits.   An
electroencephalogram showed repetitive bursts of high voltage
sharp and slow waves at intervals of three to nine seconds.   A
lumbar puncture yielded clear cerebrospinal fluid that contained
one mononuclear cell per cubic millimeter and 60 mg/dl of protein of which 30% was gamma globulin.   The antimeasles antibody titers on the serum and on the cerebrospinal fluid were
1:256 and 1:32 respectively.   A brain biopsy was performed to
confirm the clinical diagnosis.

QUESTIONS

1.   The most likely clinical diagnosis is
     A.   herpes simplex encephalitis
     B.   subacute sclerosing panencephalitis
     C.   Schilder's disease
     D.   myoclonus epilepsy

2. Significant supportive laboratory data include elevated
   A. serum measles antibody titer
   B. cerebrospinal fluid gamma globulin content
   C. cerebrospinal fluid measles antibody titer
   D. urinary coproporphyrins

3. The histological findings (Fig. 36.1) in cases of subacute sclerosing panencephalitis include
   A. intranuclear inclusion bodies
   B. demyelination
   C. perivascular polymorphonuclear leukocyte infiltrates
   D. astrocytosis

4. Fig. 36.2 is an electron micrograph prepared from the brain biopsy specimen. This shows a nuclear
   A. body
   B. inclusion composed of nucleocapsids consistent with rhabdoviruses
   C. inclusion composed of nucleocapsids consistent with herpesviruses
   D. inclusion composed of nucleocapsids consistent with myxo-paramyxoviruses

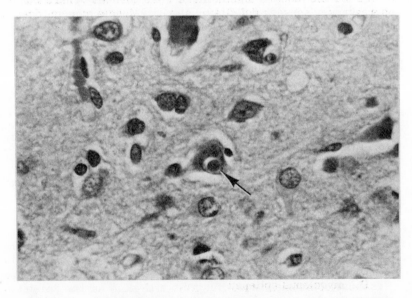

FIG. 36.1: Microscopic section showing the histological findings in the brain biopsy specimen.

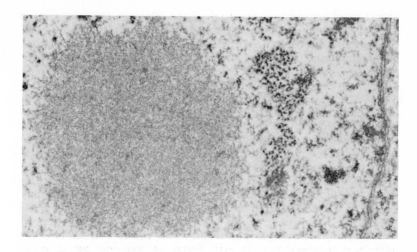

FIG. 36. 2: An electron micrograph prepared from the biopsy
       specimen.

5. So-called postinfectious encephalomyelitis is
    A. most commonly associated with measles
    B. characterized histologically by perivascular, pre-
        dominantly perivenous inflammatory cell infiltrates,
        edema and demyelination
    C. uniformly fatal
    D. probably due to an immunologic phenomenon

6. Mumps, another myxovirus
    A. is probably the most common cause of human viral
        meningoencephalitis
    B. is a common cause of fatal meningoencephalitis in
        man
    C. can be isolated from the spinal fluid
    D. produces hydrocephalus in newborn hamsters

ANSWERS AND DISCUSSION

1. (B) The most appropriate clinical diagnosis is subacute
sclerosing panencephalitis. This is a progressive neurological disease that is produced by a measles virus. The disorder
is more common in boys than girls and many of the patients
come from a rural environment. The disease has its clinical
onset at any time from very early childhood to adulthood. However, the majority of patients develop symptoms between 5 and

15 years of age.   The duration of the clinical disease ranges
from a few months to more than ten years with the majority of
the patients surviving for no more than a year. Most patients
have a history of having had measles, often at an unusually
early age. A few patients have had measles vaccine and in some,
a history of measles or measles vaccine is lacking. The clinical manifestations are protean; often the initial symptoms are
those of intellectual deterioration. This is often accompanied
by personality changes. With progression of the disease, gait
disturbances, visual impairment and various types of seizures,
including myoclonic jerks, appear. Further progression leads
to profound dementia, autonomic dysfunction, coma and eventually death.   The electroencephalographic findings, repetitive
bursts of high voltage slow and sharp waves, support the diagnosis but are not pathognomonic.

Herpes simplex encephalitis is the most common form of sporadic fatal encephalitis. It may occur at any age but is more
common in neonates and adults than children.   Early in its
course, the disease often produces personality and behavioral
changes but the disease progresses in a far more rapid and
fulminating manner than subacute sclerosing panencephalitis.

Sporadic Schilder's disease is a myelinoclastic demyelinating
disease, probably similar to multiple sclerosis, but generally
affecting individuals less than 10 years of age.   The patients
display personality changes, motor deficits and visual impairment.   The course of Schilder's disease often extends over a
one to three year period.   Unlike subacute sclerosing panencephalitis, seizures are not a usual feature and the brain scan
may show areas of abnormal radioisotope uptake.

Myoclonus epilepsy is a familial disorder that usually begins
in adolescence and progresses slowly to produce incapacitation
by the age of 20.   Mental deterioration and seizures, including
myoclonic jerks, are the characteristic clinical features.

2.   (A, B, C) Patients with subacute sclerosing panencephalitis generally have a normal or only moderately increased
total protein content in their cerebrospinal fluid.   The proportion of gamma globulin is strikingly elevated and constitutes 20 to 50% of the total protein. Furthermore, these
patients have elevated titers of antimeasles antibodies in both
the serum and in the cerebrospinal fluid. The ratio between
the levels of the serum and the cerebrospinal fluid antibodies
is somewhat lower than observed with other viral diseases and

has been interpreted as evidence of antibody production within the central nervous system itself.

3.   (A, B, D) Subacute sclerosing panencephalitis is characterized by widespread but often multifocal loss of neurons and astrocytosis in the cortex and subcortical grey matter. Demyelination and astrocytosis may be prominent in the white matter.   Cowdry type A intranuclear inclusions can be seen in neurons (Fig. 36.1), oligodendrocytes and astrocytes. Occasionally ill-defined cytoplasmic inclusions also may be present. Throughout the cortex there are often numerous "rod-cells," a particular configuration of microglia.   Perivascular inflammatory cell infiltrates are present and consist predominantly of lymphocytes with occasional plasma cells and macrophages. With the passage of time, inclusion-bearing cells may become very sparse in the cerebral hemispheres.   Many of these patients will still have inclusion-bearing cells within their brain stems.   At no time during the course of the disease are inclusion-bearing cells abundant in the cerebellum.   Some patients with subacute sclerosing panencephalitis have chorioretinitis with changes morphologically similar to those in the brain.   The chorioretinitis is responsible for some of the loss of visual acuity.

4.   (D) The electron micrograph (Fig. 36.2) illustrates a nuclear inclusion composed of a tangled skein of tubules that average 17 nm in diameter. These are morphologically consistent with the nucleocapsids of the myxo-paramyxovirus group to which the measles virus belongs. This particular inclusion body is quite small. The aggregates of nucleocapsids may be unresolvable to light microscopy, may appear as Cowdry type B inclusion or may appear as the more typical Cowdry type A inclusion. Skeins of nucleocapsids are occasionally found in the cytoplasm and comprise the ill-defined cytoplasmic inclusions that may be seen by light microscopy. The precise nature of these nucleocapsids, their interactions with the host cells and their relation to the ordinary measles virus is under active investigation.

Nuclear bodies are minute intranuclear structures composed of varying proportions of fine filaments and granules. They are found in a wide variety of cell types and are especially conspicuous under circumstances in which the cells are thought to be metabolically active, e.g., neoplasms, infections and other reactions to injury.   Rhabdoviruses have a characteristic bullet shape and are the group of viruses to which the rabies viruses belong. Negri bodies, inclusions containing these viruses, are found in the cytoplasm rather than the nucleus of neurons. Herpesviruses appear as roughly spherical nucleocapsids with cores that average 40 nm in diameter and capsids that average 120 nm in diameter. By conventional light microscopy, the intranuclear Cowdry type A inclusions produced by various herpesviruses may be indistinguishable from the intranuclear inclusions in subacute sclerosing panencephalitis.

5. (A, B, D) A small number of patients with measles develop a neurological disorder at or within a couple of weeks of the appearance of the exanthema. The frequency has been estimated to be about 1:1000. The neurological disorder is characterized by headache, lethargy, convulsions, and occasional focal neurological deficits. The mortality has been estimated to be about 10 to 15%. Histologically, the lesions consist of perivascular, predominantly perivenous, inflammatory cell infiltrates, edema and demyelination. The disorder is an immunologic phenomenon following the infection. Although this disorder is most commonly associated with measles, similar lesions have been found in association with other exanthematous infections and following vaccinations.

6. (A, C, D) Mumps is probably the most common cause of human viral meningoencephalitis. The disease is usually mild and fatal mumps encephalitis is very rare. The virus can be isolated from the spinal fluid. When the virus is injected intracerebrally in newborn hamsters, an ependymitis develops. This leads to aqueductal stenosis and hydrocephalus; however, the usual stigmata of an infectious disease are lacking. It has been suggested, but not proven, that some human cases of aqueductal stenosis and hydrocephalus may result from similar viral infections.

REFERENCES

1. Bell WE and McCormick WF: Neurologic Infections in Children. W. B. Saunders Co., Philadelphia, 1975, pp. 167-172.

2. Dubois-Dalq M, et al.: Subacute sclerosing panencephalitis. Arch Neurol 31:355-363, 1974.

3. Johnson KP, et al.: Subacute Sclerosing Panencephalitis. In: Infectious Diseases of the Central Nervous System. Thompson RA and Green JR (Eds.). Raven Press, New York, 1974, pp. 77-86.

4. Lampert PW: Autoimmune and virus-induced demyeli-
    nating diseases. Am J Path 91:175-208, 1978.

5. Lampert PW, et al.: Morphological Changes of Cells
    Infected with Measles or Related Viruses. In: Progress
    in Neuropathology. Zimmerman HM (Ed.). Grune and
    Stratton, New York, 1976, Vol. III, pp. 51-68.

6. Ohya T, et al.: Subacute sclerosing panencephalitis.
    Neurology 24:211-218, 1974.

: :

CASE 37:   A Man with Hodgkin's Disease and Progressive
Neurological Dysfunction

CLINICAL DATA

This 61-year-old man was admitted to the hospital because of
malaise, episodes of low grade fever, and increasing collar
size. Physical examination revealed a large, firm but non-ten-
der supraclavicular mass and enlarged infraclavicular, axillary
and inguinal nodes. Both the liver and the spleen were moderately enlarged. The initial neurological examination was described as being normal. A lymph node biopsy and bone marrow
biopsy were performed and both specimens revealed Hodgkin's
disease. The patient was started on chemotherapy. Two
months later the patient was readmitted to the hospital because
of hoarseness and diminished vision. At that time, the neurological examination revealed a lethargic but oriented man.
There was mild dysarthria and diminished visual acuity. Diffuse
weakness was present but no focal motor signs were detectable.
Over the next two months the patient continued to deteriorate
with further loss of vision, increasing dysarthria, a slowly developing left hemiparesis and dementia. X-rays of the skull
were normal. A brain scan revealed an area of increased isotope uptake in the right parietal region. An electroencephalogram was abnormal with focal right posterior delta activity.
A lumbar puncture yielded clear fluid with an opening pressure
of 120 mm water. There were 3-4 lymphocytes/cmm and the
protein content was 60 mg/dl. The patient continued to deteriorate rapidly and died six months after his initial hospitalization.

QUESTIONS

1.   At autopsy, the brain was found to contain multiple lesions
     like those illustrated in Fig. 37.1. The most likely diag-
     nosis in view of the clinical data and gross findings is
     A.   progressive multifocal leukoencephalopathy
     B.   multiple sclerosis
     C.   metastatic Hodgkin's disease
     D.   microglioma

2.   The histological characteristics (Figs. 37.2 and 37.3) of
     progressive multifocal leukoencephalopathy include
     A.   demyelination
     B.   enlarged bizarre astrocytes
     C.   abnormal oligodendrocytes containing nuclear inclusions
     D.   perivascular inflammatory cell infiltrates

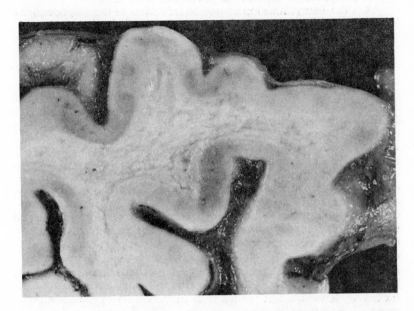

FIG. 37. 1: Photograph of some of the destructive and demye-
linative lesions.

3.   Fig. 37. 4 is an electron micrograph prepared from tissue
     removed from the margin of a demyelinated lesion. The
     ultrastructural characteristics of progressive multifocal
     leukoencephalopathy include
     A.   spherical virions in the nuclei of oligodendrocytes
     B.   tubular virions in the nuclei of oligodendrocytes
     C.   spherical virions in the nuclei of astrocytes
     D.   spherical virions in the cytoplasm of astrocytes

4.   Viruses have been isolated from the brains of patients with
     progressive multifocal leukoencephalopathy. These have
     been designated
     A.   BK virus
     B.   JC virus
     C.   SV-40 like virus
     D.   Epstein-Barr virus

5. In progressive multifocal leukoencephalopathy
    A. the demyelination is due to infection of the oligodendro-
        cytes
    B. the astrocytic changes are probably due to "transfor-
        mation" of reactive astrocytes
    C. the papovavirus must interact with a myxovirus. There-
        fore, the disease is rare
    D. both the JC and SV-40 papovaviruses must be present

ANSWERS AND DISCUSSION

1. (A) The presence of multiple foci of destruction and demyelination in the brain of a patient who developed a rapidly
evolving, ill-defined neurological disorder and who has an
underlying lymphoproliferative disorder is highly suggestive
of progressive multifocal leukoencephalopathy. This is a relatively rare disorder that has occurred in association with a wide
variety of underlying systemic disorders but lymphoproliferative
diseases have been the most common. Other associated diseases have included myeloproliferative diseases, carcinomas,
and granulomatous diseases. Very few patients appear to have
had no other disorder. The clinical manifestations are protean
including dementia and evidence of involvement of multiple regions of the central nervous system. The duration of the disease is usually two to six months; however, a few patients have
survived for over a year. Few of the reported cases have been
diagnosed antemortem. Grossly, the lesions consist of various-
sized areas of destruction and demyelination. They are more
conspicuous and extensive in the white matter but also extend
into the adjacent cortical and nuclear grey matter. The most
severely affected areas have a spongy texture, while less
severely involved areas merely appear demyelinated. All
portions of the central nervous system, cerebrum, brain stem,
cerebellum, and spinal cord can harbor the multiple lesions.

Multiple sclerosis typically shows a slowly progressive course
punctuated by exacerbations and remissions. The demyelinated
areas are multiple but tend to be more sharply circumscribed
and are especially conspicuous about the ventricular system and
in the optic pathways. The lesions are not expanding mass lesions as would be expected with a primary or metastatic neoplasm. Furthermore, Hodgkin's disease rarely involves the
neural parenchyma directly.

2. (A, B, C, D) Histologically, progressive multifocal leukoencephalopathy is characterized by multiple small focal to large
confluent areas of tissue destruction and demyelination. Within

the more severe lesions, oligodendrocytes have largely disappeared. Toward the margins of the demyelinated areas, some
of the oligodendrocyte nuclei are enlarged and contain amphophilic inclusions (Fig. 37. 2). The most conspicuous feature is
the presence of numerous, large, bizarre astrocytes. These
have hyperchromatic and multilobed nuclei and are often multinucleated (Fig. 37. 3). Although not emphasized in the earlier
descriptions, perivascular inflammatory cell infiltrates may
be prominent and contain macrophages, lymphocytes and plasma cells.

3.   (A, B) Ultrastructurally, two types of virions can be demonstrated in the nuclei of the oligodendrocytes. One type of virion
appears as spherical particles with a diameter of 35 to 40 nm.
The second type of virion appears as elongated or tubular
structures with a somewhat smaller diameter. No virions are
seen in the cytoplasm of the oligodendrocytes. The morphological similarity between these virions and other papovaviruses
was originally pointed out by Zu Rhein. The astrocytes have
large, irregular nuclei and myriads of cytoplasmic filaments
but no virions can be seen in their nuclei or cytoplasm.

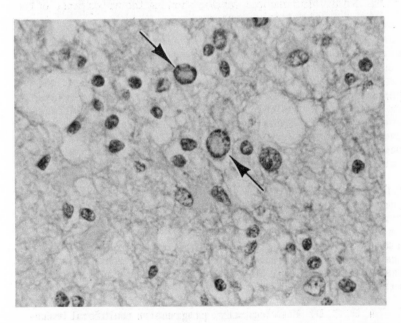

FIG. 37. 2: Microscopic section showing the appearance of the
abnormal oligodendrocytes (arrows).

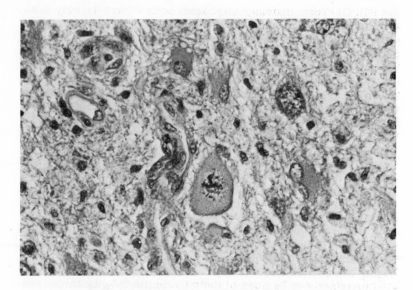

FIG. 37. 3: Microscopic section showing the appearance of the abnormal astrocytes.

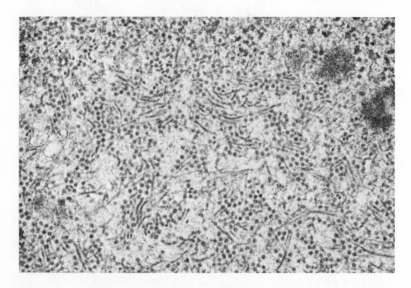

FIG. 37. 4: Electron micrograph showing spherical and tubular virions.

4.   (B, C) Two papovaviruses have been isolated from the
brains of patients with progressive multifocal leukoencephalopathy. A papovavirus antigenically indistinguishable from the
SV-40 virus had been isolated from two brains by Weiner, et
al. A second papovavirus designated as JC virus was initially
isolated by Padgett, et al. This virus appears to be the agent
that is most commonly associated with progressive multifocal
leukoencephalopathy. Although progressive multifocal leukoencephalopathy is a rare disease, antibodies against the JC
virus have been found in 69% of adults in one series. Recently,
the JC virus has been shown to be oncogenic in hamsters.

The BK virus is another papovavirus. It has been isolated from
the urine of a renal transplant recipient but to date, has not
been found in association with progressive multifocal leukoencephalopathy.

5.   (A, B) In the immunosuppressed individual, the JC or SV-
40 papovavirus infects and destroys the oligodendrocytes producing the demyelination. The astrocytic changes may repre-
sent neoplastic "transformation" of reactive glia by these oncogenic viruses. It is not known why progressive multifocal leukoencephalopathy is so rare when JC papovavirus antibodies are
so prevalent in the population.

REFERENCES

1.   McCormick WF, et al.: Progressive multifocal leuko-
     encephalopathy in renal transplant recipients. Arch Int
     Med 136:829-834, 1976.

2.   Narayan O, et al.: Etiology of progressive multifocal
     leukoencephalopathy. N Eng J Med 289:1278-1282.

3.   Richardson EP Jr.: Progressive Multifocal Leuko-
     encephalopathy. In: Handbook of Clinical Neurology.
     Vinken PJ and Bruyn GW (Eds.). North-Holland, Amster-
     dam, 1970, Vol. 9, pp. 485-499.

4.   Weiner LP and Narayan O: Progressive Multifocal Leuko-
     encephalopathy. In: Infectious Diseases of the Central
     Nervous System. Thompson RA and Green JR (Eds.).
     Raven Press, New York, 1974, pp. 87-92.

: :

CASE 38:   A 43-Year-Old Woman with Ataxia, Nystagmus
and Blurred Vision

CLINICAL DATA

This 43-year-old woman had been well until five years previously
when, following a flu-like illness, she developed a tremor of
her arms and impaired balance when standing or walking. She
was found to have an elevated protein content and 10-15 mononuclear cells/cmm in her cerebrospinal fluid. Other studies
failed to disclose any abnormalities.

She was re-evaluated six months later and was found to be "improved" but had nystagmus. Eighteen months later, she experienced another episode of ataxia and weakness and required
assistance when walking. At this time she also complained of
blurred vision. She was referred to a neurologist who found
ataxia, dysarthria, decreased vibratory sensation in her legs,
absent abdominal reflexes, increased deep tendon reflexes, and
a Babinski sign on the left. Subsequently her illness was characterized by remissions and exacerbations but overall, was
slowly progressive.

When hospitalized four years after the initial onset of her illness, she was described as alert and oriented. Her speech
was slurred. She had nystagmus but her pupils were equal and
reactive to light and her visual fields were grossly intact. She
had a severe intention tremor in her arms and was unable to
stand because of weakness in her legs. Pain perception was intact. She had a neurogenic bladder. The patient was discharged
to a nursing home. She was subsequently rehospitalized with
high fever and infected decubitus ulcers. Blood cultures grew
gram-negative bacilli. Despite antibiotics, she went into shock
and died.

QUESTIONS

1.   The clinical data are most consistent with a diagnosis of
     A.   amyotrophic lateral sclerosis
     B.   multiple sclerosis
     C.   Friedreich's ataxia
     D.   amyotonia congenita

2.   The most significant clinical laboratory finding in patients
     with multiple sclerosis is
     A.   hyperglobulinemia

  B. elevated cerebrospinal fluid protein content
  C. elevated cerebrospinal fluid IgG content
  D. cerebrospinal fluid pleocytosis

3. Multiple sclerosis is most prevalent in
  A. children
  B. young adults
  C. northern climates
  D. southern climates

4. The lesions characteristic of multiple sclerosis are called
    "plaques." These are
  A. areas of complete or partial demyelination
  B. strictly confined to the periventricular white matter
  C. found anywhere in the white matter but do not involve
      grey matter
  D. found anywhere in the white matter and also involve
      the grey matter

5. Histological characteristics of plaques include
  A. loss of myelin
  B. loss of oligodendrocytes
  C. proliferation of astrocytes
  D. lipid-laden macrophages

6. In patients with multiple sclerosis, the neurological
    deficits
  A. can be correlated closely with the distribution of the
      plaques
  B. cannot be correlated closely with the distribution of the
      plaques
  C. are due in part to impaired propagation of impulses
      along demyelinated neurites
  D. may be due in part to synaptic inhibitors

7. Multiple sclerosis has been proven to be due to
  A. an autoimmune reaction to myelin
  B. a parainfluenza virus
  C. a paramyxovirus
  D. none of the above

8. Devic's disease is a variant of multiple sclerosis char-
    acterized by involvement predominantly of the
  A. cerebellum and spinal cord
  B. cerebellum and optic pathways
  C. optic pathways and spinal cord
  D. optic pathways and auditory pathways

9.　Balo's concentric sclerosis is
　　A.　generally regarded as a rare variant of multiple
　　　　sclerosis
　　B.　characterized morphologically by concentric bands
　　　　of demyelination that alternate with bands of intact
　　　　myelin
　　C.　a form of metachromatic leukodystrophy
　　D.　due to diffusion of lecithinolytic enzyme from the
　　　　ventricular fluid

ANSWERS AND DISCUSSION

1.　(B) The clinical data are most compatible with a diagnosis
of multiple sclerosis.　The clinical manifestations of this disorder are protean and the course of the disease is usually characterized by exacerbations and remissions over a period of
years.　The most common clinical manifestations are those of
pyramidal tract involvement.　The resulting symptoms include
stiffness, weakness or even paralysis.　The lower limbs are
usually more severely affected than the upper limbs. Spasticity,
Babinski signs and weakness are eventually found in over 90%
of the patients.　Evidence of cerebellar dysfunction including
ataxia, intention tremors, incoordination and dysmetria constitute the second most common group of manifestations.　The
so-called scanning speech that is often seen in patients with
multiple sclerosis is due to a combination of cerebellar and
corticobulbar dysfunction.　Visual disturbances, including
blurred vision, field defects, and impaired ocular movement,
are very common.　Retrobulbar neuritis is often an initial manifestation of multiple sclerosis.　Internuclear ophthalmoplegia
is an uncommon but highly characteristic finding.　Bladder
dysfunction, as in the present case, is common.　Impairment
of various sensory modalities and paresthesias are also common.　Lhermitte's sign, the development of shooting pains
upon neck flexion, has often been considered pathognomonic but
can be seen with other lesions involving the cervical spinal cord.
Because of the diversity of manifestations, Schumacher, et al.
established the following diagnostic criteria for multiple sclerosis:

　　1.　Objective evidence of abnormalities attributable to
　　　　dysfunction of the central nervous system

　　2.　Evidence of involvement of two or more parts of the
　　　　central nervous system

　　3.　Evidence that the involvement is predominantly of the
　　　　white matter

4. The involvement must have occurred in two or more episodes separated by a period of one month or must have occurred in a stepwise fashion over a period of at least six months

5. The manifestations must not be better attributed to some other disease

The course of multiple sclerosis is highly variable and the prognosis of an individual case is unpredictable. Overall, one-third of the patients will be totally disabled, one-third will be moderately disabled, and one-third will have only mild or no significant disability. Death in multiple sclerosis is usually due to intercurrent infection: urinary tract infections, pneumonia or septicemia from decubiti.

2. (C) The cerebrospinal fluid from patients with multiple sclerosis usually contains a normal number of cells or only a mild mononuclear pleocytosis during exacerbations of the disease. Some authors attribute particular significance to an increased number of plasma cells in the spinal fluid. The total cerebrospinal fluid protein content is elevated in about 25% of cases of multiple sclerosis, especially during exacerbations of the disease. Of special significance is the content of IgG. Nearly 80% of all patients with multiple sclerosis have an increased proportion of IgG even when the total cerebrospinal fluid protein content is normal. It is presumed that at least a part of the cerebrospinal fluid IgG is synthesized within the nervous system of these patients. In order to be of greatest diagnostic significance, the level of cerebrospinal fluid protein must be compared with the level of serum protein and the IgG must be expressed in proportion to the total cerebrospinal fluid protein content.

3. (B, C) Multiple sclerosis is predominantly a disease of young adults with clinical manifestations usually becoming evident between the ages of 20 and 40. It is somewhat more common in women than in men. The frequency varies geographically. The prevalence of multiple sclerosis in northern climates is about 40-60/100,000 whereas the prevalence in southern climates is about 7-15/100,000. Children less than 15 years of age moving from a high risk area to a low risk area have the same chance of developing multiple sclerosis as the natives of the low risk areas. Adults migrating from a high risk area to a low risk area retain their higher risk. This type of data suggests but by no means proves that multiple sclerosis is the result of an infection with a long incubation or latent period.

Five to 20% of the patients show familial aggregation. This has been interpreted variously as evidence of a genetic predisposition or a manifestation of common exposure. Recently, several groups have reported a significantly higher prevalence of multiple sclerosis among individuals with histocompatibility antigens HL-A3 and HL-A7. Serological surveys have shown higher titers for measles and other common viral infections among multiple sclerosis patients and their families than among controls. However, higher measles antibody titers have been reported in individuals with HL-A3 regardless of whether they have multiple sclerosis.

4. (A, D) The characteristic lesions of multiple sclerosis are completely or partially demyelinated areas that are referred to as "plaques." They can be found anywhere in the white matter and also involve grey matter, since it, too, contains myelinated fibers. Plaques vary in number and size from case to case but are generally most conspicuous in the periventricular white matter about the angles of the lateral ventricles (Fig. 38.1) and beneath the floor of the fourth ventricle. The optic pathways almost invariably contain plaques and the spinal cord is frequently involved. Peripheral nerves are spared. Grossly, the demyelinated white matter closely resembles grey matter and small plaques in the grey matter are relatively inconspicuous even though they may be quite numerous. Partially demyelinated lesions are referred to as shadow plaques and tend to be less sharply demarcated. Old plaques become sparsely cellular and gliotic. In long-standing cases of multiple sclerosis, the entire brain tends to be atrophic with enlarged ventricles.

5. (A, B, C, D) Histologically, plaques appear as areas of complete or partial demyelination with relative preservation of the neurites (Fig. 38.2). Especially when appropriate myelin stains are employed, plaques are found to be far more numerous in both the grey and white matter than suspected from the appearance of the gross specimen. Along with the loss of myelin, there is a marked reduction in the number, or even absence, of the oligodendrocytes. When the plaques are undergoing active demyelination, lipid-laden macrophages are present around vessels about the periphery of the plaques. Lymphocytes and plasma cells also can be found in the plaques and about adjacent blood vessels. Astrocytosis may be pronounced and some of the astrocytes may be large and bizarre with multiple or multilobed nuclei.

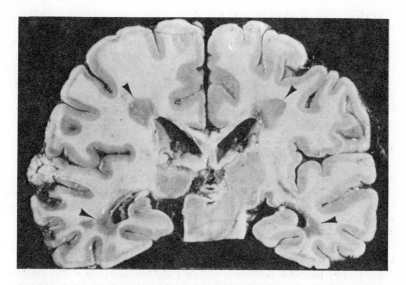

FIG. 38.1: Coronal section of the cerebral hemispheres showing multiple areas of demyelination most conspicuous about the angles of the lateral ventricles (arrows).

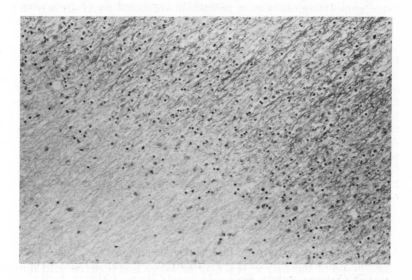

FIG. 38. 2: Microscopic section showing the margin of a plaque.
(Demyelinated plaque to the lower left, intact white
matter to the upper right.)

6. (B, C, D) The neurological deficits in patients with multiple
sclerosis are generally attributed to impaired propagation of
impulses along the demyelinated neurites. However, there is
notoriously poor correlation between the spectrum of clinical
manifestations and the distribution of the plaques. Many of the
most conspicuous plaques are in relatively "silent" areas of the
nervous system. Work by Bornstein, et al., has demonstrated
the existence of synaptic inhibitory factors; however, their significance in vivo has not been established.

7. (D) The etiology of multiple sclerosis is unknown. The
current prevalent theories include an autoimmune reaction or
a latent viral infection. These theories are not necessarily
mutually exclusive. To date, the presence of cell-mediated
immune reaction has not been proven in patients with multiple
sclerosis. There is increasing evidence for a viral infection.
The epidemiological data, including migration studies, have
been interpreted by some authors as supportive evidence of an
infectious etiology. There have been reports of viral isolation
and ultrastructural visualization of "paramyxovirus-like" structures. However, the isolated viruses have not yet been proven
to be the causative agents, and some of the "virus-like" structures actually may be alterations in chromatin.

8. (C) Devic's disease is generally regarded as a fulminating
variant of multiple sclerosis with maximal involvement in the
optic pathways and spinal cord.

9. (A, B) Balo's concentric sclerosis is generally regarded
as a very rare variant of acute multiple sclerosis that is characterized morphologically by alternating bands of demyelinating
and intact myelin. Balo originally suggested that the lesion resulted from the outward diffusion of a lecithinolytic agent from
the ventricular system; however, there is no supportive evidence for this suggestion. Hallervordan and Spatz later compared the distinctive bands to the Liesegang rings that result
from precipitation phenomena in a colloidal gel. The etiology
and pathogenesis of Balo's concentric sclerosis are currently
completely unknown.

REFERENCES

1. Kurtzke JF: Clinical Manifestations of Multiple Sclerosis.
   In: Handbook of Clinical Neurology. Vinken PJ and Bruyn
   GW (Eds.). North-Holland, Amsterdam, 1970, Vol. 9,
   pp. 161-216.

2. Lumsden CE: The Neuropathology of Multiple Sclerosis.
    In: Handbook of Clinical Neurology. Vinken PJ and
    Bruyn GW (Eds.). North-Holland, Amsterdam, 1970,
    Vol. 9, pp. 217-309.

3. Prineas J: Pathology of the early lesion in multiple
    sclerosis. Human Path 6:531-554.

4. Prineas J and Wright RG: Macrophages, lymphocytes
    and plasma cells in the perivascular compartment in
    chronic multiple sclerosis. Lab Invest 38:409-421, 1978.

5. Raine CE: The Etiology and Pathogenesis of Multiple
    Sclerosis: Recent Developments. In: Pathobiology
    Annual. Ioachim HL (Ed.). Appleton-Century-Crofts,
    New York, 1977, pp. 347-384.

6. Sever JL: Perspectives in multiple sclerosis. Neurology
    25:486-496, 1975.

7. Wolfram F, et al.: Multiple Sclerosis: Immunology,
    Virology, and Ultrastructure. Academic Press, New
    York, 1972.

: :

CASE 39: A 67-Year-Old Woman with Sudden, Painless
          Loss of Vision

CLINICAL DATA

This 67-year-old woman was hospitalized following sudden painless loss of vision in her right eye. She also complained of
severe right-sided headaches and "jaw pain" upon chewing for
the past several months.

Physical examination revealed an afebrile thin woman who appeared older than her stated age. Her scalp was tender over
the right side of her head, and the anterior branch of the right
superficial temporal artery was palpably thickened. Her carotid pulses were full but there was a loud bruit over the right
carotid artery. Her right eye was nearly blind. Funduscopic
examination showed mild arteriosclerotic changes. The right
disc had a flame-shaped hemorrhage and blurred margins.

A CTT scan was normal. A lumbar puncture yielded normal
cerebrospinal fluid. All routine laboratory studies were normal except for an erythrocyte sedimentation rate of 92 mm/hr.
The right superficial temporal artery was biopsied.

QUESTIONS

1. The clinical data are most consistent with a diagnosis of
    A. temporal arteritis
    B. systemic lupus erythematosus
    C. polyarteritis nodosa
    D. rheumatoid arteritis

2. Fig. 39.1 is a photograph of a microscopic section pre-
    pared from the temporal artery biopsy specimen. It shows
    A. intimal proliferation
    B. granulomatous inflammatory infiltrate
    C. disruption of the internal elastic lamina
    D. fibrinoid necrosis of vessel wall

3. A muscle biopsy specimen from a patient with polymyalgia
    rheumatica would be expected to show
    A. target fibers
    B. perifascicular atrophy
    C. atrophy of type 2 myofibers
    D. fibrinoid necrosis of intramuscular arteries

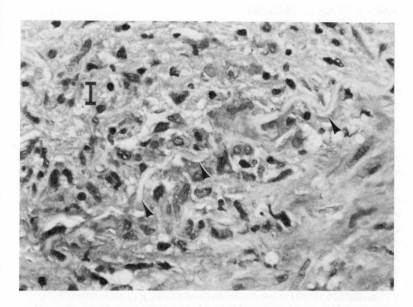

FIG. 39.1: Microscopic section prepared from the temporal artery biopsy specimen ("I" indicates intima and arrows mark fragments of elastica).

4. Neurological manifestations of polyarteritis include
    A. headaches, seizures and focal motor deficits
    B. transverse myelitis
    C. mononeuropathy multiplex
    D. myotonia

5. A muscle biopsy specimen from a patient with poly-arteritis may be expected to show
    A. fibrinoid necrosis of intramuscular arteries
    B. interstitial inflammatory cell infiltrates
    C. neurogenic atrophy
    D. focal necrosis with degenerating and regenerating myofibers

6. Granulomatous angiitis is characterized by
    A. derangement of mental function
    B. involvement of large elastic arteries
    C. involvement of small intracranial arteries
    D. thrombosis of cavernous sinus

ANSWERS AND DISCUSSION

1. (A) The clinical data are most consistent with a diagnosis
of temporal arteritis. This is an inflammatory vasculitis that
involves especially certain branches of the external and internal
carotid arteries and the vertebral arteries. The disease is encountered predominantly among the elderly and affects women
more frequently than men. The clinical manifestations reflect
the regions of maximal vascular involvement. Headaches,
typically most marked in the temporal region are often associated with focal tenderness over the temporal artery. The
vessel may be palpably nodular and pulseless. Another highly
characteristic symptom is pain upon chewing. This has been
attributed to involvement of the facial artery, another branch
of the external carotid artery, with claudication of the masseter
muscles.

Serious ocular manifestations occur in over 50% of the patients
and result from the arteritis in the ophthalmic and posterior
ciliary arteries. Varying degrees of visual loss often occur
suddenly and may be transient or permanent. Funduscopic
examination usually reveals an ischemic optic neuropathy with
a pale swollen nerve head secondary to the involvement of the
posterior ciliary arteries. Rarely, the eye shows evidence of
central retinal artery occlusion. A few patients develop
cerebral infarcts reflecting involvement of other intracranial
arteries.

There is a relation between temporal arteritis and polymyalgia
rheumatica. This condition is characterized by stiffness, pain
and tenderness in proximal limb girdle muscles. However, the
precise pathogenesis of this disorder remains controversial.

2. (A, B, C) The temporal artery biopsy specimen shows histopathological changes that are characteristic of giant cell or
temporal arteritis. This disease affects all layers of the involved arteries; however, the lesions tend to be segmental or
multifocal in distribution along the course of the vessel.

The intima generally shows marked proliferation. This narrows
the lumen and promotes thrombosis. The more characteristic
features are found in the media, especially its inner portion.
The internal elastic lamina is focally disrupted and associated
with prominent inflammatory cell infiltrates composed of lymphocytes, plasma cells, and histiocytes or epithelioid cells. Occasionally, small numbers of eosinophils and polymorphonuclear
leukocytes may be present. The most distinctive morphological

feature is the presence of multinucleated giant cells. These
are most numerous at the internal elastic lamina and often contain fragments of disrupted elastica. Infrequently, there is a
small amount of fibrinoid material along the inner surface of
the internal elastic lamina. The adventitia contains mononuclear inflammatory cells and occasional multinucleated giant
cells. Focal mineral deposits may also be present. Because
of the segmental distribution of the lesions, a "negative" biopsy
specimen does not exclude this diagnosis.

Virtually identical vascular lesions are found in the ophthalmic
and posterior ciliary arteries and account for visual complications. Involvement of the vertebral arteries, and rarely,
other intracranial cerebral arteries, accounts for the neurological deficits seen in some patients.

3.   (C) Muscle biopsy specimens from patients with polymyalgia rheumatica generally show only relatively mild and nonspecific histopathological changes. Most specimens show
atrophy of the type 2 myofibers and subtle alterations in myofiber architecture, such as moth-eaten and whorled fibers.
Necrosis and interstitial inflammatory cell infiltrates are
usually not present. Rarely, an inflammatory arteritis with
giant cells has been seen.

4.   (A, B, C) Polyarteritis nodosa is a systemic necrotizing
vasculitis that affects medium and small arteries and arterioles
throughout the body. Lesions commonly occur in the kidneys,
gastrointestinal system, heart, testes, skeletal muscles, peripheral nerves, central nervous system, and, in some forms,
the lungs. Men are affected more frequently than women. The
disease is commonly classified among the so-called collagen
vascular diseases, although the precise pathogenesis remains
controversial. In recent years, associations with serum hepa-
titis and amphetamine abuse have been emphasized.

Clinical manifestations referable to central nervous system involvement have been reported in 10-20% of cases. A much higher
prevalence has been reported in some pathological studies.
Most of the lesions are infarcts of varying sizes and ages; however, hemorrhages, even massive hemorrhages, have been reported. Rarely, extensive involvement of the spinal cord leads
to a transverse myelitis.

Clinical evidence of peripheral nerve involvement, generally in
the form of mononeuropathy multiplex, is found in about 50% of
cases and may be the initial manifestation of the disease.

Autopsy studies demonstrate involvement of the nutrient arteries in about 75% of cases. The peripheral nerves show focal ischemic lesions and Wallerian degeneration.

5. (A, B, C, D) Muscle biopsy specimens are frequently employed for establishing a morphological diagnosis of polyarteritis nodosa. When the lesions are acute, the intramuscular arteries and arterioles show fibrinoid necrosis of their walls and prominent transmural and perivascular inflammatory cell infiltrates composed of mononuclear cells, polymorphonuclear leukocytes and occasional eosinophils (Fig. 39.2). Foci of myofiber necrosis, degenerating myofibers, regenerating myofibers and interstitial inflammatory cell infiltrates may be present. When the lesions are chronic or healed, the vessels may show mural fibrosis and recanalized lumena. Reflecting the vascular involvement within peripheral nerves, the muscle may show neurogenic atrophy and/or fiber-type grouping from reinnervation.

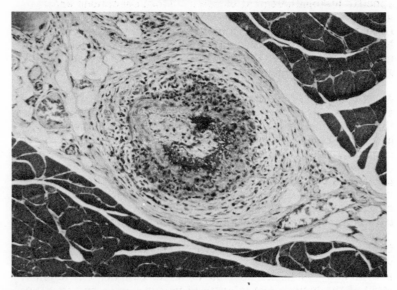

FIG. 39.2: Muscle biopsy specimen from a patient with polyarteritis nodosa showing the fibrinoid necrosis and inflammatory cell infiltrate.

6. (A, C) Granulomatous angiitis is a rare inflammatory vasculitis that is manifested clinically by derangement of mental function, focal neurological deficits, headaches, and occasionally

seizures. The disease predominantly affects the meningeal and small intracortical blood vessels. Both arteries and veins are involved. The lesions usually affect all layers of the vessels and contain lymphocytes, histiocytes and occasional giant cells. Although the inflammatory reaction is similar to temporal arteritis, the distribution of the lesions and the clinical manifestations are quite different. Several cases of granulomatous angiitis have been reported in association with lymphomas.

REFERENCES

1. Bruetsch WL: Giant Cell Arteritis (Temporal Arteritis, Cranial Arteritis, Granulomatous Angiitis). In: Pathology of the Nervous System. Minckler J (Ed.). McGraw-Hill Book Co., 1971, Vol. 2, pp. 1456-1468.

2. Bruetsch WL: Periarteritis Nodosa (Polyarteritis Nodosa, Essential Polyangiitis, Panarteritis Nodosa). In: Pathology of the Nervous System. Minckler J (Ed.). McGraw-Hill Book Co., 1971, Vol. 2, pp. 1468-1482.

3. Sole-Llenas J and Pons-Tortella E: Cerebral angiitis. Neuroradiology 15:1-11, 1978.

4. Wilkinson IMS and Russell RWR: Arteries of the head and neck in giant cell arteritis. Arch Neurol 27:378-391, 1972.

: :

CASE 40: A 60-Year-Old Man with Two "Strokes"

CLINICAL DATA

This 60-year-old man was known to have been hypertensive for
many years. Two years ago he had a stroke that began as a
sudden onset of left-sided weakness and rapidly progressed to
a complete left-sided paralysis. He recovered well and was
left with only moderate residual weakness. Three months previously he developed further weakness of his left side beginning
in his leg, progressing to his arm and eventually involving the
left side of his face. He recovered slowly and incompletely but
was able to walk with a cane upon discharge.

On the day of the present admission, the patient arose from a
nap, appeared confused and fell to the floor. He was taken to
his local hospital where he had a convulsion and was subsequently
transferred to the university hospital.

On arrival, his blood pressure was 150/100. He was unresponsive to verbal commands and responded to pain by movement of
his left arm only. There was increased tone on the left with a
Hoffman and a Babinski reflex. His pupils were equal but mio-
tic. Ciliospinal reflexes were intact. Funduscopic examination
showed no papilledema.

Carotid arteriograms revealed complete obstruction of the left
middle cerebral artery two centimeters from its origin and
severe stenosis of the right middle and anterior cerebral arteries. The patient remained in coma and died about one month
later from pneumonia.

QUESTIONS

1. By history, this patient had three "strokes." This term may
    be used to mean
    A. cerebral hemorrhage
    B. cerebral infarction
    C. an intracranial vascular occlusion
    D. all of the above

2. Fig. 40.1 illustrates a coronal section from this patient's
    brain. The lesions shown are
    A. cerebral hemorrhages
    B. old hemorrhagic infarcts
    C. old anemic infarcts
    D. acute (less than 24 hours) anemic infarcts

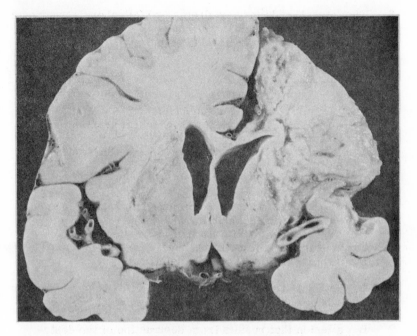

FIG. 40.1: Coronal section of the cerebral hemispheres showing bilateral infarcts.

3. Cerebral infarcts may result from
    A. thrombosis of intracranial vessels
    B. thrombosis of extracranial vessels
    C. episodes of profound hypotension
    D. cerebral embolism

4. The infarcts in the right cerebral hemisphere probably
    resulted from
    A. atheromatous emboli
    B. occlusion of the internal carotid artery
    C. thromboses of the right middle cerebral artery and
        of the right anterior cerebral artery
    D. thrombosis of the right middle cerebral artery

5. Infarcts resulting from embolization are typically
    A. hemorrhagic infarcts
    B. anemic infarcts
    C. cerebellar and/or brain stem infarcts
    D. multiple infarcts

6. The lateral medullary syndrome or Wallenberg's syndrome is usually due to occlusion of the
   A. posterior inferior cerebellar artery
   B. vertebral artery
   C. basilar artery
   D. anterior spinal artery

7. Pontine infarcts usually result from
   A. thrombosis of the posterior cerebral arteries
   B. thrombosis of the basilar artery
   C. occlusion of the paramedian and short circumflex branches of the basilar artery
   D. venous thrombosis

8. Histological characteristics of cerebral infarcts include
   A. shrinkage and acidophilia of neurons
   B. swelling and proliferation of astrocytes
   C. appearance of lipid-laden macrophages
   D. swelling of capillary endothelial cells

9. Olivary hypertrophy is
   A. a lesion that results only from destruction of the central tegmental tract
   B. a lesion that results from destruction of the dento-rubro-olivary tract
   C. most commonly encountered in patients with pontine infarcts
   D. characterized by vacuolization of the olivary neurons

ANSWERS AND DISCUSSION

1. (D) The term "stroke" is poorly defined and has different meanings to different users. It generally implies the abrupt onset of neurological deficits as the result of cerebrovascular disease. As such, it includes the manifestations of cerebral hemorrhage, cerebral infarction, intracranial thrombosis, extracranial thrombosis, cerebral embolism, etc. Collectively, cerebrovascular diseases are of enormous significance as the major cause of morbidity and the third most common cause of death in this country.

2. (C) The illustrated lesions are anemic infarcts that are old but of different ages. The usual anemic infarct does not become grossly recognizable until 12 to 18 hours have elapsed. The recently infarcted tissue is swollen, slightly softened and faintly discolored. After formalin fixation, the infarct remains softer than the surrounding uninvolved neural parenchyma. The

demarcation between the cortical grey matter or the nuclear grey matter and the adjacent white matter is obscured. Liquefaction begins after 3 to 4 days and cavitation results as the necrotic debris is removed. This is a slow process and requires about 3 months for the removal of each cubic centimeter of tissue. On this basis alone, it is evident that the infarct in the right hemisphere is older than the infarct in the left hemisphere. Eventually, the edema subsides, the necrotic tissue is removed and the glial scar contracts leaving little residua of a much larger acute lesion. Unlike abscesses, infarcts do not stimulate much collagenous tissue proliferation.

Scattered petechial hemorrhages are often found in the involved grey matter, especially along the margins of the infarct. The presence of large numbers of confluent petechial hemorrhages, i.e., hemorrhagic infarction, is more commonly associated with cerebral embolism or venous thrombosis than with arterial thrombosis.

3. (A, B, C, D) There are many recognized causes of cerebral infarction. Thrombotic occlusions of major intracranial arteries have been described in 40 to 95% of cases with large recent cerebral infarcts. The middle cerebral arteries are the most frequently involved vessels and are occluded in about 50% of cerebral infarcts. Thrombotic occlusion of the anterior cerebral arteries and of the posterior cerebral arteries are considerably less common. The posterior cerebral arteries are more commonly occluded by compression and distortion secondary to brain herniation. Severe stenosis and/or thrombosis of the extracranial vessels are responsible for more than a third of clinically significant cerebral infarcts. The carotid bifurcations are the most common sites of occlusion. Other frequently involved areas are the cavernous portions of the internal carotid arteries, the origins of the great vessels from the aortic arch and the origins of the vertebral arteries. Plaques alone must narrow the vessel lumen more than 70% to be significant but lesser degrees of stenosis can be significant if multiple vessels are involved or if complicated by hypotension. Thrombosis distal to the narrowed segments is the major complication of stenosis. Patients with significant stenosis, but without thrombosis, may develop cerebral infarcts in the border zones between the perfusion areas of adjacent cerebral arteries. These border zone infarcts are encountered most commonly between the perfusion beds of the anterior and middle cerebral arteries in the parietal lobes. They occur most often in elderly patients with multifocal atherosclerosis who suffer hypotension from myocardial infarcts, during surgery or from

overly vigorous antihypertensive therapy. Mural thrombi over
myocardial infarcts and atheromatous material from plaques in
the extracranial great vessels may embolize to the brain and
produce cerebral infarcts.

4.   (B) The massive old infarcts in the right cerebral hemisphere involving the distribution of the anterior and middle
cerebral arteries probably resulted from remote occlusion of
the internal carotid artery. Occlusion of a single internal carotid artery in the absence of significant atherosclerosis or major
anomalies of the circle of Willis usually produces no cerebral
complications. However, when complicated by severe diffuse
vascular disease, as in the present case, occlusion of the internal carotid artery produces infarction in the distribution of
the middle cerebral artery and often in the distribution of the
anterior cerebral artery as well. Occasionally, the distribution of the posterior cerebral artery is also included, producing an infarct of the entire hemisphere. In the face of a previous asymptomatic occlusion of the ipsilateral carotid artery,
infarction may result from the occlusion of the contralateral
internal carotid artery.

5.   (A, D) Infarcts resulting from embolization are typically
multiple, most numerous in the middle cerebral artery distribution and hemorrhagic. Their hemorrhagic nature has
been attributed to lysis of the embolized thrombotic material
with subsequent reestablishment of blood flow into an infarcted
area. Obviously, this explanation is inadequate to explain the
hemorrhagic nature of the infarcts when they are due to atheromatous or foreign material.

6.   (B) The lateral medullary syndrome, or Wallenberg's syndrome, is usually due to occlusion of the vertebral artery. The
resulting infarction is in the distribution of the posterior inferior cerebellar artery, which generally arises from the vertebral artery. Among the structures involved are the spinal tract
of the trigeminal, the nucleus ambiguus, the spinothalamic tract,
the lateral vestibular nucleus, part of the restiform body and
the descending sympathetic fibers. The cerebellum is also involved to a variable degree.

7.   (B, C) Small pontine infarcts are relatively common lesions and are due to occlusion of small paramedian and short
circumflex branches of the basilar artery. Thrombosis of the
basilar artery is much less common and usually results in extensive infarction of the pons (Fig. 40.2).

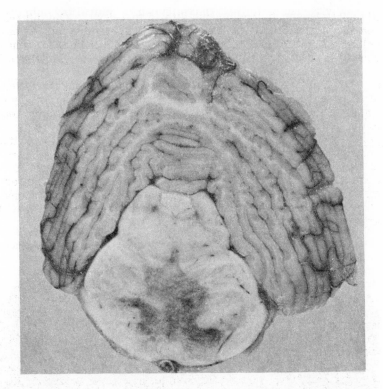

FIG. 40. 2: Transverse section of the pons showing a pontine infarct.

8.   (A, B, C, D) The histological characteristics of cerebral
infarcts change with the passage of time.   Within a few hours
after blood flow has been interrupted, the neurons show shrinkage and acidophilia of their cytoplasm and pyknosis of their
nuclei.   The astrocytes swell producing "clear spaces" about
neurons and blood vessels.   The astrocytic cytoplasm usually
contains excessive glycogen that can be demonstrated with the
periodic acid-Schiff stain.   The oligodendrocytes, especially
in the white matter, undergo cytoplasmic swelling producing
perinuclear "halos."   The capillary endothelium swells and appears to occlude the capillary lumens.   Polymorphonuclear
leukocytes can be seen around vessels, especially at the margins of the infarcts.   Within a few days lipid-laden macrophages
appear and begin to remove the necrotic debris.   Astrocytic
enlargement due to proliferation of the intracellular glial

filaments becomes conspicuous after 5 to 7 days.   Old infarcts
consist predominantly of cystic spaces traversed by blood vessels and glial fibers.   They can often be distinguished from
contusions by the preservation of a subpial band of glial tissue.

9.   (B, C, D) Olivary hypertrophy is an unusual manifestation
of transneuronal degeneration that results from lesions anywhere in the dento-rubro-olivary pathway. This uncommon lesion is usually encountered in individuals who survive for a
period of time following pontine infarcts with destruction of the
central tegmental tract, a component of the dento-rubro-olivary
pathway. Occasionally grossly, but most often in macroscopic
sections, the affected inferior olivary nucleus appears larger
than normal (Fig. 40.3). Microscopically, the olivary neurons
show distinctive enlargement, vacuolization and proliferation of
argentophilic neurofilaments (Fig. 40.4).

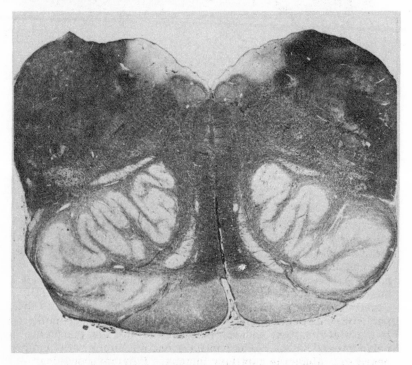

FIG. 40.3: Macroscopic section of the medulla showing hyper-
          trophy of the inferior olives. The enlargement is
          most pronounced in the ventrolateral portions of
          the nuclei.

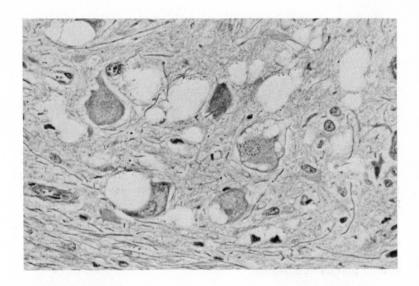

FIG. 40.4: Microscopic section showing enlargement and vacuolation of the olivary neurons.

REFERENCES

1.   Loeb C and Meyer JS: Strokes Due to Vertebro-Basilar
     Disease. Charles C Thomas, Springfield, 1965, pp. 52-79.

2.   McCormick WF and Schochet SS Jr.: Atlas of Cerebrovas-
     cular Disease. W. B. Saunders Co., Philadelphia, 1976.

3.   Sohn D and Levine S: Hypertrophy of the Olives: A Report on
     43 Cases. In: Progress in Neuropathology. Zimmerman HM
     (Ed.). Grune and Stratton, New York, 1971, pp. 202-217.

4.   Stehbens WE: Pathology of the Cerebral Blood Vessels.
     C. V. Mosby Co., St. Louis, 1972, pp. 131-206.

5.   Yates PO and Hutchinson EC: Cerebral Infarction: The role
     of stenosis of the extracranial cerebral arteries. Med Res
     Council Spec Rep 300:1-95, 1961.

6.   Zulch KJ: Hemorrhage, Thrombosis, Embolism. In:
     Pathology of the Nervous System. Minckler J (Ed.).
     McGraw-Hill Book Co., New York, 1971, pp. 1499-1536.

CASE 41:   An Elderly Man with Hypertension and Sudden
           Onset of Coma

CLINICAL DATA

This 70-year-old man, who was known to have been hypertensive for many years, suddenly fell and became unresponsive.
He was taken immediately to the hospital.

Upon admission, his blood pressure was 280/160 mm Hg, pulse
100/min and respirations 18/min.   He was quadriplegic, dys-
arthric and unable to swallow. Shortly after admission, his respirations became labored and he lapsed into deep coma.   His
pupils were pinpoint in size and minimally reactive to light.
The corneal reflexes were absent and there was no ocular
response to cold-caloric vestibular stimulation.   The patient
developed apneustic breathing, hyperthermia and died on the
second hospital day. The general autopsy disclosed pulmonary
edema and cardiomegaly.

QUESTIONS

1.   The clinical data are consistent with a
     A.   striatal hemorrhage
     B.   striatal infarct
     C.   pontine hemorrhage
     D.   medullary hemorrhage

2.   The most frequent site of hemorrhage in patients with
     hypertension and no other demonstrable lesion is
     A.   cerebral lobes
     B.   region of the basal ganglia
     C.   pons
     D.   cerebellum

3.   The most common cause of pontine hemorrhage is
     A.   hypertension
     B.   rupture of an angioma
     C.   rupture of a basilar artery aneurysm
     D.   caudal displacement of the brain stem secondary to a
          supratentorial mass lesion

4.   Important causes of massive nontraumatic intracerebral
     hemorrhages include
     A.   blood dyscrasias
     B.   ruptured aneurysms

   C. ruptured vascular malformations
   D. primary or metastatic neoplasms

5. The mechanism by which hypertension produces massive
    intracerebral hemorrhages is
   A. formation and rupture of Charcot-Bouchard aneurysms
   B. development of ischemic foci into which bleeding sub-
      sequently occurs
   C. development of angionecrosis with subsequent rupture
      of the affected vessels
   D. unknown

ANSWERS AND DISCUSSION

1. (C) The clinical data are consistent with a diagnosis of a
pontine hemorrhage. Individuals developing these lesions often
have a history of long-standing hypertension. In the present
case, evidence of hypertension is provided by the histological
information and the cardiomegaly encountered at the time of
autopsy. The elevated blood pressure recorded on admission,
immediately after the hemorrhage, cannot be used as a reliable
indicator of the preictal blood pressure.

Pontine hemorrhages typically result in the abrupt onset of coma,
quadriplegia, and impaired eye movements. The pupils are
typically small but reactive to light when the hemorrhage is mid-
pontine. The patients develop respiratory difficulties, elevated
body temperature, and generally die within a few days of the
hemorrhage. Fig. 41.1 illustrates the lesion found at autopsy.

2. (B) In patients who are hypertensive with no other demonstrable cause for their intracerebral hemorrhages, the most
common site of bleeding is the region of the basal ganglia. This
site, which includes the striatum and thalamus, harbors 50 to
80% of the hematomas found in such patients. It is important
to remember that there are many causes for intracerebral
hemorrhages and when all are considered, lobar hemorrhages
are more common than ganglionic hemorrhages.

All authors are in agreement that primary pontine hemorrhages
are relatively uncommon and account for only 5 to 15% of all
primary intracerebral hemorrhages. A relatively high proportion of these hemorrhages are found in individuals who are hypertensive and have no other demonstrable cause for the hemorrhage.

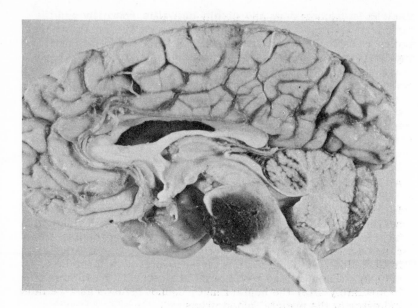

FIG. 41. 1: Sagittal section of the brain from the present case showing the primary pontine hemorrhage.

The pontine hemorrhages usually involve the midpons and extend across the midline to involve both halves. Occasionally, the hemorrhage extends rostrally into the midbrain. Less commonly, it extends caudally into the medulla. Extensions into the cerebellar peduncles are common. Blood often gains access to the cerebrospinal fluid by direct extension ventrally into the subarachnoid space or by extension dorsally through the floor of the fourth ventricle.

3.   (D) The majority of pontine hemorrhages are secondary to caudal displacement of the brain stem by an expanding supratentorial mass lesion. While the association between these hemorrhages and supratentorial masses has been known for more than a century, the immediate pathogenesis of the hemorrhages had been extensively debated.   The current evidence indicates that they are arterial in origin.   In patients with supratentorial lesions, the brain stem is displaced caudally. The basilar artery cannot be displaced to the same degree

since it is anchored by the circle of Willis rostrally and the
vertebral arteries caudally. Therefore, as the brain stem
moves caudally, the circumferential and especially the paramedian branches from the basilar artery are stretched. Because of the angle at which they enter the brain stem, the
vessels to the midbrain and rostral pons are placed under the
greatest tension. These are precisely the areas in which the
secondary brain stem hemorrhages are most numerous. They
are not limited to a region with a specific venous drainage.
The actual hemorrhages are preceded by edema and ischemic
necrosis and at times these may be present without hemorrhage.

4. (A, B, C, D) For many years, it has been assumed that
hypertension is virtually the only cause of massive nontraumatic intracerebral hemorrhage. Many factors have contrib-
uted to the development of this concept. Many of the studies
have been based on clinical observations in which the nature
of the "strokes," hemorrhages, infarcts, etc., were not determined by autopsy. Often the presence of "hypertension"was
assumed on the basis of elevated postictal blood pressure.
Furthermore, the prevalence of hypertension, now variously
estimated to affect 20 to 40% of the adult population over 35
years of age, and the opportunity for coincidental association
with other factors were not appreciated. Careful prospective
autopsy studies have shown that there are many causes for
massive nontraumatic brain hemorrhages. Aside from hypertension, McCormick and Rosenfield found leukemia, aneurysms,
angiomas and neoplasms to be the four most common causes of
hemorrhage in their series of 144 patients. In only one-fourth
of their cases was hypertension the only factor or lesion that
could be incriminated as causing the hemorrhage. Their material showed significant correlations between the number and
distribution of the hemorrhages and the cause of the hemorrhages. Multiple hemorrhages were most common in patients
with blood dyscrasias. Lobar hemorrhages were most common
in patients with recognizable lesions other than hypertension.
Among the hypertensive patients, the striatum was the most
common site of hemorrhage. However, there were also many
other causes of striatal hemorrhages.

5. (D) The mechanism by which hypertension produces massive intracerebral hemorrhages is unknown or at least currently
unproven. All authors are now in agreement that the elevated

blood pressure alone is incapable of rupturing otherwise normal
cerebral blood vessels. Some writers have taken the stand that
hypertension is responsible for the formation and subsequent
rupture of the so-called Charcot-Bouchard aneurysms. These
miliary aneurysms are found with increasing frequency with increasing age. The majority are found in the pons, thalamus and
basal ganglia. Large numbers are also present in the subcortical white matter. Although their presence is indisputable,
any relation between their formation and rupture and hypertension
is conjectural. Other authors have suggested that hypertension
produces a necrotizing angiitis that is in turn responsible for
intracerebral bleeding. However, there is considerable evidence that the angionecrosis is the result of the hemorrhage
rather than the cause of the hemorrhage. It is generally accepted
that hypertension accelerates the development of cerebral
atherosclerosis and arteriosclerosis. Furthermore, infarcts
are more common in patients with hypertension. Especially
characteristic of hypertensive patients are multiple, small, so-
called lacunar infarcts (Fig. 41.2). It has been suggested and
seems reasonable that massive intracerebral hemorrhages result from bleeding into areas of recent encephalomalacia.
Nevertheless, this rather old hypothesis remains unproven.

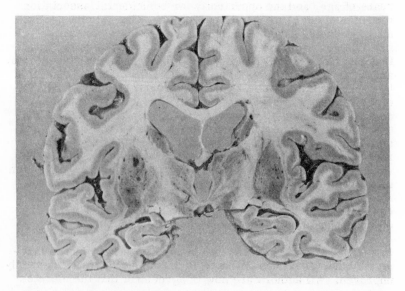

FIG. 41.2: Coronal section of the cerebral hemispheres from
a patient with long-standing hypertension. Note the
numerous, small, lacunar infarcts.

REFERENCES

1. Hassler O: Arterial pattern of human brain stem. Normal appearance and deformation in expanding supratentorial conditions. Neurology 17:368-376, 1967.

2. Klintworth GK: The pathogenesis of secondary brain stem hemorrhages as studied in an experimental model. Amer J Path 47:525-536, 1965.

3. Klintworth GK: Paratentorial grooving of human brains with particular reference to transtentorial herniation and the pathogenesis of secondary brain stem hemorrhages. Amer J Path 53:391-408, 1968.

4. Loeb C and Meyer JS: Strokes Due to Vertebro-Basilar Disease. C. C Thomas, Springfield, 1965, pp. 174-198.

5. McCormick WF and Rosenfield DB: Massive brain hemorrhage: A review of 144 cases and an examination of their causes. Stroke 4:946-954, 1973.

6. McCormick WF and Schochet SS Jr.: Atlas of Cerebro-vascular Disease. W.B. Saunders Co., Philadelphia, 1976.

7. Plum F and Posner JB: The Diagnosis of Stupor and Coma. F.A. Davis Co., Philadelphia, 1972, pp. 120-139.

8. Stehbens WE: Pathology of the Cerebral Blood Vessels. C.V. Mosby Co., St. Louis, 1972, pp. 284-350.

: :

CASE 42:   A 44-Year-Old Woman with the Sudden Onset of
           a Severe Headache and Rapid Loss of Consciousness

CLINICAL DATA

This 44-year-old woman experienced the sudden onset of severe
headache and difficulty walking. These symptoms were followed
rapidly by loss of consciousness. When initially hospitalized,
she was found to have nuchal rigidity and a positive Kernig's
sign. A lumbar puncture yielded grossly bloody cerebrospinal
fluid under increased pressure.

Thirty-six hours later, the patient was transferred to another
hospital. Physical examination on admission revealed a mildly
febrile, comatose woman with a rigid neck. The fundi showed
venous congestion. There was a full range of extraocular
movements upon the doll's head maneuver. The patient moved
all four extremities in response to pain; however, the right
side was mildly paretic. An angiogram revealed aneurysms on
the right middle cerebral artery and on the right internal carotid artery. A ventriculostomy revealed normal pressure and
a ventriculogram showed only mild enlargement of the ventricular system. A lumbar puncture needle was placed for continuous cerebrospinal fluid drainage. The following day, the
cerebrospinal fluid again became grossly bloody and the patient
died.

QUESTIONS

1.   Common clinical manifestations of a ruptured saccular
     aneurysm include
     A.   sudden onset of headache
     B.   decreased level of consciousness
     C.   ataxia
     D.   nuchal rigidity

2.   Fig. 42.1 illustrates the base of this patient's brain. On
     the basis of the pathological changes seen in this picture,
     the most appropriate diagnosis is
     A.   ruptured saccular aneurysm
     B.   subarachnoid hemorrhage
     C.   subarachnoid hemorrhage probably due to a ruptured
          saccular aneurysm
     D.   pontine hemorrhage

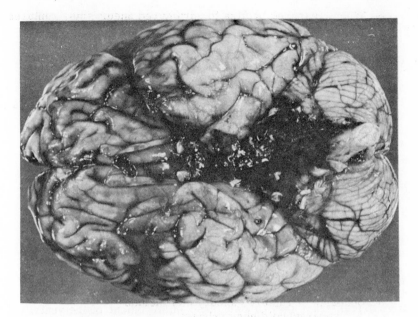

FIG. 42.1: Base of brain showing the location of the subarachnoid hemorrhage.

3. The prevalence of saccular aneurysms among patients coming to autopsy is
    A. less than 2%
    B. 2 to 3%
    C. 5 to 7%
    D. greater than 10%

4. Saccular aneurysms occur most commonly on the
    A. middle cerebral arteries
    B. anterior communicating artery
    C. posterior communicating arteries
    D. basilar artery

5. Among patients with aneurysms, multiple aneurysms are found in
    A.   5%
    B. 15%
    C. 20%
    D. 25%

6. When compared by size to unruptured aneurysms, ruptured aneurysms tend to be
    A. smaller
    B. equal in size
    C. larger
    D. much larger, so-called "giant" aneurysms

7. Histologically, saccular aneurysms are characterized by
    A. attenuation of the media
    B. a giant cell reaction to the remaining fragments of elastica
    C. severe atherosclerotic changes
    D. intralumenal thrombus

8. Conditions clearly proven to predispose to the rupture of saccular aneurysms include
    A. hypertension
    B. trauma
    C. pregnancy
    D. none of these

9. Sequelae of ruptured aneurysms include
    A. subarachnoid hemorrhages
    B. hydrocephalus
    C. cerebral infarctions
    D. intraparenchymal hematomas

10. Common systemic complications of ruptured saccular aneurysms include
    A. rhabdomyolysis
    B. cardiac abnormalities
    C. pulmonary edema
    D. renal failure

11. Complications occasionally encountered with unruptured saccular aneurysms include
    A. cerebral infarction
    B. hydrocephalus
    C. cranial nerve palsies
    D. none of these

12. Intracranial mycotic aneurysms
    A. are often found on small peripheral arteries
    B. are invariably secondary to bacterial endocarditis
    C. are more common than ordinary saccular aneurysms
    D. may be found in prepubertal individuals

13. Intracranial arteriosclerotic aneurysms
    A. are usually found in elderly individuals
    B. usually involve the vertebro-basilar system or the
       supraclinoid portion of the internal carotid arteries
    C. produce symptoms by compression of the adjacent
       neural parenchyma or by thrombosis and infarction
    D. rupture frequently

ANSWERS AND DISCUSSION

1. (A, B, D) Unruptured saccular aneurysms are generally
asymptomatic. With rupture, there is usually a dramatic onset of symptoms. Severe headache is the initial manifestation
in most cases. This is followed by a change in the level of
consciousness or even coma. Rapid loss of consciousness is
considered a grave prognostic sign. Nuchal rigidity, a positive
Kernig's sign, and other manifestations of meningeal irritation
usually develop within a few hours. Focal neurological signs
can result from hemorrhage into the neural parenchyma or
cerebral infarction. Cranial nerve palsies may develop as the
result of direct damage or secondary to increased intracranial
pressure and herniations. Papilledema and retinal hemorrhages are common manifestations of the elevated intracranial
pressure. Blood pressure, pulse, and eventually temperature
become elevated.

The cerebrospinal fluid initially is grossly bloody with concomitant elevations in the cell count and protein content. After
a few hours, the cerebrospinal fluid supernatant becomes
xanthochromic. The peripheral blood will show a mild to
moderate leukocytosis.

2. (C) On the basis of the pathological changes illustrated in
Fig. 42.1, the most appropriate diagnosis would be subarachnoid hemorrhage, probably due to a ruptured saccular aneurysm.
The hemorrhage from a ruptured aneurysm is usually most abundant on the base of the brain where it tends to obscure the major
arteries. Lesser amounts of blood may extend onto the convexities of the cerebral hemispheres and onto the superior surface of the cerebellum. Middle cerebral artery aneurysms
may produce massive hematomas in the Sylvian fissures and
anterior communicating artery aneurysms may produce hematomas between the cerebral hemispheres and on the dorsal
surface of the corpus callosum. However, merely finding
subarachnoid hemorrhage even in an appropriate location does
not establish the diagnosis of a ruptured aneurysm. Partial removal of the blood from the fresh, unfixed specimen often
facilitates actual demonstration of the ruptured aneurysm and
other unruptured aneurysms.

Trauma is the most common cause of subarachnoid hemorrhage.
Hemorrhage on this basis may be diffuse and widespread or
localized to the areas of contusion. Commonly affected are the
inferior surfaces of the frontal lobes and the anterior-inferior
portions of the temporal lobes. Other causes of subarachnoid
hemorrhage that must be considered are blood dyscrasias, including leukemia, primary and metastatic neoplasms, and
ruptured vascular malformations. Intraparenchymal hemorrhages can rupture into the ventricular system and gain access
to the subarachnoid space through the outlet foramina of the
fourth ventricle.

3. (C) Meticulous prospective studies have shown that saccular aneurysms are far more common than previously suspected
from casual examination primarily of symptomatic cases.
Aneurysms are encountered in 5-7% of all patients who are
autopsied. Aneurysms are very rare before puberty and show
no significant variation in prevalence thereafter. If only adults
are considered, the prevalence is nearly 7%. An increased
prevalence has been encountered in individuals with type 3 polycystic renal disease and a questionable increased prevalence
has been described in association with coarctation of the aorta.

Rupture of a saccular aneurysm is a relatively uncommon event
with only about 20% of aneurysms eventually rupturing. When
rupture does occur, the patients are usually between the ages
of 40 and 60.

4. (A) Virtually all major arterial junctions have been found
to be the site of aneurysms (Fig. 42.2). As determined by examination at autopsy, the most common site for aneurysms is
at the major bifurcation or trifurcation of the middle cerebral
arteries. Approximately 40% of all saccular aneurysms are
found in this location. The next most common locations are the
junctions of the anterior communicating artery with the anterior
cerebral arteries or the median artery of the corpus callosum.
These so-called "anterior communicating artery" aneurysms
comprise about 24% of the total. Third in prevalence are the
junctions of the internal carotid arteries and their branches.
These sites, collectively, harbor about 23% of all saccular
aneurysms. This last group is somewhat confusing since a
number of vessels can be regarded as branches of the internal
carotid arteries. Among these, the most important with regard
to aneurysms are the posterior communicating arteries. In the
present case (Fig. 42.3) a ruptured aneurysm (white arrows) was
present at the junction of the right internal carotid artery and the
posterior communicating artery. A second unruptured aneurysm
was present on the middle cerebral artery (black arrows).

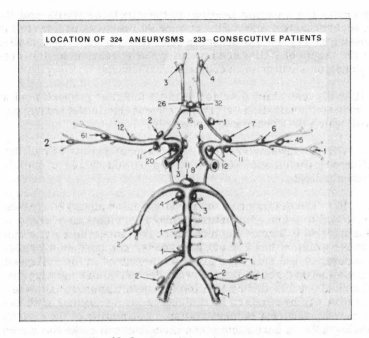

FIG. 42.2: Location of aneurysms.

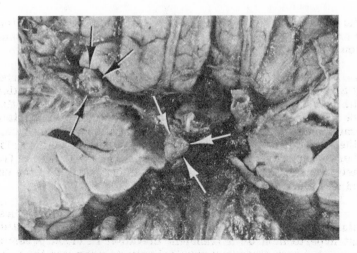

FIG. 42.3: Partially dissected brain from the present case
showing a ruptured aneurysm (white arrows) and
an unruptured aneurysm (black arrows).

Overall, the anterior portion of the circle of Willis and its
branches harbor about 85% of saccular aneurysms, while the
basilar artery and its branches harbor about 15%. Anomalies
of the circle of Willis seem to have little bearing on the prevalence or location of saccular aneurysms.

Clinically ascertained series suggest a higher proportion of anterior communicating artery aneurysms due to the frequency
with which they become symptomatic.

5. (D) Aneurysms are multiple in approximately 25% of the
affected patients and bilateral in approximately 15% of the affected patients.

6. (C) The diameter of the usual saccular aneurysm varies
from 0.2 to 5 cm. Unruptured aneurysms have an average
diameter of 0.5 cm. Ruptured saccular aneurysms are almost
always greater than 1.0 cm in diameter and have an average
diameter of 1.5 cm. The size, as measured in the collapsed,
formalin-fixed state, is somewhat deceptive since aneurysms
shrink about 10% during fixation. A better approximation of
the size can be obtained by distending the aneurysms with saline and measuring before fixation. Estimation of the size by
angiography is unreliable since thrombus can make the lumen
small and thus the aneurysm is interpreted as being spuriously
small.

The occasional, very large, so-called "giant" aneurysms tend
to produce symptoms by their mass effect but rupture is uncommon.

7. (A) Histologically, saccular aneurysms are characterized
by a marked attenuation of the media and a paucity of elastica.
The aneurysmal sac is composed predominantly of adventitia.
The lumen, especially in the larger aneurysms, often contains
laminated thrombus. Foci of mineralization are common.
Atherosclerotic changes are usually no more severe than elsewhere in the intracranial arteries and thus vary in degree from
case to case. When ruptured, necrosis of a portion of the sac
and an inflammatory cell infiltrate can be seen.

8. (D) The circumstances predisposing to the rupture of a saccular aneurysm are currently unknown. It has often been claimed
that hypertension or a transient elevation in blood pressure
associated with strenuous physical activity promotes the rupture
of an aneurysm. However, the majority of patients dying from
a ruptured aneurysm lack a history or anatomical evidence of

pre-existing hypertension. A series of 43 cases analyzed by
McCormick for activity at the time of rupture disclosed only
two patients who were engaged in strenuous activities, gym-
nastics and a fight; five were sleeping, ten were sitting quietly,
and the remainder were only moderately active. Trauma has
been mentioned as a possible cause of rupture but the evidence
is inconclusive. There is no increased risk of rupture during
pregnancy.

9. (A, B, C, D) The mortality from ruptured saccular aneurysms has been reported to range from 33 to 64%. Nearly 33%
of the deaths occur during the first two days, 40% within the
first two weeks and 75% within the first six weeks. Because
of the location of saccular aneurysms on the major cerebral
arteries, subarachnoid hemorrhages are the most common
sequelae of their rupture. The subarachnoid hemorrhage can
produce hydrocephalus by blockage of the pacchionian granulations or by eliciting meningeal fibrosis. The ruptures are
further complicated by intracerebral or intraventricular hemorrhages in 50 to 70% of the fatal cases. Cerebral infarctions
are important complications that are seen most often following
the rupture of anterior communicating artery aneurysms. Subdural hemorrhages may occur, but are rare.

10. (B, C) Common systemic complications of ruptured saccular aneurysms include cardiac abnormalities and pulmonary
edema. Cardiac abnormalities are found in nearly 50% of patients with subarachnoid hemorrhages and include arrhythmias,
bundle branch blocks and ischemic changes. Morphologically
subendocardial hemorrhages and foci of myofibrillar degeneration are common findings. The cardiac changes are thought to
be due to excessive sympathetic activity. Pulmonary edema
and gastromalacia are encountered with a variety of intracranial lesions, including ruptured saccular aneurysms.

11. (B, C) Although the majority of the complications associated with saccular aneurysms result from rupture, large
and/or strategically located aneurysms can produce symptoms
by acting as space-occupying masses. As such they can ob-
struct the intracerebral cerebrospinal fluid pathways producing
hydrocephalus or can compress one or more cranial nerves.
The oculomotor nerves are probably the most frequently involved of the cranial nerves. Compression of portions of the
visual pathways may lead to visual field defects. Aneurysms
in the region of the pituitary have been mistaken for nonfunc-
tional pituitary adenomas.

12. (A, D) Mycotic aneurysms result from inflammation of the vessel walls. They are commonly found in association with bacterial endocarditis but may occur in association with septicemia from other sources, with blood-borne fungal infections, with meningitis or with the vasculitides. They are often small, involve small peripheral arteries and may be multiple. They can be found in individuals of all ages including prepubertal individuals. As a group, they are much rarer than ordinary saccular aneurysms.

13. (A, B, C) Arteriosclerotic aneurysms are fusiform dilatations of the intracranial blood vessels that develop as a complication of atherosclerosis usually in the elderly. They involve most commonly the vertebro-basilar system and the supraclinoid portions of the internal carotid arteries. They rarely rupture but produce symptoms by compression of adjacent structures or by thrombosis with infarction, especially in the brain stem. As a group, they are less common than ordinary saccular aneurysm.

REFERENCES

1. McCormick WF: Problems and Pathogenesis of Intracranial Arterial Aneurysms. In: Cerebral Vascular Diseases. Toole JF, et al. (Eds.). Grune and Stratton, New York, 1971, pp. 219-231.

2. McCormick WF and Acosta-Rua GJ: The size of intracranial saccular aneurysms. An autopsy study. J Neurosurg 33:422-427, 1970.

3. McCormick WF and Schochet SS Jr.: Atlas of Cerebrovascular Disease. W.B. Saunders Co., Philadelphia, 1976.

4. Stehbens WE: Pathology of the Cerebral Blood Vessels. C.V. Mosby Co., St. Louis, 1972, pp. 252-293; 351-470.

5. Weintraub BM and McHenry LC Jr.: Cardiac Abnormalities in subarachnoid hemorrhage: A resume. Stroke 5:384-392, 1974.

: :

CASE 43: A 65-Year-Old Man with a Long History of
          Focal Seizures

CLINICAL DATA

This 65-year-old man had a long history of a focal seizure disorder and had had previous myocardial infarcts. There was no
history of head trauma.

On admission, the patient was having frequent focal seizures
consisting of right-sided facial twitching that lasted 30 to 60
seconds. He was fully aware of events but was unable to talk
during the seizures. A slight slurring of speech and facial
tingling persisted postictally. Physical examination was essentially normal except for gingival hypertrophy that was attributed
to Dilantin.   An isotopic brain scan and a left carotid angiogram failed to reveal any lesions.

Three days after admission, the patient developed severe chest
pain and respiratory difficulties. An electrocardiogram showed
evidence of an acute myocardial infarct. Despite supportive
measures, the patient died on the fifth hospital day.

The significant findings at autopsy were a recent myocardial infarct and the lesion illustrated in Fig. 43.1. This lesion was
confined to the inferior frontal gyrus and was the only abnormality encountered in the brain.

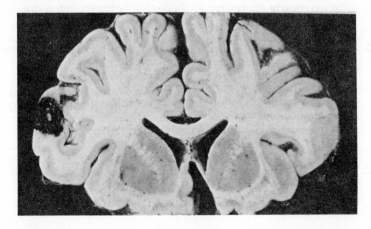

FIG. 43. 1: Coronal section of the cerebral hemispheres
             showing the lesion in the left frontal lobe.

QUESTIONS

1. Based on the clinical data and gross appearance, the most
   appropriate diagnosis for the lesion shown in Fig. 43.1 is
   A. glioblastoma
   B. metastasis
   C. vascular malformation
   D. contusion

2. Common clinical manifestations of vascular malformations
   include
   A. intracranial hemorrhage
   B. epilepsy
   C. progressive neurological deficits
   D. dystonia

3. Vascular malformations are found in the brains of about
   A. 0.5% of all patients coming to autopsy
   B. 2% of all patients coming to autopsy
   C. 5% of all patients coming to autopsy
   D. 10% of all patients coming to autopsy

4. Arteriovenous malformations are characterized by the
   presence of
   A. varying-sized arteries, veins and arterialized veins
   B. gliotic neural parenchyma between the component
      vessels
   C. essentially normal neural parenchyma between the
      component vessels
   D. virtually no neural parenchyma between the com-
      ponent vessels

5. Cavernous angiomas are characterized by the presence of
   A. varying-sized sinusoidal vessels
   B. gliotic neural parenchyma between the component
      vessels
   C. essentially normal neural parenchyma between the
      component vessels
   D. virtually no neural parenchyma between the com-
      ponent vessels

6. Venous angiomas are characterized by the presence of
   A. varying-sized veins
   B. gliotic neural parenchyma between the component
      vessels

   C. essentially normal neural parenchyma between the
       component vessels
   D. virtually no neural parenchyma between the component
       vessels

7. Telangiectases are characterized by the presence of
    A. capillary-type vessels
    B. gliotic neural parenchyma between the component
        vessels
    C. essentially normal neural parenchyma between the
        component vessels
    D. virtually no neural parenchyma between the component
        vessels

8. Varices are characterized by the presence of
    A. congeries of sinusoidal vessels
    B. single anomalous veins
    C. dilatation of the vein of Galen
    D. Congeries of capillary-type vessels

9. The syndrome of Foix-Alajouanine is due to
    A. spinal thrombophlebitis
    B. acute multiple sclerosis
    C. thrombosis of the anterior spinal artery
    D. a vascular malformation of the spinal cord

ANSWERS AND DISCUSSION

1. (C) The most appropriate diagnosis for the lesion shown
in Fig. 43.1 is a vascular malformation. The lesion is sharply
demarcated and consists of a closely packed congeries of abnormal vascular channels. The bosselated periphery is surrounded by a narrow rim of discolored, gliotic neural parenchyma. The overlying meninges are thickened and opacified.

Both glioblastomas and metastases may have a dark, hemorrhagic appearance and a porous texture due to foci of necrosis
and hemorrhage but the lesions would be accompanied by extensive cerebral edema. Furthermore, all malignant tumors
can be reasonably eliminated from consideration by the long
clinical history. Old contusions are commonly epileptogenic
foci but they tend to be shrunken, wedge-shaped and consist of
poorly vascular glial tissue. Furthermore, a large contusion
is unlikely in the absence of a history of head trauma.

2. (A, B, C) The majority of intracranial vascular malformations are probably asymptomatic. However, they may give rise
to a variety of neurological manifestations. Hemorrhages,

either intraparenchymal or subarachnoid, are the most important of these. The true incidence of hemorrhages from vascular malformations in unknown. In contrast to most clinical reports, autopsy studies indicate that hemorrhages are relatively
uncommon events occurring in only 5-10% of patients with vascular malformations. Although all types of vascular malformations can give rise to hemorrhages, they are most commonly a
complication of arteriovenous malformations. Non-traumatic
subarachnoid hemorrhages in patients under the age of 30 are
due more often to vascular malformations than aneurysms.
A significant number of the patients with symptomatic hemorrhages experience recurrence of the hemorrhage.

Epilepsy is another important manifestation of vascular malformations. Nearly one-third of patients with large vascular
malformations have focal or generalized seizures. The seizures are not restricted to any one type of vascular malformation.
but are especially common with cavernous angiomas. Surgical
removal of the vascular malformation often does not produce significant improvement in the number or severity of the seizures.

Progressive neurological deficits can result from ischemic
necrosis of the neural parenchyma surrounding the vascular
malformation. The necrosis is due to the rapid shunting of
blood by the malformation, a process designated as "steal."
With the passage of time, some malformations increase in size by
incorporating adjacent parenchymal vessels. This phenomenon
has been referred to as "recruitment." Rarely, the malformations enlarge sufficiently to act as space-occupying masses.

3.   (C) Vascular malformations are relatively common lesions in about 5% of all patients coming to autopsy. In surgical
material, arteriovenous malformations are especially heavily
represented because of their tendency to produce symptoms
from rupture (Fig. 43.2). Prospective autopsy studies reveal
a much higher proportion of venous angiomas. Thus, it would
appear that venous angiomas are the most common vascular
malformations while arteriovenous malformations are clinically the most significant. Angiography often fails to demonstrate cavernous angiomas, telangiectases or venous angiomas.

4.   (A, B) Arteriovenous malformations, as illustrated in Fig.
43.3, are characterized by the presence of varying-sized arteries,
veins and arterialized veins. The component vessels are
separated from one another by gliotic neural parenchyma that
often contains clusters of hemosiderin-laden macrophages.
Foci of mineralization, and even ossification, may be encountered within the vessel walls. Some of the vessels may be
thrombosed.

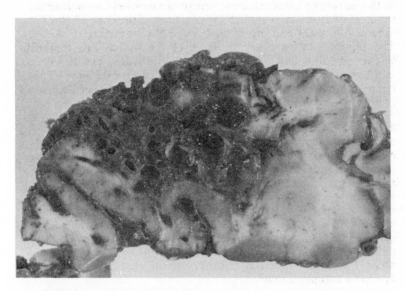

FIG. 43.2: An arteriovenous malformation surgically removed
because of recurrent hemorrhage.

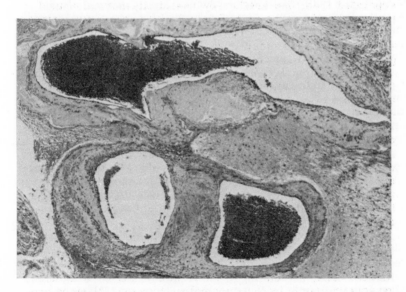

FIG. 43.3: Microscopic section showing an arteriovenous malformation.

In the cerebral hemispheres, large arteriovenous malformations are often cone-shaped with the base of the cone at the surface of the brain and the apex toward the ventricular system. The leptomeninges over the base of the lesion are typically thickened and opacified. Elsewhere in the brain, arteriovenous malformations have a discoid or ovoid configuration. They comprised about 12% of the vascular malformations encountered in a prospective autopsy study.

5. (A, D) Cavernous angiomas, as illustrated in Fig. 43.4, are composed of varying-sized sinusoidal vessels that are closely apposed to one another with virtually no intervening neural parenchyma. The vessel walls are often hyalinized and may be mineralized or even ossified. These compact vascular malformations are often surrounded by a thin rim of gliotic neural parenchyma containing foci of hemosiderin-laden macrophages. These angiomas are frequently epileptogenic but rarely give rise to massive hemorrhages. In a significant number of patients, cavernous angiomas are multiple. They comprised about 7% of the vascular malformations encountered in a prospective autopsy study.

6. (A, C) Venous angiomas, as illustrated in Fig. 43.5, are characterized by the presence of varying-sized veins that are separated from one another by essentially normal neural parenchyma. A large central vein drains to the leptomeninges or into the Galenic system. These vascular malformations are less compact than other types and are accompanied by less gliosis, mineralization or evidence of previous hemorrhage. Venous angiomas are the most common type of vascular malformations and comprised 67% of the vascular malformations encountered in a prospective autopsy study.

7. (A, C) Telangiectases, as illustrated in Fig. 43.6, are characterized by the presence of capillary-type vessels that are separated from one another by relatively normal neural parenchyma. Telangiectases may occur anywhere in the brain but are encountered most often in the pons. Hemorrhage from this type of vascular malformation is relatively rare. Telangiectases comprised about 11% of the vascular malformations encountered in a prospective autopsy study.

8. (B) Varices are rare vascular malformations that consist of single anomalous veins. The walls are usually thin and hyalinized. They are distinguished from normal, but congested, vessels primarily by their anomalous location. Varices are usually asymptomatic. They comprised about 3% of the vascular malformation encountered in a prospective autopsy study.

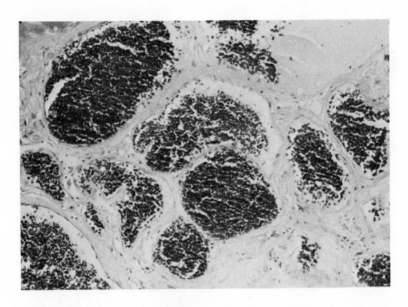

FIG. 43.4: Microscopic section showing a cavernous angioma.

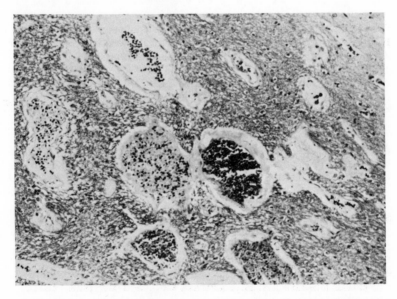

FIG. 43.5: Microscopic section showing a venous angioma.

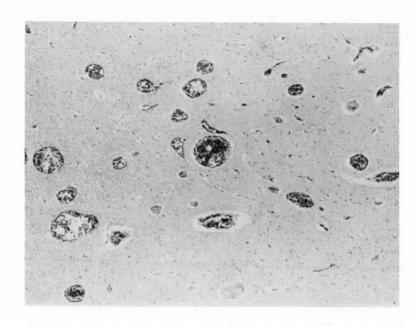

FIG. 43.6:   Microscopic section showing a telangiectasis.

9.   The syndrome of Foix-Alajouanine is a necrotizing myelitis due to the presence of a vascular malformation. Formerly
it was thought to be a form of thrombophlebitis.

REFERENCES

1.   McCormick WF: The pathology of vascular ("arterio-
     venous") malformations. J. Neurosurg 24:807-816, 1966.

2.   McCormick WF, et al.: Vascular malformations ("angio-
     mas") of the brain, with special references to those
     occurring in the posterior fossa. J Neurosurg 28:241-
     251, 1968.

3.   McCormick WF and Nofzinger JD: "Cryptic" vascular
     malformations of the central nervous system. J Neuro-
     surg 24:865-875, 1966.

4.   McCormick WF and Schochet SS Jr.: Atlas of Cerebrovas-
     cular Disease. W. B. Saunders Co., Philadelphia, 1976.

: :

CASE 44: An Infant with Tachypnea, Cyanosis and an Intracerebral Vascular Malformation

CLINICAL DATA

This 4-day-old boy was the product of an uncomplicated pregnancy, labor and delivery. His birth weight was 8 lbs, 4 oz.
He breathed and cried spontaneously and, for the first three
days, did well except for decreased sucking. Early on the
morning of the fourth postnatal day, he began having tachypnea
and developed cyanosis. A chest x-ray revealed cardiomegaly.
He was digitalized and transferred to the university hospital.

On admission, the child had a pulse rate of 140/min and respiratory rate of 80/min. His neck veins were distended and there
was generalized edema. Even with face mask oxygen, his color
was dusky and there were retractions of the costal margins.
Rales were heard over the entire chest and a systolic murmur,
thought not to have been present previously, was heard over
the precordium. The liver extended 6 cm below the costal margin. There were no definite neurological abnormalities.

An electrocardiogram was interpreted as showing right atrial
and biventricular hypertrophy. A cardiac catheterization revealed nearly equal pressures in the left and right ventricles
and 99% oxygen saturation in the innominate and jugular veins.
An angiogram revealed dilatation of the carotid arteries and a
vascular malformation in the area of the vein of Galen. The
child died later the same day.

QUESTIONS

1. The most appropriate diagnosis is
    A. atrial septal defect
    B. vein of Galen aneurysm
    C. dolichoectasia
    D. Sturge-Weber disease

2. Common clinical manifestations of vein of Galen aneurysms
    include
    A. congestive heart failure
    B. intracranial hemorrhage
    C. hydrocephalus
    D. blindness

3. The vascular malformations that give rise to vein of Galen
    aneurysms are
    A. cavernous angiomas
    B. venous angiomas
    C. varices
    D. arteriovenous malformations

4. Other manifestations of the massive vascular shunt in pa-
    tients with vein of Galen aneurysms include
    A. meningeal angiectasia
    B. enlargement of feeding arteries
    C. calcification of the aneurysm wall
    D. enlargement of scalp veins

5. Carotid-cavernous fistulas also produce intracranial
    shunting of blood. These lesions
    A. are usually the result of head trauma
    B. are usually the result of ruptured saccular aneurysms
        on the intracavernous portion of the carotid artery
    C. commonly produce congestive heart failure
    D. commonly produce pulsatile exophthalmos

ANSWERS AND DISCUSSION

1. (B) The most appropriate diagnosis is a vein of Galen
aneurysm. This designation is somewhat misleading since the
primary lesion does not directly involve the vein of Galen. The
aneurysmal dilatation of this structure (Fig. 44.1) is secondary
to shunting of arterial blood through a vascular malformation
into the Galenic vein system. In this patient, the angioma
was located predominantly in the thalamus and tectum of the
mesencephalon (Fig. 44.2). The vascular malformation derived its blood supply primarily from the posterior cerebral
arteries.

2. (A, C) The clinical manifestations of so-called vein of
Galen aneurysms vary with the extent of the vascular shunting
and age of the patient. When the shunt is large, a common
manifestation is intractable heart failure. As in the present
case, these infants are often misdiagnosed initially as having
congenital heart malformations. For this reason, it is often
recommended that the cerebral vessels should be examined
angiographically if no other cause for the heart failure can be
identified.

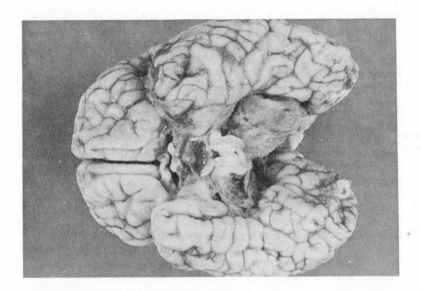

FIG. 44.1: Base of brain showing the vein of Galen aneurysm.

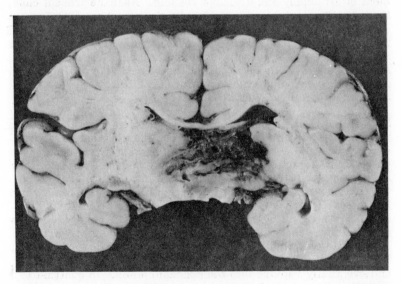

FIG. 44.2: Coronal section of cerebral hemispheres showing
the vascular malformation responsible for the dilatation of the Galenic vein.

If the vascular shunting is somewhat less extensive, the patient may present as an older infant or child with hydrocephalus. This is due to the mass effect of the progressively enlarging vein of Galen aneurysm with compression and deformation of adjacent structures including the aqueduct. The onset of clinical manifestations from the hydrocephalus may be quite sudden.

Subarachnoid or intracerebral hemorrhage in association with vein of Galen aneurysms is uncommon and is probably derived from the underlying vascular malformation rather than the dilated Galenic vein. Various focal neurological deficits may develop occasionally from ischemic necrosis of neural parenchyma secondary to the diversion of blood, the "steal," by the vascular malformation.

3. (D) The vascular malformations that give rise to vein of Galen aneurysms are arteriovenous malformations. This is probably the only type of vascular malformation through which there is adequate shunting of blood to produce the secondary Galenic vein dilatation.

4. (A, B, D) The massive shunting of blood is reflected not only by enlargement of the vein of Galen but also be enlargement of all supply and drainage vessels. As in the present case, the carotid arteries and occasionally the vertebral arteries are enlarged. The pial vessels may become abnormally ectatic and tortuous, so-called "meningeal angiectasia." The dural sinuses and jugular veins regularly become dilated and the scalp veins may become dilated. The wall of the dilated vein of Galen becomes thickened and may even mineralize but this is probably not a manifestation of the shunting.

5. (A, D) Carotid-cavernous fistulas are abnormal connections between the internal carotid artery and the adjacent cavernous sinus. The majority are the result of head trauma, usually a basilar skull fracture involving sphenoid bone. Less often they have been attributed to the rupture of a saccular aneurysm on the cavernous portion of the internal carotid artery. In a very few cases, they have been associated with Ehlers-Danlos disease. As a result of the shunting of blood, the cavernous sinus and draining veins, especially the ophthalmic veins, enlarge. A pulsatile exophthalmos commonly develops. In some cases, the enlarged veins erode the sella turcica and sphenoid bone and eventually rupture into the sphenoid sinus. In contrast to patients with vein of Galen aneurysms, these patients usually do not develop congestive heart failure. Surgical repair or closure of carotid-cavernous fistulas is complicated and not very satisfactory at the present time.

REFERENCES

1. McCormick WF and Schochet SS Jr.: Atlas of Cerebro-
    vascular Disease. W. B. Saunders Co., Philadelphia,
    1976.

2. Montoya G, et al.: Arteriovenous malformation of the
    vein of Galen as a cause of heart failure and hydro-
    cephalus in infants. Neurology 21:1054-1058, 1971.

3. Stehbens WE: Pathology of the Cerebral Blood Vessels.
    C.V. Mosby Co., St. Louis, 1972, pp. 493-495; 529-
    534.

4. Stehbens WE, et al.: Aneurysm of vein of Galen and
    diffuse meningeal angiectasia. Arch Path 95:333-335,
    1973.

: :

CASE 45: An 81-Year-Old Woman with Leukemia and Rapid
         Deterioration of her Neurological Status

CLINICAL DATA

This 81-year-old woman was evaluated because of progressive
weakness. She had had no recurrent infections or episodes of
bleeding. Physical examination disclosed no significant abnormalities; she had no lymphadenopathy, hepatomegaly or splenomegaly. Laboratory studies revealed a hemoglobin of 11.8 g/dl,
a hematocrit of 35% and a white blood cell count of 1600 consisting of 87% lymphocytes, 10% neutrophils and 3% blasts. A bone
marrow aspiration yielded hypocellular marrow with 20 to 25%
blasts. The patient was considered to be preleukemic and no
treatment was given.

Four months later, the patient was hospitalized because of weakness and "bruising" without any precipitating injuries. Physical examination revealed multiple ecchymoses on her arms,
chest and back and multiple petechiae on her lower legs. She
had a soft systolic heart murmur, and both the liver and spleen
were moderately enlarged. Neurological examination revealed
no abnormalities. Laboratory studies revealed a hemoglobin
of 8.2 g/dl, a platelet count of 130,000 platelets/cmm and a white
blood cell count of 278,000 consisting of 6% lymphocytes, 2%
neutrophils and 92% blasts. Aspirated bone marrow was interpreted as acute myelocytic leukemia. Thioguanine and cytosine
arabinoside were begun. The next day, the patient's hemoglobin
fell to 7.2 g/dl and the platelets fell to 25,000/cmm. Two days
after the initiation of chemotherapy, the patient became comatose and died without localizing neurological signs.

QUESTIONS

1. The very rapid deterioration of this patient's neurological
    status was most likely due to
    A. meningeal leukemia
    B. disseminated necrotizing leukoencephalopathy
    C. intracranial hemorrhages
    D. progressive multifocal leukoencephalopathy

2. Patients with leukemia are susceptible to a wide variety
    of opportunistic infections. These include
    A. staphylococcal meningitis
    B. "gram-negative meningitis"
    C. aspergillosis
    D. toxoplasmosis

3. Leukemic infiltration of the leptomeninges occurs most
    often in
    A. acute lymphocytic leukemia
    B. acute myelocytic leukemia
    C. adults
    D. children

4. The clinical manifestations of meningeal leukemia, i.e.,
    leukemic infiltration of the leptomeninges and their intra-
    cerebral perivascular extensions include
    A. headaches
    B. vomiting
    C. meningeal irritation
    D. cerebellar ataxia

5. A combination of intrathecal methotrexate and irradiation
    is commonly employed for the treatment or prevention of
    central nervous system involvement in acute lymphocytic
    leukemia. A recently delineated complication of this
    regimen is
    A. progressive multifocal leukoencephalopathy
    B. disseminated necrotizing or subacute leukoencephalo-
        pathy
    C. the Gordon phenomenon
    D. choroid plexitis

6. Vincristine, an alkaloid employed in the chemotherapy of
    leukemia, is known to produce
    A. peripheral neuropathy
    B. toxic myopathy
    C. bone marrow depression
    D. choroid plexitis

ANSWERS AND DISCUSSION

1. (C) The very rapid deterioration of this patient's neurological status was due to subarachnoid and intracerebral hemorrhages, as illustrated in Fig. 45.1. Intracranial hemorrhages
constitute one of the most common and serious complications of
leukemia. The prevalence of intracranial hemorrhage has ranged
from 11 to 70% among the various reported series. Hemorrhages
have been described in association with all types of leukemia but
occur most often with acute leukemias and during acute exacerbations (blastic crises) of the chronic forms. Hemorrhages are
distinctly less common in association with chronic lymphocytic
leukemia.

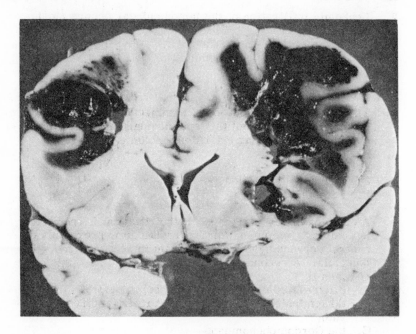

FIG. 45.1: Coronal section of the cerebral hemispheres show-
             ing the multiple intraparenchymal and subarachnoid
             hemorrhages in this patient.

Characteristically, the hemorrhages tend to be multiple and can
involve all parts of the brain with only a slight predilection for
the white matter.   The subarachnoid and subdural spaces also
can be affected.   The intraparenchymal hemorrhages may have
a distinctive gross appearance when they accompany leukemic
infiltrates. As illustrated in Fig. 45.2, the lesions may appear
as irregular aggregates of greyish neoplastic tissue surrounded
by hemorrhage.

The development of intraparenchymal hemorrhages has been
correlated by various authors with the degree of leukocytosis
or with the severity of thrombocytopenia.   Fritz, et al., reported fatal hemorrhages to be five times more frequent among
patients with leukocyte counts of 300,000 or greater than in patients with lesser degrees of leukocytosis. Moore, et al., con-
cluded that the majority of intracerebral hemorrhages in patients with acute leukemia were related to the blastic crises
but regarded the regularly associated thrombocytopenia as an

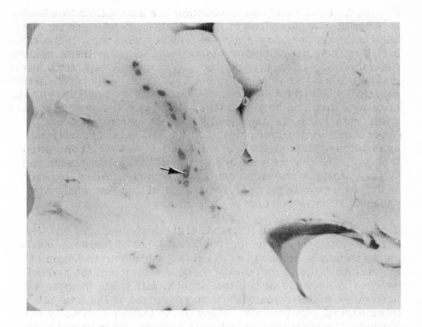

FIG. 45. 2: Close-up photograph showing the characteristic ap-
            pearance of hemorrhage in association with leuke-
            mic infiltrates. Note the central nidus of leukemic
            infiltrate (arrow). These lesions may be large or
            small as illustrated here.

important contributory factor. Other authors, such as McCormick and Rosenfield, felt that thrombocytopenia was the major
factor predisposing to hemorrhage regardless of the types of
leukemia. Even those workers who emphasized leukostasis in
the production of intracerebral hemorrhage, accepted thrombocytopenia as the underlying factor for subarachnoid hemorrhage.
In contrast to most other authors, Price and Warren attributed
the intracerebral hemorrhages in their patients with acute lymphocytic leukemia to ischemic changes from perivascular infiltrates or infectious vasculopathy. None of their patients had
terminal leukocyte counts over 200,000 cells/cmm and the degree of thrombocytopenia was essentially the same in both the
patients with and without hemorrhage. These latter interpre-
tations do not appear applicable to all cases, since hemorrhages
can be seen with minimal leukemic infiltration.

2. (B, C, D) Patients with leukemia are susceptible to a host
of opportunistic infections of the nervous system. Among the
bacterial infections, meningitis caused by gram-negative enteric
bacilli is the most common. In part due to better therapeutic
control of the bacterial infections, opportunistic mycotic infections have become more prevalent. Of these, aspergillosis is
especially important in patients with leukemia. Other fungal
infections that may be encountered in the nervous system of patients with leukemia are candidiasis and cryptococcosis.
Opportunistic toxoplasma encephalitis has been encountered
most often with Hodgkin's disease but also has accompanied
leukemia. Of the viruses, infections with varicella-zoster and
cytomegalovirus have been especially common. About one-half
of the patients with progressive multifocal leukoencephalopathy
have had either lymphoma or leukemia.

3. (A, D) Leukemia infiltration of the leptomeninges and the
perivascular spaces can occur with all types of leukemia but is
most frequently encountered in acute lymphocytic leukemia of
childhood. Without aggressive therapy directed at the central
nervous system, 60-80% of the patients with acute lymphocytic
leukemia would eventually develop meningeal and perivascular
intracerebral involvement. Many of the lesions commonly regarded as leukostasis and leukemic nodules are interpreted as
deep arachnoidal extensions by Price and Johnson. They feel
that true intraparenchymal invasion is relatively uncommon
and when present, results from destruction of the pial-glial
membrane with extension of cells from deep arachnoidal infiltrates. This is in contrast to the older concepts of transmural
migration of leukemic cells through capillaries.

4. (A, B) Until very recently, the incidence of meningeal leukemia had been increasing as a result of the extended survival
of children with acute lymphocytic leukemia treated by chemotherapy. The main clinical features are those of increased intracranial pressure including headache, vomiting, irritability,
and lethargy. Cranial nerve palsies and seizures are not uncommon and papilledema can usually be demonstrated. Meningeal irritation, i.e., nuchal rigidity, Kernig's sign and Brudzinski's sign, is usually not present unless there is a coexistent
infection. Cerebrospinal fluid examination usually reveals a
normal or only slightly reduced glucose content and a normal
or only slightly elevated protein content. The cell count is generally increased but the precise identification of the cells as
leukemic cells is often difficult.

5.   (B) The combination of intrathecal methotrexate and irradiation has been found to be an effective means for the treatment or prevention of central nervous system involvement by
acute lymphocytic leukemia.   Recently, a necrotizing leukoencephalopathy, variously described as disseminated necrotizing
leukoencephalopathy or subacute leukoencephalopathy, has been
recognized as a complication of this combined therapy.   Similar lesions also have been reported following the use of intraventricular methotrexate and radiation for the therapy of posterior
fossa neoplasms. Thus, the leukoencephalopathy appears to be
a complication of the therapy rather than another manifestation
of the leukemia. The lesions consist predominantly of confluent
or multiple discrete foci of necrosis in the cerebral white
matter. Reactive axons and mineralized debris are found within the lesions. The inflammatory reaction is minimal, vascular
changes are inconstant, but gliosis is prominent.

The Gordon phenomenon was originally described as the destruction of Purkinje cells in animals that had been given intracerebral injections of emulsified tumor from patients with
Hodgkin's disease. Later, it was shown that the Purkinje cell
destruction also resulted from intrathecal injections of bone
marrow and especially eosinophil extracts.

Choroid plexitis and destruction of cerebellar granule cells have
been produced experimentally in rats by administration of high
doses of cyclophosphamide.

6.   (A, B) Vincristine is unique among the present cancer
chemotherapy agents inasmuch as neurotoxicity is the major
complication. In man, the most prominent complication is
peripheral neuropathy. Paresthesias are early subjective manifestations of the toxicity. Motor involvement, preceded by depression of the deep tendon reflexes, is the most disabling manifestation.   The cranial nerves may be involved with ptosis as
the most conspicuous manifestation. In experimental animals,
myopathy is more severe than the peripheral neuropathy, but
in man, only minor changes have been demonstrated in muscle.
Inappropriate intrathecal administration of vincristine has been
reported to cause an ascending paralysis accompanied by the
formation of intraneuronal microtubule crystals.

REFERENCES

1.   Azzarelli B and Roessmann U: Pathogenesis of central
      nervous system infiltration in acute leukemia. Arch Path
      Lab Med 101:203-205, 1977.

2. Fritz RD, et al.: The association of fatal intracranial hemorrhage and "blastic crisis" in patients with acute leukemia. N Eng J Med 261:59-64, 1959.

3. McCormick WF and Rosenfield DB: Massive brain hemorrhage: A review of 144 cases and an examination of their causes. Stroke 4:946-954, 1973.

4. Meyer RD, et al.: Aspergillosis complicating neoplastic disease. Amer J Med 54:6-15, 1973.

5. Moore EW, et al.: The central nervous system in acute leukemia. Arch Int Med 105:451-468, 1960.

6. Price RA and Birdwell DA: The central nervous system in childhood leukemia: III. Mineralizing microangiopathy and dystrophic calcification. Cancer 42:717-728, 1978.

7. Price RA and Jamieson PA: The central nervous system in childhood leukemia: II. Subacute leukoencephalopathy. Cancer 35:306-318, 1975.

8. Price RA and Johnson WW: The central nervous system in childhood leukemia: I. The arachnoid. Cancer 31:520, 533, 1973.

9. Rubinstein LJ, et al.: Disseminated necrotizing leukoencephalopathy: A complication of treated central nervous system leukemia and lymphoma. Cancer 35:291-305, 1975.

10. Weiss HD, et al.: Neurotoxicity of commonly used antineoplastic agents. N Eng J Med 291:75-80, 127-133, 1974.

: :

CASE 46:   A 56-Year-Old Woman with a Left Frontal Lobe
           Metastasis

CLINICAL DATA

This 56-year-old woman was admitted to the hospital because
of progressive dizziness and confusion. Shortly after admission,
she developed a right hemiparesis and dysphagia. A brain scan
showed increased isotope uptake in the left fronto-temporal area.
A left carotid angiogram demonstrated a left frontal lobe lesion. A craniotomy was performed and the resected tissue was
interpreted as metastatic undifferentiated carcinoma. She was
treated with systemic chemotherapy and radiation to her head.

The patient did well for nine months, at which time she experienced increased ataxia. On the day of rehospitalization, she
had a seizure followed by post-ictal confusion. The patient was
given additional radiotherapy and chemotherapy and improved
temporarily. She eventually died one year after her initial
hospitalization.

QUESTIONS

1.   The most likely sources for this woman's cerebral meta-
     stases are carcinoma of the
     A. cervix
     B. lung
     C. breast
     D. pancreas

2.   Fig. 46.1 illustrates some of the metastases found in this
     patient's brain. Cerebral metastases are typically
     A. solitary
     B. focally to extensively necrotic
     C. confined to the perfusion area of the basilar artery
     D. surrounded by severely edematous neural parenchyma

3.   Patients with cerebral metastases from carcinoma of the
     lung generally survive
     A. 3-6 months
     B. 6-12 months
     C. 1-3 years
     D. more than five years

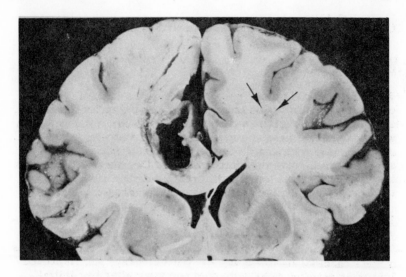

FIG. 46. 1: Coronal section of this patient's brain showing a large
cystic metastasis in the left frontal lobe and a smaller metastasis in the right frontal lobe (arrows).

4. Occasionally, metastatic carcinoma will diffusely infiltrate
    the leptomeninges rather than forming discrete intraparen-
    chymal masses. The clinical manifestations observed in
    patients with this pattern of metastasis usually include
    A. headaches
    B. changes in mental status
    C. dysfunction of multiple cranial nerves
    D. inappropriate ADH syndrome

5. Cerebrospinal fluid findings characteristic of meningeal
    carcinomatosis include
    A. normal glucose content
    B. elevated protein content
    C. negative cultures
    D. atypical or frankly malignant cells

6. Neurological syndromes described in patients with car-
    cinomas, but in the absence of central nervous system
    metastases, include
    A. subacute cerebellar degeneration
    B. carcinomatous neuropathy
    C. Eaton-Lambert syndrome
    D. parkinsonism

ANSWERS AND DISCUSSION

1. (B, C) Metastases constitute the largest single group of intracranial neoplasms encountered at autopsy. The most common sources of cerebral metastases are carcinoma of the lung and carcinoma of the breast. As many as 65% of cerebral metastases have been reported to come from carcinoma of the lung. This high figure is due to the prevalence of carcinoma of the lung and to the propensity of this malignancy to metastasize to the central nervous system. As many as 38% of lung carcinomas have been reported to be accompanied by cerebral metastases at autopsy. There is little or no correlation between the histological type of lung carcinoma and the occurrence of cerebral metastases. In the present case, the patient was found to have a carcinoma of the left upper lobe bronchus and metastases to the liver, adrenals, lymph nodes, kidney and brain. Carcinoma of the breast is generally found to be the second most common source of cerebral metastases. Other common sources include carcinomas of the kidney, colon, ovary and pancreas. Sarcomas rather infrequently metastasize to the central nervous system. Although melanomas are relatively uncommon lesions, a very high percentage have cerebral metastases.

2. (B, D) Metastases are usually multiple and can involve any part of the central nervous system. The cerebral and cerebellar hemispheres are sites of predilection due to their volume and pattern of blood supply. Metastases in the brain stem and spinal cord are relatively infrequent but often escape clinical detection despite their critical locations. Apparently solitary cerebral metastases occur in less than 25% of the cases and even these often prove to be multiple upon meticulous examination. The metastases often have a granular texture and contain focal to extensive areas of necrosis. As illustrated in Fig. 46.1, metastases may be so extensively necrotic that the lesions mimic abscesses. Grossly, this type of metastasis is best distinguished from an abscess by the absence of a hyperemic border. Even a smear of material aspirated from the interior of the lesion may be confusing, since both will contain necrotic material and inflammatory cells. Quite often, metastases are hemorrhagic and have a dark color. Occasionally, the hemorrhage may be massive and dominates the clinical manifestations. The neural parenchyma surrounding a metastasis is usually severely edematous. This is due to increased vascular permeability, i.e., vasogenic edema, and the edema fluid spreads widely through the white matter. Histologically, the metastatic nature of the lesion usually can be recognized with ease (Fig. 46.2), but the source of the metastasis is rarely evident from the microscopic appearance alone.

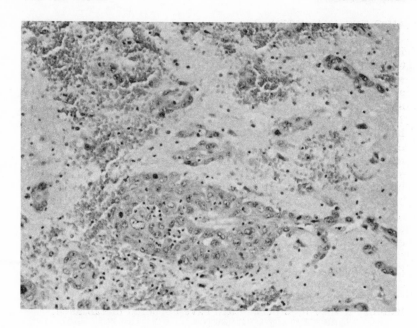

FIG. 46.2: Microscopic section showing some of the small me-
          tastases. The metastatic nature of the lesion is
          obvious, but the origin is not evident histologically.

3. (A) Patients with cerebral metastases from carcinoma of
the lung have an average survival of 3 months when the lesions
are untreated. When surgical extirpation of apparently solitary
metastases, radiation therapy to the head or chemotherapy are
used alone or in combination, the patients generally survive
for 3-6 months. The one-year survival in the present case is
somewhat longer than usual. To date, only six patients have
been reported to survive for more than five years.

4. (A, B, C) Diffuse infiltration of the leptomeninges, or meningeal carcinomatosis, is a relatively uncommon pattern of intracranial metastasis. The meninges become thickened and
infiltrated with tumor and the surface of the brain is obscured
(Figs. 46.3 and 46.4). As with the usual cerebral metastases,
carcinomas of the lung and breast are the most common sources
for meningeal carcinomatosis. The clinical manifestations in
these patients include headache, changes in mental status or
dementia, dysfunction of multiple cranial nerves and ataxia.

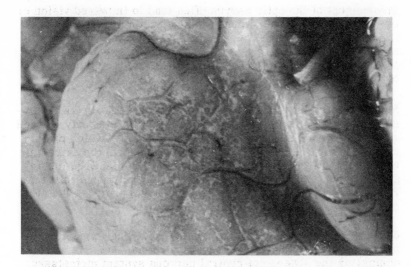

FIG. 46. 3: Close-up photograph of the ventral surface of the
right cerebellar hemisphere from a patient with leptomeningeal carcinomatosis. Note the reticulated
pattern and the complete obscuration of the cerebellar folia.

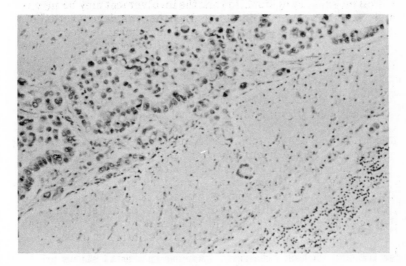

FIG. 46. 4: Microscopic section showing the neoplasm in the leptomeninges over the cerebellum.

Involvement of the optic nerves often lead to impaired vision or even blindness. Involvement of the acoustic nerves may lead to impaired hearing or vestibular dysfunction. Ocular movements are frequently impaired. Initially, these patients are often misdiagnosed as having meningitis, either tuberculous or fungal.

5. (B, C, D) The cerebrospinal fluid from patients with meningeal carcinomatosis characteristically has a markedly reduced glucose content, an elevated cell count and an elevated protein content. Cultures are obviously negative except in the extremely uncommon case where there is a concurrent infectious meningitis. Demonstration of atypical or frankly malignant cells may require multiple spinal fluid examinations but provides the most convincing evidence for the diagnosis.

6. (A, B, C) A number of syndromes have been described in patients with carcinomas, especially ovarian and lung carcinomas, in the absence of central nervous system metastases. Patients with the subacute cerebellar degeneration show ataxia, dysarthria, dysphagia and mental changes. Histologically, there is a striking loss of Purkinje cells, a moderate to mild meningeal lymphocyte infiltration and degeneration of various spinal tracts, especially the spinocerebellar tracts. The patients with carcinomatous neuropathy may have predominantly motor or sensory dysfunction and the involvement may be proximal, distal or focal. Histologically, there is degeneration of sensory ganglia, posterior roots and peripheral nerves. The patients may also have demyelination of the posterior columns of the spinal cord and loss of Purkinje cells. Patients with the Eaton-Lambert syndrome have muscular weakness and fatigability superficially resembling myasthenia gravis. Electromyography demonstrates facilitation of the response upon supramaximal stimulation in contrast to the decay in classical myasthenia gravis. No histological abnormalities can be demonstrated by the conventional techniques. A rare but interesting phenomenon is the occurrence of opsoclonus in patients with occult malignancies. Opsoclonus is a form of ocular dyskinesia in which the eyes display rapid erratic but conjugate movement. This disorder of eye movement has also been observed in some patients with encephalitis. Limited pathological studies have demonstrated loss of Purkinje and granular cells from the cerebellum and mild cell loss from the inferior olivary nuclei.

REFERENCES

1. Bellur SN: Opsoclonus: Its clinical value. Neurology
    25:502-507, 1975.

2. Brain WR and Norris FH Jr.: The Remote Effects of
    Cancer on the Nervous System. Grune and Stratton,
    New York, 1965.

3. Halpert B, et al.: Intracranial involvement from car-
    cinoma of the lung. Arch Path 69:93-103, 1960.

4. Little JR, et al.: Meningeal carcinomatosis. Arch
    Neurol 30:138-143, 1974.

5. Modesti LM and Feldman RA: Solitary cerebral meta-
    stasis from pulmonary cancer. JAMA 231:1064, 1975.

6. Newman SJ and Hansen HH: Frequency, diagnosis and
    treatment of brain metastases in 247 consecutive patients
    with bronchogenic carcinoma. Cancer 33:492-496, 1974.

7. Olson ME, et al.: Infiltration of the leptomeninges by
    systemic cancer. Arch Neurol 30:122-137, 1974.

8. Ross A and Zeman W: Opsoclonus, occult carcinoma and
    chemical pathology in dentate nuclei. Arch Neurol 17:
    546-551, 1967.

: :

CASE 47: An Elderly Man with Focal Seizures and Hemiparesis

CLINICAL DATA

This 78-year-old man developed focal seizures that initially involved his left arm and later progressed to involve his left leg also. The seizures were accompanied by weakness but no loss of consciousness or incontinence.

When seen two months later, the patient had a left hemiparesis but no sensory deficits. The cranial nerves were intact. The deep tendon reflexes on the left were hyperactive and a left Babinski sign was present. A radioisotopic brain scan showed increased uptake in the right hemisphere. A carotid arteriogram showed a midline shift from right to left and a "tumor stain" in the right parietal lobe. Formal neuro-ophthalmological examination disclosed a subtle left hemianopic visual field defect. A chest x-ray was normal.

A right frontoparietal craniotomy was performed and a highly vascular, subcortical neoplasm was biopsied. The patient tolerated the procedure well but became febrile and died from pneumonia ten days later.

QUESTIONS

1. Clinical findings that are pathognomonic of a brain tumor include
   A. headaches
   B. seizures
   C. papilledema
   D. none of these

2. Among the intracranial tumors that are especially common in elderly patients are
   A. cerebellar astrocytomas
   B. meningiomas
   C. ependymomas
   D. glioblastomas

3. Figs. 47.1 and 47.2 illustrate the appearance of the tumor in the present case as seen in the intact brain and after the coronal sectioning. Gross features indicative of a glioblastoma include
   A. involvement of the surface of the brain
   B. hippocampal and cingulate gyrus herniation
   C. apparent circumscription
   D. variegated appearance due to foci of hemorrhage and necrosis

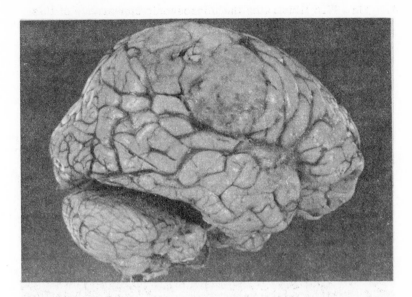

FIG. 47.1: Lateral view of the brain showing the tumor presenting at the surface.

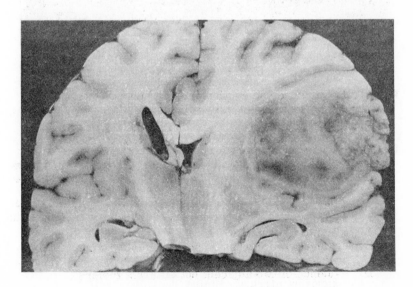

FIG. 47.2: Coronal section of the cerebral hemispheres showing the neoplasm.

4.   Fig. 47.3 illustrates the microscopic appearance of this
     neoplasm. Features characteristic of glioblastoma that
     are seen in this photograph include
     A.   foci of necrosis surrounded by pseudopalisades
     B.   nuclear pleomorphism
     C.   vascular proliferation and glomeruloid formation
     D.   abundant mitoses

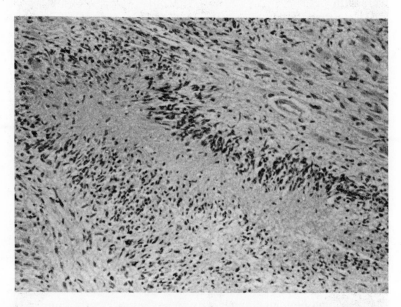

FIG. 47. 3: Microscopic section showing some of the histologi-
             cal features of this neoplasm.

5.   At the time of surgery, a frozen section was prepared
     and the specimen was diagnosed as an astrocytoma. In view
     of the findings at autopsy, this discrepancy is best explain-
     ed as
     A.   an error in interpretation of the findings in the frozen
          section
     B.   a sampling problem
     C.   evidence of progression of the lesion to a more malig-
          nant form
     D.   evidence of two adjacent but different tumors

6. Feigin tumors consist of
   A. an underlying glioblastoma
   B. an overlying fibrosarcoma
   C. nodular masses of glial tissue within the peritoneal
      cavity
   D. glial tissue in ovarian teratomas

7. Extracranial metastases have been reported in patients
   with
   A. medulloblastomas
   B. glioblastomas
   C. meningiomas
   D. none of these

8. The majority of patients with glioblastomas survive
   A. less than one month
   B. less than nine months
   C. more than two years
   D. more than five years

ANSWERS AND DISCUSSION

1. (D) There are no signs or symptoms that can be regarded
as truly pathognomonic of a brain tumor. Headaches are a
common complaint and are often severe but intermittent. They
are often aggravated by activities that increase the intracranial
pressure. The headaches are of little localizing value since
they tend to be generalized, but they may be accompanied by
head tenderness in the vicinity of the tumor. Nausea and vomiting are less frequent complaints in adults than in children.
Papilledema develops especially in association with tumors that
directly or indirectly impede the circulation of the cerebrospinal fluid. Slowly growing, non-obstructing neoplasms may
become quite large without producing papilledema. The onset
of seizures in a non-traumatized individual beyond the second
decade of life is suggestive of a tumor of the cerebral hemispheres. Clinical differentiation from a vascular lesion must
be based on angiography. Alterations in the patient's mental
status may occur in association with tumors.

2. (B, D) The three tumors that are most commonly encountered in elderly patients are meningiomas, metastases,
and glioblastomas. Meningiomas are more common in women
than in men, and many are found as incidental lesions at the
time of autopsy. They are predominantly surface lesions that
displace rather than invade the underlying neural parenchyma.

Metastases constitute the largest group of intracranial neoplasms encountered at autopsy in elderly individuals. Most
common are metastases from carcinoma of the lung or breast.
Glioblastomas are the most common glial neoplasms and the
most common primary intracranial neoplasms. They may arise
in any part of the central nervous system but are found most
often in the frontal or temporal lobes and rarely in the cerebellum or spinal cord. They are most prevalent in adult men
between the ages of 45 and 60. Glioblastomas of the pons constitute a special category and are often found as a component of
pontine gliomas in children. Multiple discrete glioblastomas
are found in a small number of patients; between 2.5 and 5% of
patients with primary gliomas. Extensions from one part of
the brain to another, e.g., across the corpus callosum, are
more frequently encountered.

3. (C, D) The most characteristic gross feature of glioblastomas is the variegated appearance that results from foci of
hemorrhage and necrosis within the tumor. Cysts containing
blood or proteinaceous fluid also may be present. The tumors
often appear to be sharply circumscribed; however, this is
readily shown to be spurious upon microscopic examination of
the surrounding tissue. Although glioblastomas appear to arise
from deep within the brain, they often extend to the pial surface
and invade the leptomeninges or even become attached to the
dura. The resulting fibroblastic proliferation may mimic the
gross appearance of a meningioma. The prominent hippocampal and subfalcial herniation are largely the result of the
associated edema and are common to any appropriately located space-occupying masses.

4. (A, B) Foci of necrosis surrounded by pseudopalisades, as
seen in Fig. 47.3, are the most characteristic histological features of glioblastomas and must be present in order to warrant
this diagnosis. The palisades are composed of both neoplastic
cells and reactive microglia. Various vascular changes, including endothelial proliferation, proliferation of small vessels
forming glomeruloids and proliferation of perivascular fibrous
tissue, are typically found in glioblastomas but are not illustrated in this photograph. Glioblastomas are highly cellular
and often show marked nuclear and cytoplasmic pleomorphism.
Mitotic figures are variable in number. Some glioblastomas
contain exceedingly bizarre giant cells with large atypical nuclei.
These tumors are designated most appropriately as giant cell
glioblastomas although some writers had previously interpreted
them as sarcomas derived from blood vessels and called them
monstrocellular sarcomas. The glial nature of these giant cells
has been confirmed by electron microscopy.

5. (B) Tissue remote from the center of the neoplasm often appears less malignant. For this reason, the grading of gliomas on the basis of biopsy specimens is often misleading. Glioblastomas are often so extremely anaplastic and dedifferentiated that their derivation from astrocytes is not readily evident. Nevertheless, Rubinstein feels that the majority of glioblastomas arise from anaplasia of smaller pre-existing astrocytomas. However, some glioblastomas may arise de novo.

6. (A, B) Glioblastomas readily invade the leptomeninges. However, similar invasion of the subarachnoid space is encountered frequently with more benign gliomas. Glioblastomas also may become adherent to, and invade, the dura. In some cases, especially those with dural attachment, an overlying fibrosarcoma develops from neoplastic transformation of endothelial cells and/or fibroblasts. These lesions have been designated as Feigin tumors. The exact pathogenesis of these tumors is unclear. Other cases have been reported in which a fibrosarcoma was thought to have induced a glial tumor.

7. (A, B, C) Extracranial metastases are very rare but have been described with medulloblastomas, meningiomas, and all types of gliomas. They are found almost exclusively in patients who have been treated surgically. The most common sites of metastases are the cervical lymph nodes, lungs, and bone marrow.

8. (B) The majority of patients with glioblastomas survive less than nine months and virtually all die within two years.

REFERENCES

1. Manuelidis EE and Solitare GB: Glioblastoma Multiforme. In: Pathology of the Nervous System. Minckler J (Ed.). McGraw-Hill Book Co., New York, 1971, Vol. 2, pp. 2026-2071.

2. Rubinstein LJ: Tumors of the Central Nervous System. Armed Forces Institute of Pathology, Washington, 1972, pp. 7-15, 55-85.

3. Russell DS and Rubinstein LJ: Pathology of Tumors of the Nervous System. Williams and Wilkins Co., Baltimore, 1977, pp. 226-244.

: :

CASE 48: A 13-Year-Old Boy with a Two-Year History
of Episodic Headaches and Vomiting

CLINICAL DATA

This 13-year-old boy had a two-year history of episodes of headaches and vomiting. During the six weeks prior to admission,
these complaints had become much more severe.

On admission, the patient was irritable and apprehensive. The
general physical examination was within normal limits. The
pupils were equal and reacted normally to light. Funduscopic
examination revealed early papilledema. Evaluation of extraocular movements elicited nystagmus to the right. Finger to
nose testing demonstrated a mild intention tremor, and tandem
walking and hopping were done poorly. Evaluation of motor
function revealed a full range of motion and normal strength.
Deep tendon reflexes were normal and sensation was intact.

A brain scan was performed and interpreted as showing abnormal isotope uptake in the vermis and possibly the right cerebellar hemisphere. Ventriculography demonstrated moderate
dilatation of the lateral and third ventricles and anterior displacement of the aqueduct.

A suboccipital craniectomy was performed and revealed a cystic
reddish-yellow mass in the vermis and a cyst in the right cerebellar hemisphere.

QUESTIONS

1. Included in the differential diagnosis of posterior fossa
   tumors in childhood are
   A. medulloblastomas
   B. cerebellar astrocytomas
   C. ependymomas
   D. pontine gliomas

2. Clinical features that favor the diagnosis of a cerebellar
   astrocytoma rather than a medulloblastoma in this patient
   are
   A. long history of symptoms
   B. absence of cranial nerve palsies

    C.   evidence of involvement of cerebellar hemispheres
    D.   hydrocephalus

3.   The presence of a cystic lesion in the cerebellar hemis-
     phere, as found at surgery, favors a diagnosis of
    A.   medulloblastoma
    B.   cerebellar astrocytoma
    C.   ependymoma
    D.   hemangioblastoma

4.   Fig. 48.1 is a photograph of a microscopic section pre-
     pared from this neoplasm. The microscopic features
     support a diagnosis of
    A.   medulloblastoma
    B.   cerebellar astrocytoma
    C.   ependymoma
    D.   hemangioblastoma

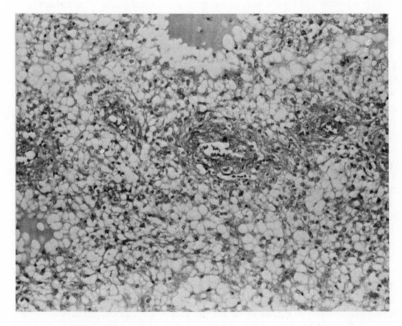

FIG. 48. 1: Microscopic section showing the histological features
in this posterior fossa neoplasm.

5. Rosenthal fibers are
   A. eosinophilic, rounded or elongated structures
   B. associated with and probably derived from astrocytic
      microfilaments
   C. diagnostic of astrocytic neoplasms
   D. condensation products of the proteinaceous cyst fluid
      in cerebellar astrocytomas

6. Patients with surgically resectable cerebellar astrocyto-
   mas generally survive
   A. more than 10 years
   B. more than 5 years
   C. less than 2 years
   D. less than 6 months

7. Morphologically similar neoplasms may be found in the
   A. spinal cord
   B. diencephalon
   C. optic nerves
   D. pons

ANSWERS AND DISCUSSION

1. (A, B, C, D) All of these neoplasms must be considered in
the differential diagnosis of posterior fossa tumors in children.
Medulloblastomas and cerebellar astrocytomas are the most
common, occur with about equal frequency, and together comprise about 60% of the posterior fossa tumors in children.
Ependymomas and pontine gliomas are less common, and
hemangioblastomas of the cerebellum are unusual in children.

2. (A, C) The clinical manifestations of medulloblastomas
and cerebellar astrocytomas are quite similar, i.e., evidence
of a posterior fossa neoplasm. Although medulloblastomas can
be found in older children and even adults, they are most commonly encountered between the ages of 4 and 10 years and present as midline lesions. The cerebellar astrocytomas tend to
have a longer history of symptoms, many months to a year or
more; they occur predominantly in older children and often display evidence of cerebellar hemisphere involvement. Ependymomas can mimic either of these neoplasms. Definitive diagnosis of these neoplasms must be made morphologically.

3. (B) Cerebellar astrocytomas commonly contain cysts or
even occur as small mural nodules in the wall of a large cyst.
They may involve the cerebellar hemispheres, the vermis or
both. Hemangioblastomas are also commonly cystic and may

occur as small, highly vascular nodules in the wall of a large,
often hemorrhagic cyst. Hemangioblastomas usually involve
the cerebellum but may arise from the medulla or spinal cord.
Medulloblastomas usually involve the cerebellar vermis but
may involve the cerebellar hemispheres. They are homogeneous, solid tumors that rarely show cyst formation or extensive
hemorrhage. Posterior fossa ependymomas usually arise within the fourth ventricle and compress adjacent structures. They
tend to be granular, solid masses. Cysts are less common in
the posterior fossa ependymomas than in the large supratentorial lesions.

4.   (B) Histologically, this is a typical cerebellar astrocytoma.
The distinctive morphological features include the loosely associated stellate astrocytes that become more compactly aggregated about the blood vessels, and the extensive areas of microcystic degeneration. The astrocytes may show a moderate degree of pleomorphism but mitoses are very rarely encountered.
The blood vessels may show endothelial hyperplasia.   The
microcystic areas are filled with a proteinaceous fluid. Rosenthal fibers may be found about the blood vessels and are often
very numerous in the walls of large cysts that contain mural
nodules. Some of the European authors designate these tumors
as spongioblastomas.

5.   (A, B) Rosenthal fibers are rounded or fusiform structures
that form within astrocytes in association with, and probably
from, the astrocytic microfilaments.   They stain red with eosin,
red with the Movat pentachrome stain and deep purple with the
phosphotungstic acid-hematoxylin stain.   They were first described in the walls of syringomyelic cavities. Although they
are commonly found in cerebellar astrocytomas, diencephalic
gliomas and spinal cord gliomas, they are not restricted to
astrocytomas or even neoplasms. They are commonly found
in the glial walls of cysts associated with hemangioblastomas,
adjacent to craniopharyngiomas, in the glia within the center
of the normal pineal gland, within ependymal granulations and
occasionally in old infarcts or other destructive lesions. They
are especially widespread and abundant in the brains of children with Alexander's disease. Alexander's disease is generally
classified among the leukodystrophies but is probably a metabolic disorder of astrocytes.

6.   (A) The cystic cerebellar astrocytomas located in the cerebellar hemispheres are surgically accessible and generally have
a favorable prognosis. Eighty to 90% of these patients have been
reported to survive for more than 10 years.

7.   (B, C) Morphologically similar tumors, variously designated as juvenile astrocytomas or pilocystic astrocytomas of
the juvenile type, occur in the diencephalon and optic nerves of
children. The location of these neoplasms determines their
poor prognosis.

REFERENCES

1.   Bell WE and McCormick WF: Increased Intracranial Pres-
     sure in Children. W. B. Saunders Co. , Philadelphia, 1978,
     pp. 356-379.

2.   Davis RL: Astrocytomas. In: Pathology of the Nervous
     System. Minckler J (Ed.). McGraw-Hill Book Co. , New
     York, Vol. 2, 1971, pp. 2007-2026.

3.   Ross ER: Neural Tumors of Infancy and Childhood. In:
     Pathology of the Nervous System. Minckler J (Ed.).
     McGraw-Hill Book Co. , New York, Vol. 2, 1971, pp.
     2196-2219.

4.   Rubinstein LJ: Tumors of the Central Nervous System.
     Armed Forces Institute of Pathology, Washington, 1972,
     pp. 19-50.

: :

CASE 49:   A Young Girl with Vomiting, Staggering and Falls

CLINICAL DATA

This 3-1/2-year-old girl was admitted to the hospital with a
two-month history of early morning vomiting and a six-week
history of staggering and frequent falls when walking. She had
become increasingly irritable and had episodes of crying. Her
mother noticed a change in the child's facial expression and
quality of her speech.   For one week, the child was having
difficulty in swallowing food.

The general physical examination on admission was within normal limits. The child's head circumference was 48 cm.   The
pupils were equal and reacted normally to light.   The fundi
were normal.   A right lateral gaze palsy and bilateral ptosis
were noted. There was intermittent nystagmus to the left. The
right corneal reflex was diminished and hearing was impaired
on the right.   Examination of motor function revealed a full
range of motion and normal strength in all extremities. The
deep tendon reflexes were hyperactive with bilateral extensor
plantar responses.

Plain skull x-rays were normal. A brain scan revealed abnormal uptake in the midline of the posterior fossa.   Pneumoencephalography demonstrated that the fourth ventricle appeared
flattened and was shifted posteriorly. The prepontine cistern
was narrowed and the pons appeared enlarged.

Two days later, the child developed a cardiorespiratory arrest
and died.

QUESTIONS

1.   The most appropriate clinical diagnosis in this patient is
     A.   medulloblastoma
     B.   cerebellar astrocytoma
     C.   ependymoma
     D.   brain stem glioma

2.   Fig. 49.1 is a photograph of a sagittal section of this child's
     brain. The gross pathological diagnosis is
     A.   medulloblastoma
     B.   cerebellar astrocytoma
     C.   ependymoma
     D.   brain stem glioma

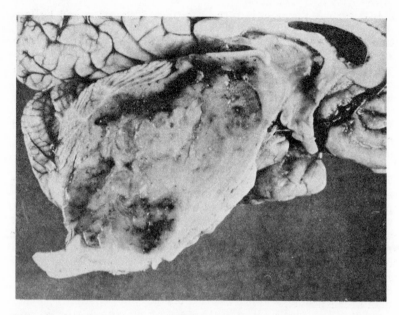

FIG. 49.1: Sagittal section of the brain showing the neoplasm.

3. Histologically, brain stem gliomas are usually
    A. oligodendrogliomas
    B. polar spongioblastomas
    C. pilocystic astrocytomas
    D. glioblastomas

4. The usual therapy for brain stem gliomas is
    A. radiation
    B. chemotherapy
    C. surgical extirpation
    D. shunting

5. Polar spongioblastomas are rare neoplasms that
    A. occur in children
    B. occur in adults
    C. involve the cerebral hemispheres
    D. involve the brain stem

ANSWERS AND DISCUSSION

1.   (D) The combination of an ataxic gait, long tract signs, and multiple cranial nerve palsies in a child is highly suggestive of a brain stem glioma. Signs and symptoms referable to hydrocephalus occur late, if at all, in patients with pontine gliomas but may occur earlier if there is significant mesencephalic involvement. The pneumoencephalographic demonstration of the displacement of the fourth ventricle and enlargement of the pons further support the diagnosis of brain stem glioma. These are relatively uncommon tumors and constitute only 5 to 10% of tumors in children. They occur most often between the ages of 3 and 8 years.

2.   (D) The gross pathological diagnosis is brain stem glioma. The tumor primarily involves the pons but also extends caudally into the medulla and rostrally into the mesencephalon.   These tumors typically produce a diffuse or nodular enlargement of the pons with flattening and posterior displacement of the fourth ventricle. By contrast, medulloblastomas commonly extend into the fourth ventricle from the vermis and ependymomas fill and expand the fourth ventricle. In the past, the neoplastic enlargement of the pons has been erroneously designated as "hypertrophy of the pons." The basilar artery may be deeply invaginated into the ventral surface of the enlarged pons. The rostral extension of the tumor into the mesencephalon probably accounts for the partial third nerve involvement in addition to the more typical pontine cranial nerve palsies. This brain stem glioma contains extensive areas of hemorrhage and necrosis; however, many consist predominantly of rubbery, homogeneous grey-white tissue.

3.   (C, D) Brain stem gliomas are predominantly pilocytic astrocytomas.   This term refers to the tendency for elongated fibrillary astrocytes to insinuate themselves among the pre-existing brain stem structures (Fig. 49.2).   Tumors of this nature are usually homogeneous, grey-white in color and rubbery in consistency. With the passage of time, these tumors become more anaplastic and less well differentiated.   By the time of autopsy, nearly half of these brain stem gliomas contain at least focal areas of glioblastoma. Grossly, these are indicated by areas of hemorrhage and necrosis, as seen in the present case.

4.   (A) The usual therapy for brain stem gliomas is radiation. A few patients who are obstructed may benefit from shunting. The tumor is invariably lethal, but survival may range from a few months to a few years.

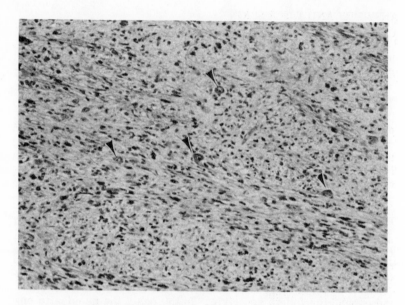

FIG. 49.2: Microscopic appearance of the neoplasm. Note the
persistence of neurons (arrows) within the neural
tissue infiltrated by the neoplasm. Other areas of
the tumor showed glioblastoma multiforme.

5. (A, D) Polar spongioblastoma as defined by Russell and
Cairns is a rare malignant neoplasm of childhood that is usually
located in the brain stem. The tumor has a distinctive morphological appearance consisting of palisades of fusiform cells alternating with bands of cytoplasmic processes. The restricted
use of the term polar spongioblastoma for this distinctive morphological pattern should be noted. Other authors apply similar
terms to a wide variety of neoplasms including the cerebellar
astrocytomas, diencephalic gliomas, pontine gliomas, etc.

REFERENCES

1. Bell WE and McCormick WF: Increased Intracranial Pressure in Children. W. B. Saunders Co., Philadelphia, 1978,
   pp. 356-379.

2. Rubinstein LJ: Tumors of the Central Nervous System.
   Armed Forces Institute of Pathology, Washington, 1972,
   pp. 19-50, 53-55.

: :

CASE 50: A Middle-Aged Man with Dysphagia, Dysphonia
          and Occipital Headaches

CLINICAL DATA

This 59-year-old man experienced the insidious onset of dysphagia and dysphonia. These symptoms fluctuated from day to
day but became progressively more severe. He also developed
occipital headaches that occurred predominantly in the morning
and were made worse by neck flexion or extension and by straining. Neurological examination a few months after the onset of
these symptoms revealed dysphagia, dysphonia, a marked decrease in the gag reflex, an equivocal intention tremor and an
equivocal decrease in pain perception over the C_2 dermatomes.
Plain skull and cervical spine x-rays and a "barium swallow"
study were normal. Brain scan, electromyography, nerve
conduction studies and a Tensilon test were all normal.   An
otolaryngological evaluation and a pharyngeal biopsy specimen
were normal. A pneumoencephalogram was recommended but
refused by the patient.

Six months later, the patient was rehospitalized because of persistent severe dysphagia and a 70-pound weight loss. Bilateral
carotid arteriograms were normal. Two months later, a gas-
trostomy feeding tube was inserted. The patient died a short
time later from pulmonary complications.

QUESTIONS

1.   Fig. 50.1 illustrates the major findings in the central
     nervous system encountered at autopsy. The most
     appropriate gross diagnosis is
     A.   medulloblastoma
     B.   cerebellar astrocytoma
     C.   ependymoma
     D.   hemangioblastoma

2.   Fig. 50.2 is a photograph of a microscopic section pre-
     pared from this neoplasm. The appropriate histological
     diagnosis is
     A.   oligodendroglioma
     B.   ependymoma
     C.   glioblastoma
     D.   hemangioblastoma

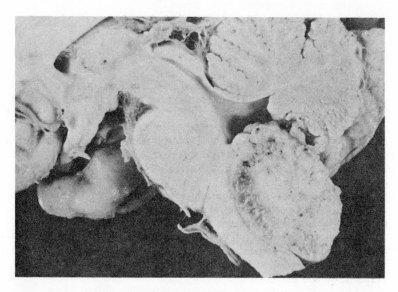

FIG. 50. 1: Sagittal section of the brain showing the neoplasm within the fourth ventricle.

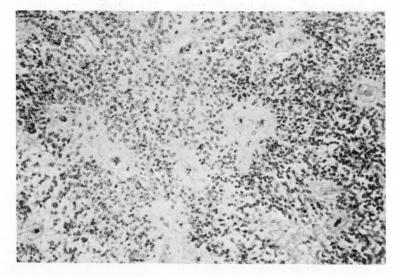

FIG. 50.2: Microscopic section showing the histological characteristics of the neoplasm.

3. Intracranial ependymomas are
   A. usually cytologically benign
   B. usually highly anaplastic
   C. usually diffusely invasive neoplasms
   D. circumscribed expansive lesions

4. Choroid plexus papillomas are derived from the specialized
   ependymal cells of the choroid plexi. They are distinguished
   from ependymomas by their
   A. fibrovascular stroma
   B. papillary configuration
   C. location in the ventricular system
   D. mucus secretion

5. Subependymomas are small, grey-white nodular lesions
   attached to the walls of the ventricles. They are
   A. regarded as a type of ependymoma
   B. regarded as a type of astrocytoma
   C. usually found in children
   D. usually associated with trauma

6. The most common gliomas involving the spinal cord are
   A. glioblastomas
   B. astrocytomas
   C. oligodendrogliomas
   D. ependymomas

7. Myxopapillary ependymomas are found in the
   A. conus medullaris and filum terminale
   B. cerebellum
   C. fourth ventricle
   D. cerebral hemispheres

ANSWERS AND DISCUSSION

1. (C) The most appropriate gross diagnosis is an ependymoma. These are relatively uncommon tumors that comprise
only 5-6% of all intracranial gliomas. Since they are derived
from the ependyma, they are often found in, or in continuity
with, the ventricular system or the central canal of the spinal
cord. About 70% of the intracranial ependymomas arise in the
fourth ventricle, and the majority of these are encountered during the first decade of childhood. By contrast, cerebral ependymomas are more evenly distributed among all age groups. Ependymomas are usually well demarcated masses that compress the
surrounding structures. The infratentorial lesions are usually
solid but may contain small cysts and foci of mineralization. The
supratentorial tumors often contain large cysts. Occasionally,

the tumor may extend out of the fourth ventricle into the cere-
bello-pontine angle and over the dorsolateral aspects of the medulla and upper spinal cord. These lesions have been termed
"plastic ependymomas." Medulloblastomas are very rare in
this patient's age group and would be expected to show evidence
of origin from the cerebellum. Similarly, cerebellar astrocytomas are predominantly tumors of childhood, and ventricular
extension would be associated with an obvious cerebellar mass.
Hemangioblastomas are more common posterior fossa tumors in
adults but usually involve the cerebellum, spinal cord or medulla
rather than the cavity of the fourth ventricle. These tumors are
often cystic and have a distinctive yellow or reddish color.

2.   (B) The appropriate diagnosis is ependymoma. The diagnosis is based on the presence of perivascular pseudorosettes
that surround virtually every vessel within the neoplasm. The
anuclear zone of the perivascular pseudorosette is composed of
cytoplasmic processes that extend toward the blood vessel.
True ependymal rosettes with patent lumens and ependymal
canals are highly characteristic structures in which the neoplastic ependymal cells reflect the relation of normal ependymal
cells to the ventricular system. In our experiences these structures are encountered far less commonly than perivascular
pseudorosettes. The cells surrounding the lumens of ependymal
rosettes and canals may contain cilia and blepharoplasts. These
structures are demonstrated conventionally by the use of the
phosphotungstic acid-hematoxylin stain. However, these specialized structures are of limited diagnostic value since they
are not demonstrable in the majority of ependymomas, and other
organelles, such as mitochondria, can be mistaken for blepharoplasts when evaluated by light microscopy.

Histologically, oligodendrogliomas are composed of sheets of
relatively uniform cells.   Perinuclear halos produced by cytoplasmic swelling are a commonly observed artifact of diagnostic
value. The tumors are highly vascular, and the thin, but conspicuous blood vessels divide the sheets of cells into uniform nests.
Hemangioblastomas are composed of lipid-laden, vacuolated
parenchymal cells with myriads of intervening sinusoidal vessels.

3.   (A, D) Ependymomas are generally well-differentiated, cytologically benign neoplasms.   They tend to produce clinical
symptoms by obstructing cerebrospinal fluid pathways and com-
pressing adjacent structures rather than by invasions of the
neuroparenchyma.   Nevertheless, intracranial ependymomas
have a rather poor prognosis because of the operative complications associated with fourth ventricular tumors and their
poor response to radiation.

4. (A) Choroid plexus papillomas are rare tumors accounting for less than 1% of all intracranial neoplasms. They have been found in all age groups but are somewhat more common in children. The majority, and especially those in adults, occupy the fourth ventricle. Rarely, the tumors in the lateral ventricles have been regarded as responsible for producing hydrocephalus by oversecretion of cerebrospinal fluid. Microscopically, the tumors appear as papillary lesions with the fronds of fibrovascular stroma covered by a layer of columnar or cuboidal epithelium. Occasionally, mucus containing vacuoles are found within the epithelial cells. Cilia and blepharoplasts are very rarely demonstrable by light microscopy. In common with the normal choroid plexus, the endothelial cells lining the vessels within the choroid plexus papillomas are fenestrated. This may prove to be the most accurate criterion for distinguishing choroid plexus papillomas from papillary ependymomas. Occasionally, choroid plexus papillomas may invade the leptomeninges. Very rarely, frankly malignant tumors of the choroid plexus, so-called carcinomas of the choroid plexus, have been described.

5. (A) Subependymomas, also known as subependymal glomerate astrocytomas, have been regarded as a type of ependymoma or as a type of astrocytoma. Grossly they appear as small, grey-white nodules attached to the walls of the ventricles. They are found most often in the fourth ventricle and are more common in older individuals. They rarely, if ever, produce clinically recognizable symptoms and are not associated with any specific antecedent condition or disease. Microscopically, they consist of cellular nests scattered widely in a dense fibrillary stroma. The abundance of glial fibers had been the basis for regarding them as a form of astrocytoma. However, the presence of occasional rosettes, perivascular pseudorosettes and blepharoplasts favors an origin from ependymal cells. Their ultrastructure also supports this interpretation.

6. (D) Although ependymomas are relatively uncommon intracranial gliomas, they are the most common intraspinal gliomas. In contrast to the intracranial tumors, the intraspinal ependymomas are more common in adults with a peak incidence during the fourth decade. The tumors may be intramedullary, in which case they are commonly accompanied by a syrinx, or they may be extramedullary, in which case they commonly involve the conus medullaris or filum terminale.

7. (A) The histologically distinctive tumors designated as myxopapillary ependymomas are largely restricted to the conus

medullaris and filum terminale. These tumors consist of connective tissue stroma and cuboidal to columnar ependymal cells with conspicuously vacuolated cytoplasm. The blood vessels are surrounded by abundant hyalin material. Both the cytoplasmic vacuoles and the connective tissue contain abundant mucin. The tumors are highly vascular and are prone to spontaneous hemorrhage. Some of the patients even present clinically with subarachnoid hemorrhages.

REFERENCES

1. Azzarelli B, et al.: Subependymoma. Acta Neuropath 40:279-282, 1977.

2. Dohrmann GJ and Collias JC: Choroid plexus carcinoma. J Neurosurg 43:225-232, 1975.

3. Kernohan JW: Ependymomas. In: Pathology of the Nervous System. Minckler J (Ed.). McGraw-Hill Book Co., New York, 1971, Vol. 2, pp. 1976-1992.

4. Rawlinson DG, et al.: The fine structure of a myxopapillary ependymoma of the filum terminale. Acta Neuropath 25:1-13, 1973.

5. Rubinstein LJ: Tumors of the Central Nervous System. Armed Forces Institute of Pathology, Washington, 1972, pp. 104-126.

6. Russell DS and Rubinstein LJ: Pathology of Tumors of the Nervous System. Williams and Wilkins Co., Baltimore, 1977, pp. 203-224.

7. Shuman RM, et al.: The biology of childhood ependymomas. Arch Neurol 32:731-739, 1975.

: :

CASE 51: A 7-Year-Old Boy with Headaches and Clumsiness

CLINICAL DATA

This 7-year-old boy was admitted to the hospital with a 9-month history of headaches and clumsiness. The patient's mother stated that his unsteadiness had increased markedly during the month prior to admission.

Physical examination revealed an alert, oriented boy. His pupils were equal and reacted normally to light. Funduscopic examination revealed early papilledema. He had bilateral lateral rectus palsies. Examination of his motor function revealed a full range of motion and normal strength. His deep tendon reflexes were increased bilaterally. His gait was broad-based and ataxic. Tests reflecting cerebellar function, such as tandem walking, hopping and Romberg, were all done poorly. Plain skull x-rays revealed widened sutures. A brain scan was normal. Ventriculography revealed dilatation of the lateral ventricles, third ventricle, aqueduct and rostral portion of the fourth ventricle. A suboccipital craniectomy was performed exposing a tumor filling the fourth ventricle. The tumor was biopsied and the specimen was interpreted as a medulloblastoma. A shunt was inserted and postoperatively, x-ray was administered. The child died 11 months after completion of his radiation therapy.

QUESTIONS

1.   The differential diagnosis of a posterior fossa neoplasm in a child must include
     A.   medulloblastoma
     B.   astrocytoma
     C.   ependymoma
     D.   oligodendroglioma

2.   Fig. 51.1 is a photograph of the biopsy specimen. The histological characteristics of medulloblastomas include
     A.   perivascular pseudorosettes
     B.   hyperchromatic nuclei with scanty cytoplasm
     C.   Homer Wright rosettes
     D.   Flexner-Wintersteiner rosettes

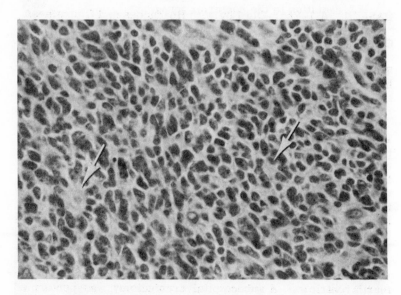

FIG. 51. 1: Microscopic section of the biopsy specimen. Two ro-
    settes are indicated by arrows.

3. Medulloblastomas are currently regarded as being derived
    from
    A. cell nests in the anterior or posterior medullary vela
    B. embryonal mesenchymal cells
    C. the internal granular layer
    D. remnants of the fetal external granular layer

4. Medulloblastomas commonly show
    A. local invasion of meninges
    B. dissemination along cerebrospinal fluid pathways
    C. extracranial metastases to lungs
    D. intracranial metastases to the cerebrum

5. "Cerebellar sarcomas" are
    A. malignant meningiomas of the posterior fossa
    B. arachnoidal sarcomas of the posterior fossa
    C. desmoplastic medulloblastomas
    D. carcinomas metastatic to the leptomeninges of the
        posterior fossa

6. Currently recommended therapy for medulloblastoma is
   A. radiation to the posterior fossa
   B. radiation to the entire neuraxis
   C. radical surgical extirpation followed by local irradiation
   D. chemotherapy alone

7. Fig. 51.2 is a photograph of the autopsy specimen. As a manifestation of the radiation therapy, one sees
   A. no residual tumor
   B. hemorrhage
   C. radiation necrosis
   D. mineralization within the tumor

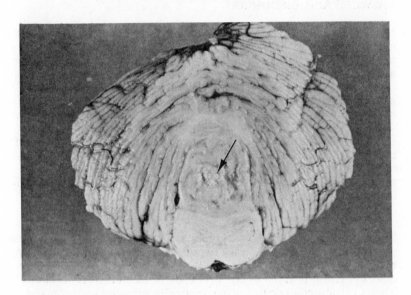

FIG. 51.2: Transverse section of cerebellum and brain stem. Note the foci of mineralization (arrow).

8. Medulloepitheliomas are
   A. primitive multipotential neoplasms derived from the components of the neural tube
   B. primitive ependymal neoplasms
   C. composed of well-differentiated neurons and glial cells
   D. primitive neoplasms of the sympathetic nervous system

9. Cerebral neuroblastomas are
   A. tumors of late adult life
   B. tumors of childhood
   C. characterized by spongioblastic differentiation
   D. primitive tumors that show neuronal differentiation

10. Esthesioneuroblastomas are
    A. encountered predominantly in young adults
    B. derived from the olfactory bulbs and tracts
    C. often first manifested by epistaxis and nasal
       obstruction
    D. radioresistant

ANSWERS AND DISCUSSION

1.   (A, B, C) In children, approximately 70% of all intracranial
neoplasms are infratentorial and of these, the vast majority are
neuroglial. Medulloblastomas and cerebellar astrocytomas are
about equally common and together account for about 60% of posterior fossa tumors in children. Medulloblastomas are most
prevalent during the second half of the first decade, although
some occur during late childhood or even adult life. Cerebellar
astrocytomas are more often found in older children. Ependymomas are the third most common posterior fossa neoplasm of
childhood but are considerably less common than medulloblastomas or astrocytomas. Brain stem gliomas usually produce
multiple cranial nerve palsies and rarely hydrocephalus. Oligodendrogliomas occur predominantly during the fourth and fifth
decades and are usually found in the cerebral hemispheres.

2.   (B, C) The medulloblastomas are highly cellular neoplasms
composed of small cells with hyperchromatic nuclei and scanty
cytoplasm. Mitotic figures are variable in number. A highly
characteristic feature is the presence of Homer Wright rosettes.
These structures consist of peripherally situated nuclei about
eosinophilic fibrillary central zones. Unfortunately, these
rosettes are found in less than one-third of medulloblastomas
and when present are often poorly formed. Flexner-Wintersteiner
rosettes have a clear central lumen and are typically found in
retinoblastomas. Perivascular pseudorosettes are a feature of
ependymomas.

3.   (A, D) Current evidence favors a derivation of the medulloblastoma from residual germinative cells that populate the external granular layer of the fetal cerebellum. During the course
of normal development, multipotential cells arise from the germinal bud in the rhombic roof of the fourth ventricle. These

cells migrate into the anterior and posterior medullary vela
and give rise to the external granular layer of the cerebellum.
Later in the course of development, cells migrate from the external granular layer to populate the internal granular layer.

4.   (A, B, D) Local invasion of the cerebellar leptomeninges
is a very common finding and may stimulate a marked desmoplastic reaction.   Dissemination along the cerebrospinal fluid
pathways is common and is seen in over one-half of the patients
studied at autopsy.   Involvement of the spinal leptomeninges
may be especially pronounced. The tumor may invade the cerebrum as a result of subarachnoid or intraventricular spread.
Extraneural metastases have been reported but are relatively
uncommon.   Among the extraneural sites, bone, lymph nodes,
and liver have been involved most frequently.   The lungs are
usually spared for reasons that are unknown.

5.   (C) The so-called "cerebellar sarcomas" are medulloblastomas that have invaded the leptomeninges and stimulated
an especially marked desmoplastic response.   The fibroblastic
proliferation alters the morphology of the neoplasm so that
nests of more rounded cells are separated by reticulin-rich
bands of elongated cells.   This pattern is somewhat more common among the medulloblastomas of the cerebellar hemispheres
in older individuals.

6.   (B) Medulloblastomas are highly radiosensitive and are
currently treated by radiation to the entire neuraxis.   The entire
neuraxis must be treated because of the frequency of metastases
along the cerebrospinal fluid pathways.   The same therapy should
be given for the so-called "cerebellar sarcomas," the laterally
situated medulloblastomas in older individuals.   Chemotherapy
may be used as an adjuvant but not in place of radiation.

7.   (D) The tumor largely fills the fourth ventricles. Within
the tumor, one sees numerous grey-white granules that are
mineralized.   Extensive hemorrhage, cyst formation, and
mineralization are all uncommon findings among untreated
medulloblastomas. However, after radiation therapy, necrosis
and mineralization may be extensive.

8.   (A) Medulloepitheliomas are rare primitive multipotential
neoplasms derived from the components of the neural tube. The
tumors are found most often in the cerebral hemispheres of
young children.   They appear as papillary or sinusoidal arrays
of columnar cells with evidence of both neuronal and glial differentiation.   Mitoses may be common.

9. (B, D) Cerebral neuroblastomas are rare cerebral neoplasms of children. Morphologically, they are highly cellular
tumors composed of small cells with pleomorphic nuclei and
scanty cytoplasm. Mitotic figures are often abundant. Ill-
defined rosettes and cells showing neuronal differentiation are
important diagnostic features. The tumors may be accompanied by pronounced reactive gliosis and fibroblastic proliferation.

10. (A, C) Esthesioneuroblastomas, otherwise known as olfactory neuroblastomas, are rare neuroblastic neoplasms generally considered to be derived from the olfactory receptor
cells. They are encountered predominantly in adults and often
present with nasal obstructions and epistaxis. Some present
initially as intracranial masses. They are radiosensitive and
have a more favorable prognosis than the extracephalic neuroblastomas of childhood.

REFERENCES

1. Bailey OT: Medulloblastoma. In: Pathology of the Ner-
    vous System. Minckler J (Ed.). McGraw-Hill Book Co.,
    New York, 1971, Vol. 2, pp. 2071-2081.

2. Chatty EM and Earle KM: Medulloblastoma. A report
    of 201 cases with emphasis on the relationship of histo-
    logical variants to survival. Cancer 28:977-983, 1971.

3. Hamilton AE, et al.: Primary intracranial esthesio-
    neuroblastoma (olfactory neuroblastoma). J Neurosurg
    38:548-556, 1973.

4. Kadin ME, et al.: Neonatal cerebellar medulloblastoma
    originating from the fetal external granular layer. J
    Neuropath Exp Neurol 29:583-600, 1970.

5. Lewis MB, et al.: Extra-axial spread of medulloblastoma.
    Cancer 31:1287-1297, 1973.

6. Rubinstein LJ: Tumors of the Central Nervous System.
    Armed Forces Institute of Pathology, Washington, 1972,
    pp. 127-167.

7. Rubinstein LJ: Presidential address: Cytogenesis and
    differentiation of primitive central neuroepithelial
    tumors. J Neuropath Exp Neurol 31:7-26, 1972.

8. Schochet SS, et al.: Intracranial esthesioneuroblastoma.
    Acta Neuropath 31:181-188, 1975.

9. Smith CE, et al.: Medulloblastoma: An analysis of time-
    dose relationships and recurrence patterns. Cancer 32:
    722-728, 1973.

: :

CASE 52: A 58-Year-Old Man with Headache, Slurred Speech
          and a Tendency to Fall to the Right

CLINICAL DATA

This 58-year-old man was admitted to the hospital with a one-
month history of persistent headache, slurred speech, impaired
handwriting, and a tendency to fall to the right.

Physical examination on admission revealed a mildly obese man
in no acute distress. The general physical examination disclosed no abnormalities. Neurological examination revealed
mild disorientation and decreased strength in the right arm.
Skull and chest x-rays, brain scan, an electroencephalogram,
and audiometry were all interpreted as normal. While in the
hospital, his condition improved.

Six weeks later, the patient was readmitted to the hospital complaining of nausea, vertigo, slurred speech, and paralysis of
his right hand.

Physical examination disclosed paralysis of the entire right
arm and horizontal nystagmus. The general physical examination remained non-contributory. His condition progressively
deteriorated and he developed weakness of the right leg, devi-
ation of the tongue, and uvula to the right and a right homonymous hemianopsia.   Extensive evaluation, including multiple
spinal fluid cultures, failed to disclose any infectious process.
A left carotid arteriogram revealed elevation of the proximal
segment of the left middle cerebral artery, mild ventricular
dilatation, and displacement of the internal cerebral veins.
Four months later, the patient developed papilledema, a left
oculomotor paralysis, and eventually died of bronchopneumonia.
A careful autopsy revealed no systemic infections or visceral
neoplasm.

QUESTIONS

1.   Fig. 52.1 illustrates one of the lesions found within the
     brain. Similar-appearing lesions were present in the
     mesencephalon and in the left cerebellar hemisphere.
     The appropriate gross diagnosis is
     A. reticulum cell sarcoma or microglioma
     B. meningioma
     C. astrocytoma
     D. glioblastoma

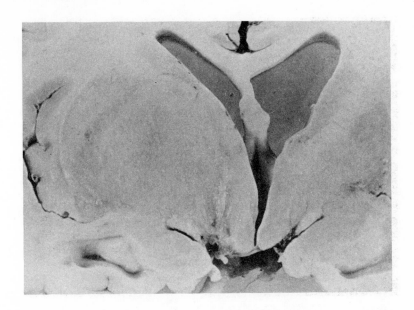

FIG. 52. 1: Coronal section of cerebral hemispheres showing
one of the three lesions in the present case.

2. Fig. 52.2 illustrates the microscopic appearance of the
    tumor. The characteristic histological features include
    A. preponderance of neoplastic lymphoreticular cells
    B. perivascular arrangement of the neoplastic cells
    C. Rosenthal fibers within neoplastic cells
    D. proliferation of perivascular connective tissue

3. Microgliomas are
    A. more common in middle-aged individuals
    B. more common in children
    C. more common in women
    D. exceptionally common among renal transplant
        recipients

4. Hodgkin's disease most often involves the central nervous
    system by
    A. producing nodular infiltrates in the cerebral parenchyma
    B. producing diffuse infiltrates in the leptomeninges
    C. producing spinal cord compression from extradural
        infiltrates
    D. infiltrating cranial nerve and spinal nerve roots

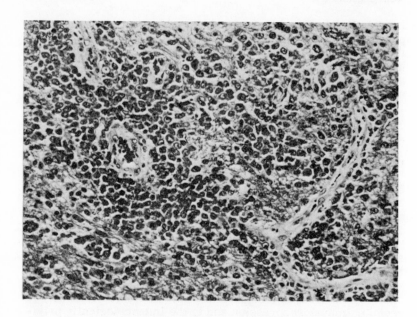

FIG. 52.2: Microscopic section showing the perivascular arrangement of the neoplastic cells.

5. Plasmacytomas, including multiple myeloma, may involve
    the central nervous system by
    A. producing spinal cord compression from extradural
        infiltrates and collapse of affected vertebrae
    B. forming solitary intracerebral mass lesions
    C. producing amyloid angiopathy
    D. producing amyloid deposits in fiber tracts

ANSWERS AND DISCUSSION

1. (A) The terms reticulum cell sarcoma of the brain and
microglioma are now used interchangeably to designate lymphoreticular neoplasms that arise within the nervous system.
These tumors are generally poorly demarcated infiltrative lesions of the cerebral hemispheres. They may be multifocal, as
in the present case. The neoplastic tissue is soft and has a
distinctly granular texture. The color ranges from white to
tan or grey. The lesions rarely appear as necrotic and hemorrhagic as glioblastomas and are more granular than the usual
astrocytomas. Meningiomas are predominantly surface lesions
that compress and displace the adjacent neural parenchyma.

2.   (A, B, D) These tumors are densely cellular lesions composed of neoplastic lymphoreticular cells that closely resemble
the constituents of extracerebral lymphomas. Especially toward
the periphery of the lesions, the neoplastic cells are often
aggregated as perivascular infiltrates. When these areas are
stained for reticulin, a prominent concentric perivascular proliferation of connective tissue can be demonstrated. The
involved neural parenchyma may show a pronounced hyperplasia and hypertrophy of reactive astrocytes. In some of
the cases, the meninges are heavily infiltrated by the neoplastic cells.

3.   (A, D) Microgliomas are relatively rare tumors that probably comprise no more than 1% of all primary central nervous
system neoplasms. They usually become clinically apparent
during the fifth or sixth decades and are more common in men
than in women. They have been exceptionally prevalent among
renal transplant recipients. Organ transplant recipients have
an incidence of tumors approximately 80 times greater than the
general population, and many of their neoplasms are microgliomas. The increased incidence has been attributed variously to
uremia, immunosuppression and to the immunologically privi-
leged status of the central nervous system.

4.   (C) The distinction between microgliomas or reticulum
cell sarcomas of the brain and systemic lymphomas is not an
absolute one. However, most systemic lymphomas, including
Hodgkin's disease, do not produce intraparenchymal infiltrates
within the central nervous system. They may produce limited
leptomeningeal or nerve root infiltration. The usual central nervous system involvement from Hodgkin's disease is
spinal cord compression secondary to spinal extradural infiltrates.

5.   (A, B) Plasmacytomas can affect the nervous system in
several ways. By far the most common is compression of the
spinal cord from collapsed vertebrae and spinal extradural
deposits in patients with multiple myeloma. Patients with
multiple myeloma may also have cranial lesions that secondarily
affect the brain by acting as space-occupying masses. A peripheral neuropathy due to amyloid deposition is commonly encountered in the patients with multiple myeloma, but these
individuals usually do not have amyloid deposits within the
central nervous system. Rarely, intracranial solitary plasmacytomas have been observed in the absence of multiple
myeloma.

REFERENCES

1. Penn I and Starzl TE: Malignant tumors arising de novo in immunosuppressed organ transplant recipients. Transplantation 14:407-417, 1972.

2. Rubinstein LJ: Tumors of the Central Nervous System. Armed Forces Institute of Pathology, Washington, 1972, pp. 215-234.

3. Zimmerman HM: Malignant Lymphomas. In: Pathology of the Nervous System. Minckler J (Ed.). McGraw-Hill Book Co., New York, Vol. 2, 1971, pp. 2165-2178.

: :

CASE 53:   A 48-Year-Old Woman with Headaches, Right-Hand
           Weakness and Ataxia

CLINICAL DATA

This 48-year-old woman was hospitalized with headaches that
had been increasing in severity and frequency over the past six
months.   The headaches were fronto-parietal in location and
were exacerbated by coughing, bending or straining.   The patient also complained of right-hand weakness for the past three
weeks. The family had noticed an unsteady gait and personality
changes over the past five to six weeks.

On admission, the general physical examination was within normal limits.   The patient was somewhat lethargic but oriented.
Her gait was broad-based and slightly ataxic.   She was unable
to tandem walk.   Examination of the eyes revealed bilateral
papilledema and a congruent right superior quadrantanopsia.
Her pupils responded poorly to light.   Extraocular muscle
movements were intact.   Facial sensation, corneal reflexes
and masseter strength were normal. There was a mild central
facial weakness.   Perception of pain, touch and position were
normal.   Muscle strength was normal.   Deep tendon reflexes
were brisk and there was an equivocal Babinski sign on the
right.

Routine laboratory studies were normal. A brain scan showed
increased uptake in cerebellum and left occipital area. Cerebral angiography demonstrated a vascular mass in the cerebellar and left occipital region.

A suboccipital craniectomy was performed and a neoplasm was
partially resected. The patient expired on the second postoperative day.

QUESTIONS

1.   Fig. 53.1 illustrates the brain with the neoplasm attached
      to the left leaf of the tentorium, deeply indenting and dis-
      torting the left occipital lobe and the left cerebellar hemis-
      phere. The most likely diagnosis is
      A. glioblastoma multiforme
      B. acoustic nerve tumor
      C. meningioma
      D. "plastic" ependymoma

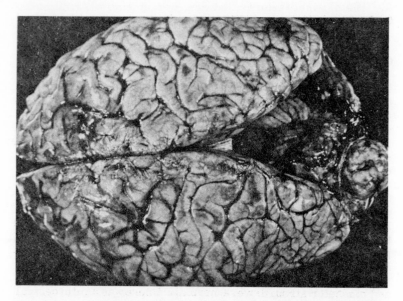

FIG. 53.1: Photograph of the brain. The neoplasm attached to
the tentorium is indenting and deforming the left
occipital lobe and the left cerebellar hemisphere.

2. Sites where meningiomas may be found include the
    A. dura over the cerebral hemispheres
    B. falx cerebri
    C. ventricular system
    D. orbit

3. Histological features that are characteristic of meningo-
    theliomatous meningiomas include
    A. ill-defined cell boundaries
    B. vacuolated nuclei
    C. psammoma bodies
    D. abundant collagenous stroma

4. Histological features that are characteristic of transitional
    meningiomas include
    A. ill-defined cell boundaries
    B. vacuolated nuclei
    C. psammoma bodies
    D. prominent whorls

5. Histological features that are characteristic of fibrous
    meningiomas include
    A. ill-defined cell boundaries
    B. vacuolated nuclei
    C. psammoma bodies
    D. abundant collagenous stroma

6. Fig. 53.2 is a photograph of a microscopic section pre-
    pared from this case. This lesion can be described as
    A. meningiotheliomatous meningioma
    B. transitional meningioma
    C. fibrous meningioma
    D. hemangiopericytoma variant of angioblastic
        meningioma

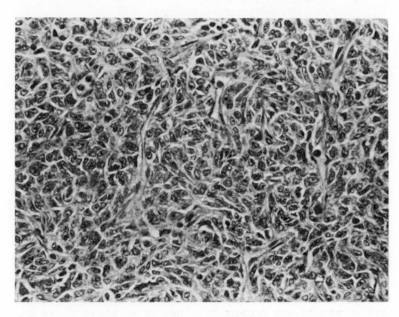

FIG. 53.2: Photomicrograph of the neoplasm encountered in the
            present case.

7. Prognosis in a patient with a meningioma is most clearly
    related to
    A. thoroughness of removal
    B. histological classification
    C. cellular pleomorphism
    D. vascularity

8. Extracranial metastases are associated with
    A. meningiomas of the spinal canal
    B. hemangiopericytoma variants of angioblastic
        meningiomas
    C. multiple attempts at surgical extirpation
    D. radiation therapy

9. Ultrastructural characteristics of meningiomas include
    A. interdigitating cellular processes
    B. desmosomes between cells
    C. cytoplasmic filaments
    D. prominent basement membranes

10. Hemangioblastomas are
    A. infratentorial neoplasms
    B. found predominantly in infancy
    C. commonly found in association with Sturge-Weber
        disease
    D. characteristically reddish-yellow in color

ANSWERS AND DISCUSSION

1. (C) The gross appearance and description are most consistent with a meningioma. These tumors account for about
15% of intracranial neoplasms and are most prevalent in adult
women. Characteristically, they are well-circumscribed
masses that indent and distort rather than invade the adjacent
neural parenchyma. The tumors are commonly attached to the
dura or a dural fold such as the falx or the tentorium. The neoplasms are generally firm and rubbery to palpation. Cystic
degeneration, necrosis and hemorrhage are infrequently encountered but calcification and ossification are occasionally
present. The skull adjacent to a meningioma may be thickened.
This hyperostosis is not necessarily associated with actual invasion of the bone by the neoplastic cells.

2. (A, B, C, D) Meningiomas can arise anywhere meninges
are found and are especially numerous in areas where the
arachnoidal villi are normally abundant. They are most frequently attached to the meninges over the cerebral hemispheres,
either parasagittally or over the lateral convexities. When
they are attached to the dural folds such as the falx and tentorium, they are often bilobed, involving both sides of these
structures. Rarely, meningiomas may be present within the
ventricular system. These arise from the meningeal folds or
invaginations that give rise to the fibrovascular stroma of the
choroid plexi. Most intraventricular meningiomas are found

within the lateral ventricles. Meningiomas also may be found
in the orbits arising from the meninges that invest the optic
nerves. Spinal meningiomas usually arise where the spinal
nerves exit from their meningeal sleeves. Very rarely, ectopic meningiomas have been reported completely outside of
the central nervous system.

3. (A, B) Meningiomas display a wide variety of histological
patterns to which a number of descriptive terms are applied.
These variations reflect the multipotential nature of the arachnoid cells and the variable contribution by other meningeal
components such as fibroblasts and blood vessels. Most of
these subtypes have little or no biological significance. Meningotheliomatous meningiomas are characterized by masses of
arachnoidal cells with ill-defined cytoplasmic boundaries and
vesicular, often vacuolated nuclei. The collagenous tissue is
largely restricted to the vascularized trabeculae that divide
the tumor into lobules.

4. (B, C, D) Transitional meningiomas (Fig. 53.3) are
characterized by prominent, well-defined whorls. The component cells are often somewhat better demarcated from
one another than in the meningiotheliomatous meningiomas.

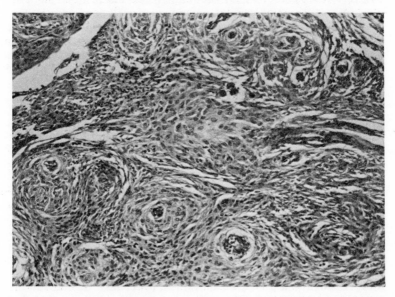

FIG. 53.3: Photomicrograph of a typical transitional meningioma.

The nuclei may still be vesicular and contain vacuoles. The centers of the whorls usually contain a capillary or a psammoma body. The psammoma bodies are laminated concretions that arise from mineralization of a vessel or degenerating cells. The whorls are often separated from one another by collagenous stroma. When the psammoma body formation is especially florid, the neoplasm may be designated as a psammomatous meningioma. The intraspinal meningiomas are often of this nature.

5.   (D) The fibrous meningiomas are characterized by elongated arachnoid cells that are accompanied by abundant collagenous stroma. Meningiomas with this pattern may be confused with Schwannomas. Many of the intraventricular meningiomas are fibrous meningiomas.

6.   (D) Another less common but morphologically distinctive group of meningiomas are the angioblastic meningiomas. These have been subdivided into two types. The hemangioblastoma variant of angioblastic meningioma is a supratentorial neoplasm that is histologically identical to the hemangioblastoma of the posterior fossa and spinal cord. The hemangiopericytoma variant of angioblastic meningioma is a histologically distinctive neoplasm with somewhat different biological behavior. As illustrated, these tumors are highly cellular neoplasms with the tumor cells surrounding the lumens of collapsed capillaries or sinusoids. They resemble the hemangiopericytomas in other organs and have been referred to simply as meningeal hemangiopericytomas. They tend to recur and metastasize somewhat more frequently than the other more common types of meningiomas.

7.   (A) The most significant feature in determining prognosis of a patient with a meningioma is the thoroughness of removal. Regardless of histological classification, recurrence will follow incomplete removal. Often because of location and involvement of vital structures only partial removal is feasible.

8.   (B, C) Extracranial metastases are uncommon and when present are often found in patients who have had multiple operations. The hemangiopericytoma variant of the angioblastic meningioma seems to be somewhat more prone to metastases than the other histological variants.

9.   (A, B, C) Ultrastructural characteristics of meningiomas include marked interdigitation of cell processes that are interconnected by desmosomes. The cytoplasm contains abundant

filaments but sparse rough endoplasmic reticulum. Some meningiomas, especially the meningotheliomatous and transitional
meningiomas, have cytoplasmic invaginations in the nuclei. By
light microscopy, these appear as vacuoles or eosinophilic nuclear inclusions.

10. (A, D) Hemangioblastomas are relatively uncommon tumors accounting for only 1-2% of all intracranial neoplasms.
Most are found in the cerebellum, but they may arise from
other infratentorial structures such as the medulla and spinal
cord. They are most commonly encountered in young to middle-
aged adults and may be associated with von Hippel-Lindau disease. Grossly, they have a distinctive reddish-yellow color
and may contain cysts (Fig. 53.4). Microscopically they are
composed of lipid-laden stromal cells and myriads of thin-
walled blood vessels (Fig. 53.5). Histologically, they are
identical to the supratentorial hemangioblastoma variant of
angioblastic meningiomas.

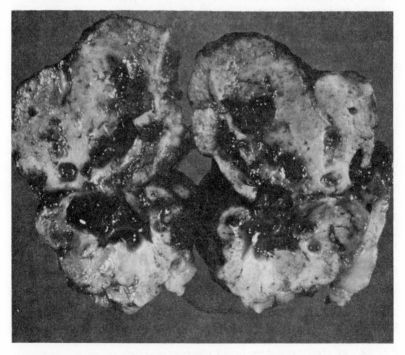

FIG. 53.4: Photograph of a surgically excised hemangioblastoma.

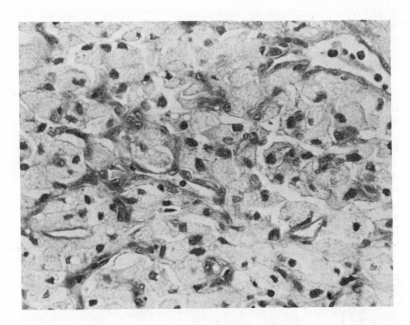

FIG. 53.5: Photomicrograph of the hemangioblastoma.

REFERENCES

1. Boldrey E: The Meningiomas. In: Pathology of the Ner-
    vous System. Minckler J (Ed.). McGraw-Hill Book Co.,
    New York, 1971, Vol. 2, pp. 2125-2144.

2. Horton WA, et al.: Von Hippel-Lindau disease. Arch Int
    Med 136:769-777, 1976.

3. Jellinger K and Slowik F: Histological subtypes and prog-
    nostic problems in meningiomas.   J Neurol 208:279-
    298, 1975.

4. Rubinstein LJ: Tumors of the Central Nervous System.
    Armed Forces Institute of Pathology, Washington, 1972,
    pp. 169-190.

5. Russell DS and Rubinstein LJ: Tumors of the Nervous
    System. Williams and Wilkins Co., Baltimore, 1977,
    pp. 65-100, 116-127.

: :

CASE 54: A Middle-Aged Woman with Progressive Loss of
          Hearing

CLINICAL DATA

This 59-year-old woman was hospitalized for evaluation of progressive loss of hearing over the past three years. Initially,
this was accompanied by numbness and tingling at the right cor-
ner of her mouth. Later, paresthesias gradually spread to involve the right maxillary region and eventually, the right mandibular area. During the past year there were episodes of loss
of balance. Three months prior to admission, the patient noted
decreasing taste and dysesthesias on the right side of her tongue. She had occasional headaches but no nausea or vomiting.

Physical examination confirmed a mild decrease in taste perception on the right side of the patient's tongue. There was a
moderate decrease in pain perception over the distributions of
the maxillary and mandibular branches of the right trigeminal
nerve. The corneal reflex was markedly reduced. There was
no papilledema and extraocular movements were normal.
There was mild sway with the Romberg test.

Audiometric evaluation revealed severe sensorineural hearing
loss on the right. Skull laminograms disclosed enlargement of
the right internal auditory meatus. Posterior fossa contrast
study demonstrated a 2 cm mass in the right cerebellopontine
angle.

A craniectomy was performed and a 4 x 2 x 2 cm round, yellow tumor was found extending from the internal auditory meatus to the base of the pons. The tumor was densely adherent to
the seventh nerve which was sacrificed during removal of the
neoplasm.

QUESTIONS

1.   The most appropriate clinical diagnosis is
     A.   acoustic neurinoma
     B.   meningioma of the cerebellopontine angle
     C.   metastasis to the cerebellopontine angle
     D.   ependymoma

2. Fig. 54.1 illustrates the microscopic appearance of this
    neoplasm. Appropriate histological diagnoses are
    A. neuroma
    B. neurofibroma
    C. neurilemoma
    D. schwannoma

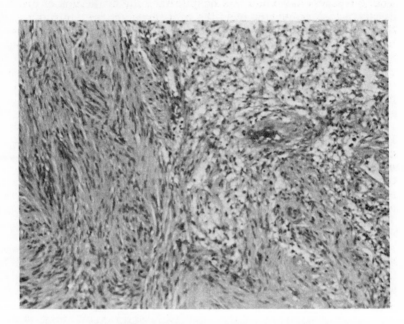

FIG. 54. 1: Histological appearance of this cerebellopontine an-
             gle tumor. Note the compact tissue (Antoni type-A)
             to the left and the looser tissue (Antoni type-B) to
             the upper right.

3. Electron microscopy of this neoplasm would be expected to
    reveal
    A. prominent basement membranes around the majority
        of the neoplastic cells
    B. fibrous long-spacing collagen
    C. tubules, 22 nm in diameter, that constrict to a dia-
        meter of 10 nm at 80 nm intervals
    D. fenestrated capillaries

4. Acoustic neurilemomas
   A. are encountered predominantly in middle-aged or
      elderly adults
   B. are twice as common in men as in women
   C. account for 5-10% of all intracranial neoplasms
   D. are treated by radiation

5. Bilateral acoustic neurilemomas
   A. are characteristic of von Hippel-Lindau disease
   B. are commonly encountered in Bourneville's disease
   C. may be encountered in von Recklinghausen's disease
   D. may constitute Gardner's syndrome

ANSWERS AND DISCUSSION

1. (A) The history, physical findings and operative findings
are consistent with an acoustic neurinoma. These tumors arise
from the vestibular branch of the eighth nerve but produce predominantly tinnitus and progressive loss of hearing. The vestibular symptoms are generally less striking and take the form
of mild vertigo. With growth of the tumor, additional symptoms arise from compression of the facial nerve. In many patients, this is initially in the form of hypesthesia of the posterior wall of the external auditory canal but later includes impaired taste and weakness of facial muscles. Further growth
with involvement of the trigeminal nerve commonly results in
a decreased corneal reflex and paresthesias in the distribution
of the trigeminal nerve. Compression of the cerebellar hemispheres may produce an unsteady gait and ataxia. Over 75% of
the patients will show enlargement of the internal auditory meatus on x-ray. The cerebrospinal fluid characteristically shows
an elevated protein content.

Grossly, as observed at the time of surgery, the tumors are
well encapsulated and have a yellowish-grey color. The interior is often partially cystic.

2. (C, D) These tumors are derived from Schwann cells, the
cells that ensheath peripheral nerves. Schwann cells are generally regarded as giving rise to two morphologically and bio-
logically distinct groups of benign neoplasms, the neurofibromas and the neurilemomas which are also called schwannomas.
The intracranial nerve sheath tumors that arise from the vestibular branch of the acoustic nerve, the acoustic neurinomas,
and the less common nerve sheath tumors that arise from the
trigeminal or other cranial nerves, are neurilemomas or
schwannomas. Morphologically identical tumors can arise from

spinal nerve roots, usually the dorsal roots, and from peripheral nerves. They may occur as solitary tumors or may be
part of a spectrum of lesions in patients with von Recklinghausen's disease. Characteristically, neurilemomas are well-en-
capsulated ovoid or fusiform masses. The nerves from which
they arise are largely confined to the periphery or capsule of
the neoplasm. The interior of these tumors has a grey to yellow color and often contains cysts. Microscopically, two histological patterns can be recognized within these neoplasms. The
so-called Antoni type-A pattern (seen to the left of Fig. 54.1)
is produced by compact fascicles of elongated cells with spindle-
shaped nuclei. Often the nuclei are in register producing
palisades. The Antoni type-B pattern (seen to the upper right
of Fig. 54.1) is produced by loosely aggregated stellate cells.
These often contain large, dark and occasionally bizarre nuclei.
The cytoplasm of stellate cells contain lipid that accounts
for the yellow color noted grossly. Congeries of blood vessels
with thickened, often hyalinized walls are found within these
neoplasms. Scattered macrophages containing lipid and hemosiderin may be found about the abnormal vessels as the result
of previous hemorrhage.

Neurofibromas are poorly circumscribed, loosely aggregated
neoplasms composed of Schwann cells and fibroblasts with a
collagenous and myxomatous stroma. The involved nerve is
expanded by the tumor and neurites can be demonstrated within
these neoplasms. Neurofibromas constitute the majority of the
cutaneous and peripheral nerve tumors that are found in patients
with von Recklinghausen's disease. (See Case 57 for further
discussion of von Recklinghausen's disease.)

The term neuroma should be reserved for non-neoplastic lesions that develop in response to nerve injury. These lesions
are composed of Schwann cells, fibroblasts and myriads of
tortuous neurites. The commonly employed term acoustic
"neuroma" should be regarded as a misnomer.

3.   (A, B, D) Since these tumors are derived from Schwann
cells, the majority of the neoplastic cells are surrounded by a
prominent basement membrane. This characteristic surface
feature readily distinguishes Schwann cells from fibroblasts,
ependymal cells and arachnoidal cells with which they might be
confused by light microscopy. The intracellular matrix contains collagen fibers, the majority of which have the normal 64
nm periodicity. Occasionally, distinctive cross-banded masses
of fibrous long-spacing collagen with a periodicity of 128 nm

are encountered. When originally described, these "Luse-
bodies" were thought to be diagnostic of acoustic neurilemomas.
Subsequently, they have been found in a number of unrelated
neoplasms, traumatized peripheral nerves and non-neoplastic
disorders. The blood vessels in acoustic neurilemomas have
fenestrated endothelial cells. The enhanced permeability of
these fenestrated capillaries may account for the elevated cerebrospinal fluid protein level noted in most patients with acoustic
neurilemomas.

4. (A, C) Acoustic neurilemomas are encountered predominantly in middle-aged or elderly adults. They account for
about 5-10% of all intracranial neoplasms. In common with
meningiomas, they are more frequent in women than men. By
contrast, the spinal neurilemomas are more common in men.
Acoustic neurilemomas are not radiosensitive and are treated
surgically. Since the morbidity and mortality increase with
size, early diagnosis is important. Complete removal of the
larger tumors is often not feasible.

5. (C, D) Patients with the central form of von Recklinghausen's disease often have multiple schwannomas. Especially
characteristic of this disease is the presence of bilateral acoustic neurilemomas. Some patients have bilateral acoustic
neurilemomas in the absence of other stigmata of von Recklinghausen's disease. When familial, some authors designate these
patients as examples of Gardner's syndrome.

REFERENCES

1. Minckler J: Supporting Cell Tumors of Peripheral Nerves.
    In: Pathology of the Nervous System. Minckler J (Ed.).
    McGraw-Hill Book Co., New York, 1971, Vol. 2, pp.
    2093-2114.

2. Rubinstein LJ: Tumors of the Central Nervous System.
    Armed Forces Institute of Pathology, Washington, 1972,
    pp. 206-214.

3. Russell DS and Rubinstein LJ: Pathology of Tumors of the
    Nervous System. Williams and Wilkins Co., 1977, pp.
    372-401.

4. Urich H: Pathology of Tumors of Cranial Nerves.
    Spinal Nerve Roots, and Peripheral Nerves. In:
    Peripheral Neuropathy. Dyck PJ, et al. (Eds.). W.B.
    Saunders Co., Philadelphia, 1975, pp. 1370-1403.

5. Weller RO and Cervos-Navarro J: Pathology of Peri-
    pheral Nerves. Butterworths, London, 1977, pp. 154-
    188.

: :

CASE 55: A 16-Year-Old Girl with Amenorrhea and Rapidly
          Decreasing Visual Acuity

CLINICAL DATA

Approximately 6 weeks prior to hospitalization, this 16-year-
old girl noted the onset of decreased visual acuity.   This progressed rapidly to virtual blindness over a 3-4 week period.
She had also experienced amenorrhea for a number of months.

Physical examination revealed an immature-appearing girl, 59
inches tall with scanty axillary and pubic hair.   Funduscopic
examination disclosed slight disc pallor, but normal vessels
bilaterally. Visual acuity was reduced to light perception only.
No other cranial nerve abnormalities were noted. Motor and
sensory examinations were within normal limits. Deep tendon reflexes were symmetrical and brisk. No pathological reflexes were elicited.

A CTT scan revealed a mass in the sellar and parasellar regions. The tumor showed prominent homogeneous enhancement
with intravenous contrast medium. No hydrocephalus was evident. Plain skull x-rays showed a normal sella turcica and no
suprasella mineralization. Arteriography revealed stretching
of the thalamoperforating arteries. A pneumoencephalogram
demonstrated a 2.5 x 3 cm suprasellar mass deforming the
interpeduncular and chiasmatic cisterns. The anterior portion
of the third ventricle proximal to the foramen of Monro was
obliterated.

Endocrine studies showed low levels of cortisol, luteinizing
hormone, follicle stimulating hormone, and keto- and hydroxy-
steroids.

A right frontotemporal craniotomy was performed and a tumor
was resected subtotally.

QUESTIONS

1.   The clinical data are most consistent with
     A.   suprasellar meningioma
     B.   craniopharyngioma
     C.   suprasellar germinoma
     D.   pituitary adenoma

2. Fig. 55.1 illustrates the histopathology of the resected
    neoplastic tissue. The diagnosis is
    A. craniopharyngioma
    B. germinoma
    C. astrocytoma
    D. pituitary adenoma

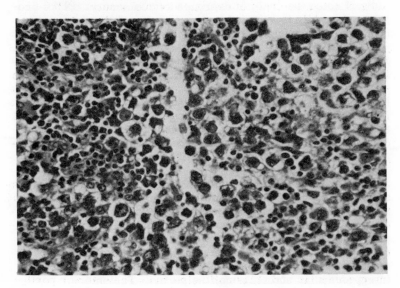

FIG. 55.1: Microscopic section of the partially resected neo-
          plasm.

3. Histologically identical neoplasms may be found in the
    A. pineal
    B. testes
    C. ovaries
    D. mediastinum

4. The most common pineal neoplasms are
    A. diktyomas
    B. pineoblastomas
    C. germinomas
    D. gliomas

5. Common non-neoplastic changes in the pineal include
    A. cyst formation
    B. Rosenthal fiber formation

C. mineralization
D. hemosiderin deposition

ANSWERS AND DISCUSSION

1. (B, C) The clinical data indicate that this girl's severe
visual and endocrine dysfunction is due to a hypothalamic or
suprasellar tumor. Tumors in this region account for 10-15%
of all childhood intracranial neoplasms. Many different entities
must be considered clinically, but the definitive diagnosis can
be established only by histopathological examination of the tumor.
On the basis of age alone, large, symptomatic pituitary adenomas and meningiomas would be unlikely. In children, craniopharyngiomas are the most common neoplasms in this region.
However, the absence of mineralization, and, to a lesser extent, the apparent lack of cyst formation, argue against this
diagnosis. Hypothalamic gliomas and germinomas must be
considered; however, both of these commonly produce diabetes
insipidus, a feature not reported in this patient.

2. (B) The partially resected neoplasm is a germinoma.
These tumors have also been designated as "ectopic pinealomas."
As illustrated, germinomas characteristically contain two distinct types of cells in varying proportions. One type, the neoplastic cells, are sharply demarcated, large, spheroidal to
polygonal cells with relatively large, vesicular nuclei and
prominent nucleoli. The cytoplasm often contains abundant
glycogen that is stainable with the periodic acid Schiff reaction.
The second type of cells are small with scanty cytoplasm and
pycnotic nuclei; these cells are apparently lymphocytes. In
addition to these major components, two types of multinucleated
giant cells occasionally may be present. Typical Langhan's
giant cells may be associated with foci of granuloma formation.
The presence of both the granulomas and the lymphocytic infiltrates are considered to be manifestations of the body's reaction
toward the neoplasm. Very rarely, syncytiotrophoblastic giant
cells may be present. The presence of these cells alone does
not justify a diagnosis of choriocarcinoma. In order for that
diagnosis to be valid, both syncytiotrophoblastic and cytotro-
phoblastic cells must be present.

Suprasellar germinomas commonly extend into the floor of the
third ventricle and the optic pathways. They may also dissemi-
nate widely along the cerebrospinal fluid pathways.

3. (A, B, C, D) Histologically identical neoplasms may be
found in the testes (seminomas), the ovaries (dysgerminomas)

and various midline sites, including the retroperitoneum, the mediastinum, the suprasellar region ("ectopic pinealomas") and the pineal. These are all neoplasms of germ cells, cells ultimately derived from the yolk sac of the embryo. The extra-gonadal germ cell tumors result, presumably, from aberrations in the migration of these cells from the yolk sac to the gonads.

4. (C) Pineal neoplasms are relatively rare, accounting for less than 1% of all intracranial tumors. Because of their location, pineal neoplasms often produce rather characteristic clinical manifestations. Increased intracranial pressure results from distortion and obstruction of the aqueduct. The most distinctive manifestation is a paralysis of upward conjugate gaze, commonly known as Parinaud's syndrome. This has been attributed to damage to the superior colliculus, but recent evidence has implicated the pretectum or posterior commissure. Ataxia results from pressure on the superior cerebellar peduncle, and hearing loss may result from involvement of the inferior colliculi.

The most common pineal neoplasms are germinomas, also known as atypical teratoid tumors. They arise in males more often than in females and generally become manifested during the second or third decade. These tumors are radiosensitive, but highly malignant, lesions that infiltrate surrounding structures and spread along the cerebrospinal fluid pathways.

The pineal also may be the site of other teratomatous neoplasms, such as mature teratomas, teratocarcinomas, embryonal carcinomas, yolk-sac carcinomas and choriocarcinomas. These may occur as pure neoplasms but are more commonly admixed with one another or with germinomas.

Nonteratomatous pineal neoplasms are very rare. Pineoblastomas and pineocytomas are derived from pineal parenchymal cells; others are glial neoplasms.

5. (A, B, C) The pineal undergoes a variety of changes with advancing age. The most prominent of these is mineralization. The mineral deposits are in the form of small, partially crystalline aggregates. They are composed of biological apatite (calcium hydroxyphosphate) and carbonates. The calcification is rarely sufficient to be seen by skull x-rays before the age of 10. When conspicuous at an earlier age, the possibility of a pineal neoplasm must be considered.

The glial core of the pineal frequently develops small cysts. Rosenthal fibers are encountered with great regularity in the glial tissue and the walls of the cysts.

REFERENCES

1. Costa E: Function and Diseases of the Pineal Gland.
    In: Scientific Approaches to Clinical Neurology.
    Goldensohn ES and Appel SH (Eds.).   Lea and Febiger,
    Philadelphia, 1977, pp. 905-916.

2. Jellinger K: Primary intracranial germ cell tumors.
    Acta Neuropath 25:291-306, 1973.

3. Rubinstein LJ: Tumors of the Central Nervous System.
    Armed Forces Institute of Pathology, Washington, 1972,
    pp. 269-284.

4. Simson LR, et al.: Suprasellar germinomas. Cancer
    22:533-544, 1968.

: :

CASE 56: A 63-Year-Old Woman with Decreased Visual
          Acuity and Headaches

CLINICAL DATA

This 63-year-old woman was hospitalized because of marked
deterioration of her vision. She had had bifrontal "sinus" headaches for several years that were more severe during the past
year. She had had no nocturia or polydypsia.

On examination, she was alert and oriented. Olfaction was intact. Her pupils were equal, but bilaterally the light reflex was
sluggish. There was no papilledema. The patient could only
count fingers with her right eye and had a visual acuity of
20/900 in her left eye. A temporal hemianopsia was demonstrable. The remainder of the neurological and general physical examination were normal.

A complete blood count and a urinalysis, including urine specific
gravity, were normal. X-rays of the skull showed that the
sella was intact and not enlarged. The posterior clinoid processes were demineralized. A brain scan was normal. Bilateral carotid angiography revealed symmetrical elevation of
the proximal segments of the anterior cerebral arteries.

A right frontal craniectomy was performed, and a partially
cystic neoplasm was removed from between the optic nerves.
Additional tumor was evident behind the chiasm but was judged
surgically inaccessible. Postoperatively, the patient's visual
fields and acuity improved.

QUESTIONS

1. Based on the clinical data and operative findings, the most
    likely diagnosis is
    A. an aneurysm
    B. a pituitary adenoma
    C. a craniopharyngioma
    D. a chordoma

2. Craniopharyngiomas in patients over 20 years of age are
    A. exceedingly rare
    B. relatively common
    C. usually associated with von Recklinghausen's
        disease
    D. more common in women

3. Features that are more common in craniopharyngiomas
   of childhood than adulthood are
   A. papilledema
   B. optic atrophy
   C. suprasellar calcification
   D. unilateral blindness

4. Gross characteristic of craniopharyngiomas include
   A. irregular lobulated surface
   B. invasion of the adjacent neural parenchyma
   C. variable-sized cysts containing clear fluid
   D. variable-sized cysts containing dark greenish-brown
      fluid

5. Histological characteristics of craniopharyngiomas include
   the presence of
   A. a basal layer of cuboidal to columnar cells
   B. expanses of stellate cells
   C. foci of keratinization
   D. psammoma bodies

6. Proposed origins for craniopharyngiomas include
   A. mucosa of the sphenoid sinus
   B. Erdheim rests
   C. metaplasia of adenohypophyseal cells
   D. remnants of Rathke's pouch

7. The majority of pituitary adenomas without obvious clinical
   evidence of hormone production are now regarded as
   A. chromophobe adenomas
   B. oncocytomas
   C. heavily granulated acidophilic adenomas
   D. poorly granulated acidophilic adenomas

ANSWERS AND DISCUSSION

1. (C) Based on the clinical data and operative findings, the
most likely diagnosis is a craniopharyngioma. The combination
of bitemporal hemianopsia and headaches with or without pituitary dysfunction is indicative of a "tumor" of the sella region.
Many different "tumors" can occur in this area and often a
specific diagnosis can be made only histologically. Craniopharyngiomas usually arise in a suprasella location and are
typically at least partially cystic, as in the present case. Pituitary adenomas usually arise from within the pituitary and, in
contrast to the present case, "balloon" the sella as they enlarge.
An aneurysm can act as a space-occupying mass in the sella

region. These must be identified by angiography before surgery is undertaken. Chordomas usually arise from the clivus
and are accompanied by bone destruction. They often produce
multiple cranial nerve palsies. Meningiomas can occur in this
region but are rarely cystic. Gliomas of the optic nerve and
chiasm usually occur in children and commonly produce enlargement of the optic foramina.

2.   (B) Although craniopharyngiomas are one of the most common supratentorial tumors of childhood, at least half of them
first become clinically apparent in individuals who are over 20
years of age. Collectively, craniopharyngiomas account for
about 3% of all intracranial neoplasms.

3.   (A, C) Craniopharyngiomas in childhood and adulthood differ somewhat in their clinical manifestations. During childhood, craniopharyngiomas are almost always calcified, whereas this feature is often absent from those presenting during
adulthood. Suprasella calcification in a child is virtually diagnostic of craniopharyngioma. Ocular abnormalities are common in both age groups; however, papilledema is more common
in childhood, whereas optic atrophy is more common in adulthood. Unilateral blindness, bitemporal scotomas or incongru-
ous homonymous hemianopsia may be present in place of the
classical bitemporal hemianopsia associated with "pituitary
tumors." Partial hypopituitarism, specifically gonadotrophin
failure, is more common in adults than children.

4.   (A, D) Grossly, craniopharyngiomas appear as irregular
lobulated masses that compress, but do not invade, the adjacent
neural structures. The third ventricle may be sufficiently dis-
torted as to produce hydrocephalus. The tumors are almost
always partially cystic. The fluid within the cysts is characteristically dark greenish-brown in color and is sometimes described as being like "machine oil." Small, glistening crystals
of cholesterol are usually suspended in the dark fluid.

5.   (A, B, C) Histologically, craniopharyngiomas are composed of a complex mixture of various types of cells (Fig. 56.1).
The periphery of the irregular cell masses consists of a basal
layer of cuboidal or columnar cells. Within the epithelial
masses are typical squamous cells and loosely aggregated
stellate cells. These are attached to one another by desmosomes. Degenerative changes among the stellate cells give
rise to the various-sized cysts. Scattered among the squamous
and stellate cells are foci, often whorls, of keratinizing cells.
These keratinizing foci often undergo subsequent calcification

or even ossification. The basal cell layer is encircled by a
layer of connective tissue. This is usually thin but focally may
be quite thick. The adjacent compressed neural parenchyma
shows pronounced gliosis and may contain abundant Rosenthal
fibers. Occasionally, biopsy specimens will consist almost
entirely of keratinized epithelium.

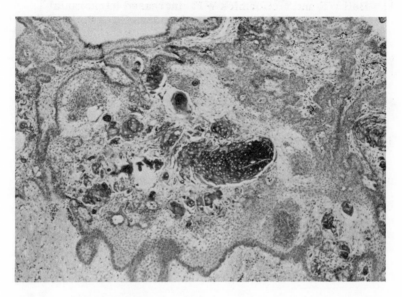

FIG. 56. 1: Microscopic section showing the histology of the partially resected tumor.

6.   (B, C, D) Craniopharyngiomas are generally regarded as
being derived from small nests of squamous cells that are
found on the surface of the infundibular stalk. These nests of
cells, the so-called Erdheim rests, are variously regarded as
remnants of Rathke's pouch or the result of metaplasia of
adenohypophyseal cells. Erdheim rests are more abundant
in older patients but have occasionally been described even in
newborn infants.

7.   (D) Pituitary adenomas without obvious evidence of hormone production comprise the majority of adenohypophyseal
neoplasms. When fixed in formalin and stained with hematoxylin-eosin only, most of these tumors appear to contain unstained,
i.e., chromophobic cells. By the use of more suitable fixatives,

e.g., Heidenhain's Susa solution and more sophisticated stains, e.g., periodic acid-Schiff-hematoxylin-light green-orange G, the majority of these tumors appear to be poorly granulated acidophilic adenomas.

REFERENCES

1. Bell WE and McCormick WF: Increased Intracranial Pressure in Children. W.B. Saunders Co., Philadelphia, 1978, pp. 393-402.

2. Landolt AM: Ultrastructure of human sella tumors. Acta Neurochir Suppl 22:104-119, 1975.

3. Petito CK, et al.: Craniopharyngiomas. Cancer 37: 1944-1952, 1976.

4. Rubinstein LJ: Tumors of the Central Nervous System. Armed Forces Institute of Pathology, Washington, 1972, pp. 292-294.

: :

CASE 57: An Elderly Woman with Subcutaneous Nodules and
          Pigmented Skin Lesions

CLINICAL DATA

This mentally retarded 60-year-old woman was seen because
of pruritis and enlargement of the lymph nodes on the right
side of her neck. She had no other complaints.

On physical examination, she was found to have multiple subcutaneous nodules and multiple pigmented cutaneous lesions
(Fig. 57.1). She had an enlarged liver and spleen in addition
to the enlarged cervical lymph nodes. A lymph node biopsy
was performed and the specimen was interpreted as a mixed
cell type of malignant lymphoma. A biopsy specimen from
one of the subcutaneous nodules was interpreted as a neurofibroma. The patient was treated with nitrogen mustard, vincristine, prednisone, and procarbazine.

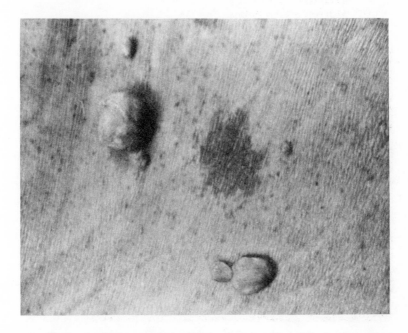

FIG. 57. 1: A close-up photograph showing the skin lesions that
          were present in great numbers on this patient's
          neck, chest, abdomen and back.

Six months later, she was readmitted with diffuse lymphadenopathy and further enlargement of her liver and spleen. She
was given further chemotherapy and developed severe bone
marrow depression. She died shortly thereafter from bronchopneumonia.

QUESTIONS

1. In addition to the malignant lymphoma, this patient
    had
    A. tuberous sclerosis
    B. von Hippel-Lindau disease
    C. von Recklinghausen's disease
    D. Bourneville's disease

2. Fig. 57.2 illustrates a peripheral nerve tumor from
    this patient. This lesion is a
    A. plexiform neurofibroma
    B. neurilemoma
    C. granular cell tumor
    D. Morton's neuroma

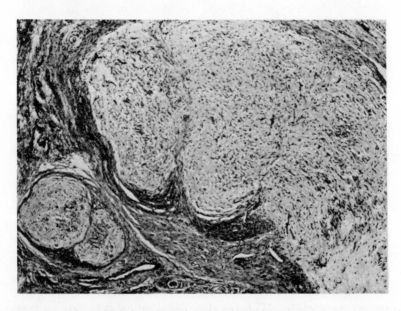

FIG. 57. 2: Photomicrograph of a peripheral nerve tumor from
             this patient.

3. Malignant peripheral nerve tumors, i.e., malignant
    schwannomas or neurofibrosarcomas develop in
    A. 45-60% of patients with von Recklinghausen's disease
    B. 31-45% of patients with von Recklinghausen's disease
    C. 16-30% of patients with von Recklinghausen's disease
    D.   3-15% of patients with von Recklinghausen's disease

4. Tumors of the central nervous system that are encountered
    with increased frequency in patients with von Recklinghau-
    sen's disease include
    A. meningiomas
    B. acoustic neurinomas
    C. gliomas
    D. choristomas

5. Other lesions that are encountered in association with von
    Recklinghausen's disease include
    A. kyphoscoliosis
    B. tumors of the stomach and small intestine
    C. cardiac rhabdomyomas
    D. pheochromocytomas

6. The prevalence of von Recklinghausen's disease has been
    estimated to be about one in
    A. 300
    B. 3,000
    C. 30,000
    D. 300,000

7. Von Recklinghausen's disease is regarded as one of the
    phakomatoses. This term is used to designate a group
    of disorders that
    A. have spots or patches on the skin
    B. are characterized by dislocation of the lens
    C. are genetically determined
    D. have peripheral nerve tumors

ANSWERS AND DISCUSSION

1. (C) In addition to the malignant lymphoma, this patient obviously had von Recklinghausen's disease. This genetically determined disorder is characterized by hamartomas and neoplasms that involve predominantly the skin, peripheral nervous
system and central nervous system. The pigmented macular
lesions seen in Fig. 57.1 are the so-called cafe-au-lait spots.
These pigmented lesions vary in size, have distinct margins
and are most numerous on the neck and trunk. They are present

in over 95% of patients with von Recklinghausen's disease. The presence of six or more cafe-au-lait spots, each greater than 1.5 cm in diameter, is generally regarded as diagnostic of this disorder even in the absence of family history or other manifestations of the disease. Microscopically, cafe-au-lait spots are unimpressive and merely show increased melanin in the basal layer of the epidermis. Axillary freckles, generally regarded as variants of the cafe-au-lait spots, are found in about 30% of the patients.

The cutaneous and subcutaneous nodules, as seen in Fig. 57.1, are sessile or pedunculated neurofibromas derived from branches of dermal nerves. These tumors are usually multiple and are most numerous on the trunk. While some neurofibromas may be present at birth, most do not develop until after puberty. Microscopically, they consist of loose aggregates of Schwann cells, fibroblasts and neurites. They are often incorrectly designated as fibromas. Highly organized areas that resemble tactile corpuscles, nevus cells and adipose tissue may be incorporated in the cutaneous and subcutaneous neurofibromas.

2.   (A) The tumor illustrated in Fig. 57.2 is a plexiform neurofibroma. These tumors characteristically involve the larger peripheral nerves in patients with von Recklinghausen's disease. Grossly, the affected nerve is markedly tortuous and has multiple irregular or fusiform enlargements along its length. Often the involved nerve cannot be dissected readily from the surrounded connective tissue. Microscopically, the normally compact nerve structure is replaced by masses of loosely aggregated fusiform nerve sheath cells with varying amounts of collagenous and myxomatous stroma. Neurites can be demonstrated within the tumor. Focal areas that resemble Meissner's corpuscles may be found in plexiform neurofibromas but are more common in cutaneous neurofibromas.

Neurilemomas, otherwise known as schwannomas, are also nerve sheath tumors. As peripheral nerve tumors, they are often solitary and can occur in the absence of von Recklinghausen's disease. These tumors are distinctly encapsulated, ovoid or fusiform masses. Many are partially or extensively cystic and often have a characteristic grey-yellow color. Microscopically, two histological patterns can be recognized within the lesions which resemble acoustic neurinomas (see Fig. 54.1, page 340). The so-called Antoni type-A pattern is produced by fusiform cells with nuclei in register resulting in palisades. The Antoni type-B pattern is produced by loosely arranged stellate cells. Congeries of vessels with thick, often

hyalinized walls are often present. Neurites are largely confined to the periphery or capsule of the tumor. Granular cell
tumors, formerly called granular cell myoblastomas, are now
commonly regarded as nerve sheath tumors. The tumor cells
have abundant granular-appearing cytoplasm and relatively small,
dark nuclei. Ultrastructurally, the cytoplasm is filled with autophagic vacuoles. These autophagic vacuoles account for the
staining that can be obtained with the periodic acid-Schiff and
acid phosphatase techniques.

Morton's neuromas are reactive lesions that develop on the in-
terdigital plantar nerves. Collagenous, elastic and fibrinoid
material accumulates in the perineurium and epineurium of the
affected nerves.

3. (D) Malignant peripheral nerve tumors, otherwise known
as malignant schwannomas or neurofibrosarcomas, probably
occur in no more than 3-15% of patients with von Recklinghausen's disease.   While it is clear that all types of soft tissue
sarcomas are more common in patients with von Recklinghausen's disease, precise figures are difficult to obtain since many
mild cases of von Recklinghausen's disease go undiagnosed.
It has also been reported that malignant schwannomas have
a worse prognosis in patients with von Recklinghausen's
disease than in patients who are not afflicted with this disorder.

4. (A, B, C) A wide variety of central nervous system tumors
have been encountered with increased frequency in patients with
von Recklinghausen's disease. Schwannomas, often multiple,
are found on spinal and cranial nerve roots. Sensory roots are
more commonly affected than motor roots. Among the cranial
nerve tumors, acoustic nerve schwannomas, otherwise known
as acoustic neurinomas, are the most common. Bilateral acoustic nerve tumors are considered characteristic of von Recklinghausen's disease or Gardner's syndrome. (See Case 54 for
further discussion of acoustic neurinomas.) Patients with von
Recklinghausen's disease commonly have intracranial and intraspinal meningiomas. As with the schwannomas, these tumors
are frequently multiple.   Various gliomas have been observed
with increased frequency. Ependymomas of the spinal cord are
common and may be accompanied by a syrinx.   Optic nerve
gliomas, especially bilateral optic nerve gliomas, may be an
early manifestation of von Recklinghausen's disease (Fig. 57.3).
These tumors are usually found in children and are histologically pilocytic astrocytomas.

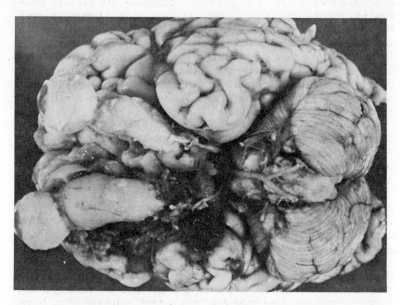

FIG. 57. 3: Bilateral optic nerve gliomas in a child with von
Recklinghausen's disease.

Choristomas are small neurohypophyseal tumors that are composed of cells that resemble granular cell tumors elsewhere
in the body. Although they are apparently derived from nerve
sheath cells, no increased prevalence has been reported in patients with von Recklinghausen's disease.

In general, patients with prominent cutaneous and peripheral
nerve manifestations of von Recklinghausen's disease have
minimal involvement of the central nervous system, while
those individuals with prominent central nervous manifestations
have minimal peripheral manifestations. Mental retardation
is common among patients with von Recklinghausen's disease,
but there are no known morphological correlates for this manifestation.

5. (A, B, D) Numerous skeletal and visceral lesions have been
encountered in patients with von Recklinghausen's disease.
Skeletal lesions are found in over a third of the patients. Kypho-
scoliosis is the most common. Other common skeletal lesions

include pseudoarthroses and fibrous defects in the skull. Tumors
of the gastrointestinal tract have been described in about 10% of
patients with von Recklinghausen's disease. The tumors most
commonly involved the stomach or jejunum and are both neurofibromas and leiomyomas. Various endocrine gland tumors
have been encountered in patients with von Recklinghausen's
disease. The most common of these are pheochromocytomas
and medullary carcinomas of the thyroid. The pheochromocytomas may be multiple and may be found in association with
the thyroid carcinomas. Rarely, other endocrine tumors have
been reported.

6. (B) The prevalence of von Recklinghausen's disease has been
estimated to be about one in 2,500 to 3,000 persons. The disorder occurs in all races and is inherited as an autosomal
dominant trait with a high degree of penetrance. There is, however, marked phenotypic variation among the cases.

7. (A, C) The term phakomatosis was introduced by Van der
Hoeve in 1923 to characterize tuberous sclerosis and von Recklinghausen's disease. The term was merely descriptive and
did not imply a common pathogenetic basis. This group of disorders has now been expanded to include von Hippel-Lindau disease. Sturge-Weber disease, neurocutaneous melanosis, etc.
In general, these are genetically determined disorders with
cutaneous manifestations and hamartomas or neoplasms of the
nervous system, peripheral or central.

REFERENCES

1. Abell MR, et al.: Tumors of the peripheral nervous system. Human Path 1:503-551, 1970.

2. Asbury AK and Johnson PC: Pathology of Peripheral Nerve.
   W.B. Saunders Co., Philadelphia, 1978, pp. 206-226.

3. Canale DJ and Hebin J: von Recklinghausen's Disease of
   the Nervous System. In: Handbook of Clinical Neurology.
   Vinken PJ and Bruyn GW (Eds.). North-Holland, Amsterdam, 1972, Vol. 14, pp. 132-162.

4. de Recondo J and Haguenau M: Neuropathologic Survey
   of the Phakomatoses and Allied Disorders. In: Handbook
   of Clinical Neurology. Vinken PJ and Bruyn GW (Eds.).
   North-Holland, Amsterdam, 1972, Vol. 14, pp. 19-100.

5. Harkin JC and Reed RJ: Tumors of the Peripheral Nervous System. Armed Forces Institute of Pathology, Washington, 1969, pp. 67-97.

6. Rubinstein LJ: Tumors of the Central Nervous System. Armed Forces Institute of Pathology, Washington, 1972, pp. 206-214, 302-308.

7. Urich H: Pathology of Tumors of Cranial Nerves, Spinal Nerve Roots, and Peripheral Nerves. In: Peripheral Neuropathy. Dyck PJ, et al. (Eds.). W.B. Saunders Co., Philadelphia, 1975, pp. 1370-1403.

8. Weller RO and Cervos-Navarro J: Pathology of Peripheral Nerves. Butterworths, London, 1977, pp. 154-188.

:::

CASE 58: A 16-Year-Old Boy with Mental Retardation and
          Seizures

CLINICAL DATA

This 16-year-old boy was known to have tuberous sclerosis.
Moderate mental retardation had been evident since infancy;
seizures had been present since the age of two; and characteristic facial lesions had been apparent since the age of five.

At age 11, he was hospitalized with headaches and papilledema.
Plain skull x-rays revealed scattered intracerebral calcifications. A ventriculogram revealed a lobulated tumor obstructing
the right foramen of Monro. A ventriculoatrial shunting procedure was performed. One year later, a carotid arteriogram
showed an intraventricular and ganglionic neoplasm. Following a craniotomy and biopsy, the patient was given x-ray therapy. The patient did relatively well for an additional two years
when he was readmitted for headaches, vomiting, and occasional episodes of opisthotonos. Ventriculography was repeated
and revealed an enlarged, non-communicating lateral ventricle
with no visualization of the third ventricle and a large mass beneath the anterior half of the right lateral ventricle. He was
given another course of radiation.

On the present admission, he was awake but lethargic and responded poorly to commands. He was not oriented to time or
place. His pupils were equal and reacted to light, but funduscopic examination revealed bilateral optic atrophy. Extraocular movements were of full range and the remainder of the
cranial nerves were intact. He had no obvious weakness in his
upper limbs but had weakness and marked spasticity of both legs
with sustained patellar and ankle clonus. His shunt was revised
but he subsequently died from pneumonia.

QUESTIONS

1. The classical triad of clinical manifestations encountered
    in patients with tuberous sclerosis includes
    A. mental retardation
    B. epilepsy
    C. facial cutaneous lesions
    D. cerebellar ataxia

2. Cutaneous lesions encountered in tuberous sclerosis
   include
   A. adenomata sebacea
   B. shagreen patches
   C. white patches
   D. Koenen tumors

3. The cortical tubers are characterized by their
   A. soft consistency
   B. firm consistency
   C. content of large bizarre cells
   D. normal cortical laminations

4. The term "candle gutterings" refers to
   A. linear cortical tubers
   B. linear cutaneous nerve
   C. conical intraventricular hamartomas
   D. Koenen tumors

5. A neoplasm characteristically associated with tuberous
   sclerosis is the
   A. subependymal giant cell astrocytoma
   B. subependymoma
   C. cerebellar hemangioblastoma
   D. optic nerve glioma

6. Ocular lesions associated with tuberous sclerosis include
   A. melanomas of the iris
   B. melanomas of the choroid
   C. diktyomas
   D. astrocytomas of the retina

7. The most common visceral lesions associated with tuberous
   sclerosis include
   A. cavernous angiomas of the liver
   B. angiomyolipomas of the kidney
   C. rhabdomyomas of the heart
   D. rhabdomyomas of the tongue

ANSWERS AND DISCUSSION

1. (A, B, C) Tuberous sclerosis, or Bourneville's disease,
is a rare phakomatosis that affects one in 40,000 to 100,000
live births. The disease may be sporadic or familial. All
races are affected but males are afflicted more commonly than
females. The predominant clinical manifestations include mental retardation, epilepsy and facial cutaneous lesions. Seizures

are encountered in over 90% of the patients and may be the
initial manifestation, appearing within the first two years of
life. Mental deficiency is found in 70% and ranges from idiocy
to mild retardation. Abnormal or even psychotic behavior is commonly encountered. The average life span is less than 15
years. Death results from brain tumors, status epilepticus or
intercurrent infection.

2.   (A, B, C, D) There are a variety of cutaneous lesions that
can be encountered in patients with tuberous sclerosis.   The
classical lesions found in virtually all of the patients are the
so-called "adenomata sebacea." These lesions develop early
in infancy and appear as reddish-brown nodules distributed
symmetrically over the malar area and in the nasolabial folds.
The designation of adenoma sebaceum is a misnomer, since
these lesions are actually fibrovascular hamartomas with no
special involvement of the sebaceous glands.

Another cutaneous lesion that is highly characteristic of tuberous sclerosis consists of hypopigmented, leaf-shaped macules.
The majority of these lesions, otherwise known as white patches,
are visible at birth and thus may be the earliest sign of the disorder.   These leaf-shaped macules are found in 50-60% of patients with tuberous sclerosis.

Shagreen patches are irregular areas of slightly raised, rough-
ened skin in the lumbosacral area.   These lesions are more
readily palpated than seen.   They are found in about 20% of patients with tuberous sclerosis.   Microscopically, the abnormal
skin shows increased dermal collagen.

Periungual and subungual fibromas, the so-called Koenen tumors, arise from the nailbeds and protrude onto the nail plates.
They occur more commonly on the toes than the fingers. Histologically, they appear to be fibrovascular hamartomas.   They
are found in 20 to 50% of the patients with tuberous sclerosis.
Somewhat similar lesions may occur on the gums.   Cafe-au-lait
spots have been described in patients with tuberous sclerosis
but are more characteristic of von Recklinghausen's disease.

3.   (B, C) The cortical tubers are localized neuroglial hamartomas.   They are quite firm and in fresh, unfixed brains are
more readily recognized by palpation than by visual inspection.
The tubers are generally smooth and slightly raised above the
surrounding cortex.   They may be demarcated by a circumferential sulcus or continuous with the adjacent gyri.   Tubers
vary in number and are randomly distributed in the cerebral
cortex.   In coronal sections of formalin-fixed brain, the tubers

appear as poorly demarcated pale areas, as seen in Fig. 58.1.
Microscopically, the normal cortical laminations are replaced
by cellular aggregates containing large, bizarre, polygonal
cells (Fig. 58.2). These are surrounded by dense feltwork of
glial fibers. The majority of the large cells are astrocytes but
some abnormal neurons are also present. Hirano, et al., reported an exceptional case in which the aberrant neurons displayed neurofibrillary tangles, granulovacuolar degeneration
and Pick bodies.   There is probably no relation between the
number or distribution of the tubers and the degree of mental
retardation or severity of the epilepsy.

Heterotopic collections of bizarre glial cells can also be found
in the white matter. These may occur in the cerebellum where
tubers are less common.

4.   (C) The term "candle gutterings" is used to describe the
intraventricular hamartomas.   They are firm, have a grey-
white color and are often cone-shaped.   They are found most
often along the thalamostriate sulcus, arising from the thalamus and caudate nucleus and projecting into the lateral ventricle.   They are considerably less common in the third or
fourth ventricles.   These hamartomas are composed of interwoven skeins of plump fibrillary astrocytes.   The "candle
gutterings" frequently undergo mineralization and are the site
of the calcifications seen on plain skull x-rays. They also produce distinctive filling defects in contrast studies.

5.   (A) Subependymal giant cell astrocytomas are neoplasms
that are characteristically, but not exclusively, associated with
tuberous sclerosis.   They apparently arise from the "candle
gutterings" on the walls of the lateral ventricles and present,
as in the present case, as intraventricular masses. Histologically, the neoplasms are composed of very large, bizarre
astrocytes with eccentric, vesicular nuclei. The tumors may
be highly vascular with calcification and siderosis of vessel
walls as evidence of previous hemorrhage. The tumors grow
slowly and produce symptoms by obstruction rather than invasion. Other forms of gliomas, including glioblastomas, have
occasionally been encountered in patients with tuberous sclerosis but are not characteristic of the condition.

6.   (D) Ocular lesions have been described in as many as 50%
of patients with tuberous sclerosis. The characteristic lesions
are astrocytomas of the retina. These are knobby, grey-white
tumors that rarely cause symptoms or interfere with vision.
Histologically, they resemble the intraventricular subependymal giant cell astrocytomas.

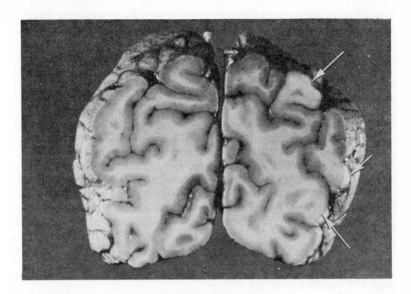

FIG. 58.1: Coronal section of the cerebral hemispheres showing cortical tubers (arrows).

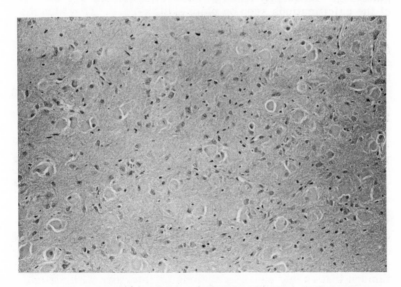

FIG. 58.2: Photomicrograph showing the histological characteristics of a cortical tuber.

7.   (B, C) Patients with tuberous sclerosis frequently have associated visceral lesions. Of these, renal tumors are the most common and have been reported in about 40% of the patients.   Most of these renal tumors are angiomyolipomas. These may be multiple but are generally relatively small and asymptomatic.   Renal tubular adenomas have also been encountered with increased frequency.   Some patients with tuberous sclerosis have subtle, but distinctive, collections of vacuolated cells in the glomeruli.

Cardiac lesions are the second most common of the visceral lesions. Cardiac rhabdomyomas have been reported in 20 to 60% of patients with tuberous sclerosis. These tumors appear as nodular, grey masses and arise most often from the wall of the left ventricle. Histologically, they are composed of large cells with glycogen-filled vacuoles. The cytoplasm compressed between the vacuoles has a stellate configuration but often retains cross-striations. These tumors may be derived from the conducting or Purkinje cells of the heart and are apparently unrelated to rhabdomyomas of skeletal muscles.

Other less common visceral lesions include cysts and fibrovascular hamartomas of the lungs and cysts and fibrous lesions of bones, especially the phalanges, metacarpals and metatarsals.

REFERENCES

1.   de Recondo J and Haguenau M: Neuropathologic Survey of the Phakomatoses and Allied Disorders. In: Handbook of Clinical Neurology. Vinken PJ and Bruyn GW (Eds.). North-Holland, Amsterdam, 1972, Vol. 14, pp. 19-100.

2.   Donegani G, et al.: Tuberous Sclerosis. In: Handbook of Clinical Neurology. Vinken PJ and Bruyn GW (Eds.). North-Holland, Amsterdam, 1972, Vol. 14, pp. 340-389.

3.   Hirano A, et al.: Neurofibrillary changes, granulovacuolar bodies and argentophilic globules observed in tuberous sclerosis. Acta Neuropath 11:257-261, 1968.

4.   Musger A: Dermatological Aspects of the Phakomatoses. In: Handbook of Clinical Neurology, Vinken PJ and Bruyn GW (Eds.). North-Holland, Amsterdam, 1972, Vol. 14, pp. 562-618.

5.   Rubinstein LJ: Tumors of the Central Nervous System. Armed Forces Institute of Pathology, Washington, 1972, pp. 40-42.
: :

CASE 59: A Mentally Retarded Woman with a "Port-Wine
          Stain"

CLINICAL DATA

This 51-year-old mentally retarded woman was transferred
from a nursing home because of feeding difficulties. She was
noted at birth to have a "port-wine stain" on the right side of
her face. At the age of six months, she began to have seizures
that diminished in frequency but have persisted over the years.
She began school at the age of nine and was able to learn to read
and write. She had been able to help with household chores but
had not been able to work outside of her home.

On physical examination, the patient appeared thin and weak,
but had normal vital signs. She had an extensive "port-wine"
nevus that roughly coincided with the distribution of the ophthalmic and maxillary divisions of the right trigeminal nerve.
Her extraocular movements were unimpaired but there was
mild weakness of the right eyelid. Her right optic nerve head
was atrophic due to old glaucoma. All of her limbs were weak
but more markedly on the left than on the right. The deep tendon reflexes were mildly hyperactive.

All clinical laboratory studies were normal. Plain skull x-rays
revealed "tram-track" calcifications in the right parietal and
occipital lobes. A radioisotopic brain scan showed increased
uptake in this area.

The patient's general physical condition improved with tube
feeding. She was discharged to a custodial care facility where
she remained for two months before dying from pneumonia.

QUESTIONS

1. The most appropriate clinical diagnosis is
    A. Sturge-Weber disease
    B. von Recklinghausen's disease
    C. von Hippel-Lindau disease
    D. Bourneville's disease

2. Characteristically, the "port-wine stain"
    A. coincides with the distribution of the facial nerve
    B. coincides with the distribution of the trigeminal nerve
    C. spares the supraorbital areas
    D. spares the eyelid

3. The characteristic intracranial lesions include
   A. a venous angioma involving the pia and arachnoid
   B. an intraparenchymal venous angioma involving the parietal and occipital lobes
   C. a venous angioma involving the cerebellum
   D. intracerebral mineralization

4. Common complications of the disorder include
   A. mental retardation
   B. epilepsy
   C. hemiplegia
   D. hemorrhage

5. The characteristic x-ray findings consist of "tram-track" or "railroad track" calcifications. These are due to mineral deposited in
   A. the angioma and in the underlying cortex
   B. superficial and deep layers of the cerebral cortex
   C. superficial layers of apposing gyri
   D. the dura and in the angioma

6. The mineral deposits are composed mainly of
   A. calcium oxalate
   B. calcium salts of fatty acids
   C. iron carbonate
   D. calcium phosphate and calcium carbonate

7. Ocular abnormalities characteristically associated with Sturge-Weber disease include
   A. cataracts
   B. glaucoma
   C. angiomas of the choroid
   D. pigmentary degeneration of the retina

8. When present, the usual associated visceral lesions are
   A. hemangiomas
   B. rhabdomyomas
   C. angiomyolipomas
   D. adrenal adenomas

9. Sturge-Weber disease
   A. has been observed only in Caucasians
   B. affects males and females equally
   C. is inherited as an autosomal recessive trait in the majority of cases
   D. is commonly sporadic but has also been described as an autosomal recessive and autosomal dominant trait in some families

10. Neurocutaneous melanosis is characterized by
    A. pigmented nerves in the skin
    B. giant pigmented nevi usually involving the trunk
    C. thickened pigmented meninges
    D. intraparenchymal pigmentation of cerebrum and cere-
       bellum

ANSWERS AND DISCUSSION

1. (A) The most appropriate clinical diagnosis is Sturge-
Weber disease. The typical clinical manifestations of this disorder include a "port-wine" nevus of the face, mental retardation, epilepsy, glaucoma, homonymous hemianopsia, hemiplegia, and distinctive intracranial calcifications that are
demonstrable on plain skull x-rays. Sturge-Weber disease is
a phakomatosis that apparently results from the abnormal differentiation of the cephalic primordial vascular plexus early
in embryogenesis.

2. (B) The mere presence of a facial angioma is not conclu-
sive evidence of this disorder. Characteristically, the vascular
nevus in Sturge-Weber disease corresponds roughly to the distribution of the trigeminal nerve, especially the ophthalmic and
maxillary divisions. Occasionally, the angioma extends into
the area of the mandibular division or even into upper cervical
nerve dermatomes. The nevus often falls short of or extends
across the midline. The lips, gums, palate, uvula and nose
also may be affected. Involvement of the eyelid and supraorbital region is especially characteristic of the nevi associated
with this disorder. Microscopically, the cutaneous angioma
consists of capillary type vessels within the dermis. The
epidermis and cutaneous adnexal structures are unaffected.

3. (A, D) The primary intracranial lesion is a meningeal
angioma, involving the pia and arachnoid over the parietal and
occipital lobes on the same side as the cutaneous vascular
nevus. The meningeal angioma is composed of abnormal
serpiginous veins with thickened or hyalinized walls (Fig. 59.1).
The intervening meninges may be quite fibrotic and in a few
cases, may contain heavily pigmented melanocytes.

The angioma does not extend into the underlying brain parenchyma. However, the subjacent parietal and occipital lobes are
usually quite atrophic. Microscopically, the cortex shows loss
of neurons, gliosis and mineralization. Fine "droplet" calcifications may be present along the intraparenchymal capillaries.
Most of the mineral is deposited in the form of small calcospherites that are most abundant in the outer two or three

layers of the cortex (see Fig. 59.1). Whether the calcospherites arise from perivascular mineralization or not is unsettled. The choroid plexus is often involved by the angioma. The involvement of this structure reflects the participation of infolded meninges in the formation of the vascular stroma of the choroid plexi. The brain stem and cerebellum are unaffected by the angioma or mineralization, but the cerebellum may show loss of Purkinje cells secondary to anoxia from the seizures.

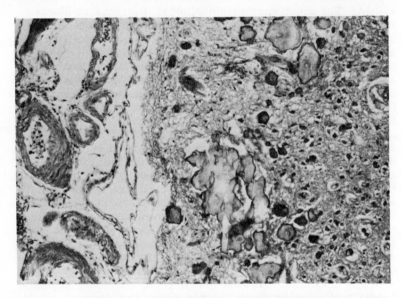

FIG. 59.1: Microscopic section through the meninges and cortex from a patient with Sturge-Weber disease. Note the venous angioma in the meninges (left of the picture) and the calcospherites in the superficial layers of the cortex (right of the picture).

4. (A, B, C) Major complications of Sturge-Weber disease include mental retardation, epilepsy, hemiplegia and loss of vision. Hemorrhage, either subarachnoid or intracerebral, is an exceptionally uncommon complication.

5. (C) The distinctive "tram-track" or "railroad track" calcifications are due to the deposits of mineral in the superficial portions of apposing gyri. Since there is only minimal mineralization within the vessels of the angioma, the sulci between the affected gyri remain radiolucent.

6. (D) The calcospherites, like most mineral deposits in the body, are composed of calcium phosphate and calcium carbonate. A variable but small quantity of iron is also present. Calcium oxalate is found in the mineral deposits within the thyroid gland and calcium salts of fatty acids, i.e., calcium "soaps," result from fat necrosis.

7. (B, C) Ocular abnormalities that are characteristically associated with the Sturge-Weber syndrome include increased intraocular tension and angiomas of the choroid. Glaucoma is found in about one-third of the patients and is probably due to an angioma of the choroid. Microscopically, the retina and sclera are usually uninvolved. Occasionally, the conjunctiva is involved by the facial angioma. Iridial heterochromia has been observed in patients with Sturge-Weber disease.

8. (A) Sturge-Weber disease is rarely accompanied by lesions in the visceral organs. When present, they are predominantly hemangiomas.

9. (B, D) Sturge-Weber disease has been encountered in all races and affects males and females equally. Many of the cases are sporadic although autosomal recessive and autosomal dominant inheritance have been described in some families.

10. (B, C, D) Neurocutaneous melanosis is a rare, but dramatic, phakomatosis. The patients usually have giant pigmented nevi that involve the lower abdomen, buttocks or back. The nevi are often hairy. The meninges are often thickened and pigmented due to an increased number of melanocytes. Intraparenchymal pigmented areas are more common in the cerebellum than the cerebrum. The intraparenchymal pigmented areas result from pigmented meningeal melanocytes along penetrating blood vessels and from pigmented macrophages. Although the lesions superficially resemble metastases from melanoma, there are no neoplastic cells. However, there is a high risk of developing a malignant melanoma from the pigmented meninges.

REFERENCES

1. Alexander GL: Sturge-Weber Syndrome. In: Handbook of Clinical Neurology. Vinken PJ and Bruyn GW (Eds.). North-Holland, Amsterdam, 1972, Vol. 14, pp. 223-240.

2. Alexander GL and Norman RM: The Sturge-Weber Syndrome. John Wright, Bristol, 1960.

3. de Recondo J and Haguenau M: Neuropathologic Survey
    of the Phakomatoses and Allied Disorders. In: Handbook
    of Clinical Neurology. Vinken PJ and Bruyn GW (Eds.).
    North-Holland, Amsterdam, 1972, Vol. 14, pp. 61-69.

4. Fox H: Neurocutaneous Melanosis. In: Handbook of
    Clinical Neurology. Vinken PJ and Bruyn GW (Eds.).
    North-Holland, Amsterdam, 1972, Vol. 14, pp. 414-
    428.

5. Slaughter JC, et al.: Neurocutaneous melanosis and
    leptomeningeal melanomatosis in children. Arch Path
    88:298-304, 1969.

6. Stehbens WE: Pathology of the Cerebral Blood Vessels.
    C.V. Mosby Co., St. Louis, 1972, pp. 519-526.

: :

CASE 60: A 2-Year-Old Jewish Boy with Psychomotor
             Retardation

CLINICAL DATA

This 2-year-old boy was the product of an uneventful pregnancy
and delivery in a 20-year-old Jewish woman. The child's birth
weight was 7 lbs, 12 oz. His growth and development were
apparently normal until the age of 8 months. Following a mild
febrile illness, he began to lose weight and was no longer able
to sit. By 11 months, he was lethargic, rarely cried, and fed
poorly. The child continued to deteriorate and was eventually
hospitalized at 22 months of age for evaluation of his psychomotor retardation.

Physical examination revealed a lethargic child with a weak
cry. His head circumference was normal and his anterior
fontanelle was closed. His eyes showed roving movements but
no tracking. The pupils reacted to light. Funduscopic examination disclosed optic atrophy with a cherry red spot in the
macula.   The child exhibited an exaggerated startle response
and episodes of decerebrate posturing. His extremities were
wasted, stiff, and displayed "clasp knife" spasticity. Deep tendon reflexes were hyperactive but there were no Babinski signs.
The thorax and abdomen were normal; there was no visceromegaly. All routine clinical laboratory studies including cerebrospinal fluid examination were normal. Plain skull x-rays,
a ventriculogram and a radioisotope brain scan were normal.
A brain biopsy was performed to confirm the clinical impression.

QUESTIONS

1.   The clinical data are most consistent with a diagnosis of
     A. Tay-Sachs disease
     B. infantile Niemann-Pick disease
     C. generalized gangliosidosis
     D. Krabbe's disease

2.   Fig. 60.1 illustrates the morphological features encoun-
     tered in the brain biopsy specimen. These can be inter-
     preted most appropriately as diagnostic of
     A. Tay-Sachs disease
     B. a sphingolipidosis
     C. a storage disorder
     D. Niemann-Pick disease

3. Fig. 60.2 is an electron micrograph illustrating the ultra-
    structure of the material stored within the neurons. These
    bodies are best described as
    A. lipofuscin granules
    B. membranous cytoplasmic bodies
    C. zebra bodies
    D. peroxisomes

4. The metabolic derangement in Tay-Sachs disease is an
    accumulation of
    A. GM-2 ganglioside due to deficiency of beta-galacto-
        sidase activity
    B. GM-1 ganglioside due to deficiency of beta-galacto-
        sidase activity
    C. GM-2 ganglioside due to deficiency of hexosaminidase
        A and B activity
    D. GM-2 ganglioside due to deficiency of hexosaminidase
        A activity

5. Sandhoff's disease differs from Tay-Sachs disease in
    regard to
    A. demography
    B. composition of material stored in the nervous system
    C. enzyme deficiency
    D. clinical course

6. So-called generalized gangliosidosis differs from Tay-
    Sachs disease in regard to
    A. demography
    B. clinical manifestations
    C. composition of stored material
    D. enzyme deficiency

7. The biochemical abnormalities in infantile Niemann-Pick
    disease are
    A. deficiency of sphingomyelinase
    B. deficiency of glucuronidase
    C. accumulation of sphingomyelin and cholesterol
    D. accumulation of glucocerebroside

8. The biochemical abnormalities in Gaucher's disease are
    A. deficiency of galactocerebrosidase
    B. deficiency of glucocerebrosidase
    C. accumulation of galactocerebroside
    D. accumulation of glucocerebroside

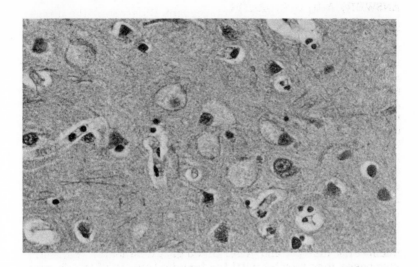

FIG. 60. 1: Microscopic section prepared from the brain biopsy specimen.

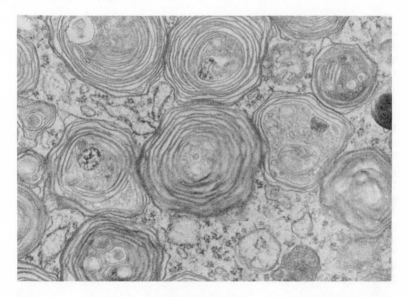

FIG. 60.2: Electron micrograph prepared from the brain biopsy specimen showing the abnormal structures within the cytoplasm of a neuron.

ANSWERS AND DISCUSSION

1. (A) The clinical data are most consistent with a diagnosis of Tay-Sachs disease. This is a rare metabolic disorder that is characterized by an increased concentration of GM-2 ganglioside, especially in nervous tissue. The disease is inherited as an autosomal recessive trait and is found predominantly in Ashkenazi Jews, among whom it occurs with a frequency of 1 in 4,000 to 6,000 live births. The onset of clinical symptoms usually becomes obvious around 6 months of age. Early symptoms include listlessness, weakness, inability to sit, and feeding difficulties. A common early or even initial sign is an exaggerated startle response that is often designated erroneously as "hyperacusis." Visual impairment is often manifested by inattentiveness, roving eye movements and a lack of tracking. Optic atrophy and a cherry red spot in the macula have been found in virtually every patient. A cherry red spot can also be found in patients with Sandhoff's disease, infantile Niemann-Pick disease and generalized gangliosidosis. Pupillary responses may persist until the terminal stages of the disease. Older children with Tay-Sachs disease may have megalencephaly. There are no skeletal abnormalities and no visceromegaly. Death usually ensues by 3 or 4 years of age.

Niemann-Pick disease is actually a group of related disorders of which the infantile form is by far the most common. Infantile Niemann-Pick disease is found predominantly among Jews and is characterized by the early onset of psychomotor retardation. Over one-third of these children have a cherry red spot in their macula. Of diagnostic significance are hepatic and splenic enlargement which develop during the first few months of life. Furthermore, many of these children are mildly jaundiced for three to four months. Death ensues by the age of 3 or 4 years.

Patients with generalized gangliosidosis often show obvious psychomotor retardation from the time of birth. They also display various facial anomalies including frontal bossing, depressed nasal bridge, hypertrophied gums and macroglossia. Numerous skeletal anomalies can be demonstrated roentgenographically. Cherry red spots can be found in the macula of about half of these patients. Hepatosplenomegaly is usually evident by six months of age. Unlike Tay-Sachs disease, this disorder shows no ethnic predilection. Death usually ensues by the age of two years.

Patients with Krabbe's disease show marked irritability, pronounced temperature lability, opisthotonic posturing and lack the cherry red spots in the macula.

2. (C) The neuronal perikarya are enlarged and have rounded
profiles. The Nissl granules and nuclei are displaced by intracytoplasmic material that appears somewhat "foamy" in
paraffin embedded sections. Similar material is found in the
distended neuronal processes. The neuronal alterations are not
diagnostic of Tay-Sachs disease or even a sphingolipidosis.
They should be interpreted merely as evidence of a storage disease. Routine histochemical techniques are of limited value in
defining the nature of the intraneuronal stored material, since
no stains are specific for the gangliosides. The cortex shows
mild to marked astrocytosis and the white matter eventually
shows demyelinization.

3. (B) Ultrastructurally, the stored material appears as myriads of concentrically laminated spheroids admixed with smaller
quantities of granular osmiophilic material. The bodies are
membrane-bounded and display intense acid phosphatase activity
suggesting a derivation from lysosomes. These bodies have
been designated as "membranous cytoplasmic bodies" and are
typically found in Tay-Sachs and Sandhoff's diseases. Unfortunately, similar cytosomes have been found in other gangliosidoses, such as generalized gangliosidosis.

Zebra bodies are typically elongated, transversely striated cytosomes. They are characteristically found in neurons in association with various mucopolysaccharidoses. Lipofuscin granules typically consist of membrane-bounded aggregate of granular osmiophilic material and homogeneous electron-lucent
lipid droplets. They may be found in normal individuals and in
patients with certain of the neuronal ceroid-lipofuscinoses.
Peroxisomes are intensely osmiophilic spheroids characteristically found in the liver and kidney.

4. (D) In 1942, Klenk demonstrated elevated levels of gangliosides, complex sphingolipids that contain sialic acid, in the
brains of patients with Tay-Sachs disease. In 1962, Svenner-
holm identified the accumulated material specifically as GM-2
ganglioside. Normally, this is a minor cerebral component
but in patients with Tay-Sachs disease, GM-2 constitutes 70 to
80% of the total gangliosides and is 100 to 300 times more abundant than in the normal brain. Lesser amounts of the asialoderivative of GM-2 ganglioside also accumulate.

In 1969, Okada and O'Brien demonstrated a profound deficiency
of hexosaminidase A activity in patients with Tay-Sachs disease.
The deficiency or absence of this lysosomal hydrolytic enzyme is
responsible for the abnormal accumulation of GM-2 ganglioside.

Assays for this enzyme can be performed on serum to identify heterozygous carriers and on amniotic cells and fluid to detect affected progeny prenatally. Although the enzyme deficiency is found throughout the body and small amounts of GM-2 ganglioside accumulate in a number of visceral organs, morphological changes are virtually limited to the nervous system and eyes in Tay-Sachs disease.

5. (A, C) Sandhoff's disease is a form of GM-2 gangliosidosis that clinically is indistinguishable from Tay-Sachs disease except for showing no ethnic predilection. The morphological changes in the nervous system by both light and electron microscopy are identical in the two conditions. The visceral organs in patients with Sandhoff's disease have been reported to show a number of features not found in Tay-Sachs disease. Most striking is vacuolation of pancreatic acinar cells and lesser degrees of vacuolation in hepatocytes and the tubular cells of the kidney. Granules that stain blue with luxol-fast blue are found in the heart, bronchial epithelium, splenic histiocytes and lymph nodes. Biochemically, both hexosaminidase A and B activity are deficient. As a result, GM-2 ganglioside and the asialoderivative of GM-2 ganglioside accumulate in the nervous system and in the viscera. In addition, globoside, an aminoglycolipid, accumulates in visceral organs.

6. (A, B, C, D) So-called generalized gangliosidosis or GM-1 gangliosidosis differs in many respects from Tay-Sachs disease. There is no ethnic predilection as in Tay-Sachs disease. Psychomotor retardation is evident sooner, beginning at or shortly after birth. The disorder is accompanied by multiple skeletal and somatic anomalies somewhat resembling those found in some of the mucopolysaccharidoses. Hepatomegaly and splenomegaly are usually evident by six months of age. GM-1 ganglioside accumulates in the nervous system and both GM-1 ganglioside and a keratan sulfate-like polysaccharide accumulate in the visceral organs. The storage of these compounds appears to be due to a profound deficiency of beta-galactosidase activity. Death usually ensues by the age of two years.

7. (A, C) The biochemical abnormalities in infantile Niemann-Pick disease are a deficiency in sphingomyelinase and an accumulation of sphingomyelin and cholesterol. By light microscopy, the neuronal alterations are virtually indistinguishable from those in Tay-Sachs disease. In the viscera, foamy cells are noted in the bone marrow, spleen, liver, lymph nodes, adrenals and lungs.

8. (B, D) The biochemical abnormalities in Gaucher's disease are a deficiency of glucocerebrosidase and an accumulation
of glucocerebroside. In the infantile form of the disease, the
enzyme deficiency is more severe and the nervous system is
involved. In the more common adult form, the enzyme deficiency is partial and the nervous system is spared.

REFERENCES

1. Aronson SM and Volk BW: The Gangliosidoses. In:
    Scientific Approaches to Clinical Neurology. Goldensohn
    ES and Appel SH (Eds.). Lea and Febiger, Philadelphia,
    1977, pp. 116-139.

2. Brady RO: Sphingomyelin Lipidosis: Niemann-Pick Dis-
    ease. In: The Metabolic Basis of Inherited Disease.
    Stanbury JB, et al. (Eds.). McGraw-Hill Book Co.,
    New York, 1978, pp. 718-730.

3. O'Brien JS: The Gangliosidoses. In: The Metabolic Basis
    of Inherited Disease. Stanbury JB, et al. (Eds.). McGraw-
    Hill Book Co., New York, 1978, pp. 841-865.

4. Volk BW, et al.: Clinic, Pathology and Biochemistry of
    Tay-Sachs Disease. In: Handbook of Clinical Neurology.
    Vinken PJ and Bruyn GW (Eds.). North-Holland, Amster-
    dam, 1970, Vol. 10, pp. 385-426.

: :

CASE 61: A 9-Month-Old Girl with Psychomotor Retardation,
Increased Muscle Tone and Seizures

CLINICAL DATA

This 9-month-old girl was the product of a normal pregnancy
and delivery.   Her neonatal growth and development were unremarkable except for a tendency to keep her fists clenched and
her arms and legs extended.   At the age of three months, the
child seemed overly irritable and cried excessively.   At four
months of age, she began to have generalized seizures that were
poorly controlled by anticonvulsants.   She had recurrent respiratory infections but also had marked temperature fluctuations
even when apparently well.   By seven months, the child showed
severe motor retardation and was deaf and blind.   Her pupils
reacted poorly to light and there were only random eye movements with no tracking.   The fundi were pale.   Muscular tone
was increased moderately in the arms and markedly in the legs.
She withdrew her extremities upon painful stimulation.   Her
head circumference was 42 cm and there was no visceromegaly.
Examination of the cerebrospinal fluid revealed a glucose of
53 mg/dl and a protein of 270 mg/dl.   Motor nerve conduction
velocity was markedly reduced.   A right frontal lobe biopsy was
performed and a morphologic diagnosis was established.   The
child died two months later.

QUESTIONS

1.   The clinical data are most consistent with a diagnosis of
     A.   Krabbe's disease
     B.   Canavan's disease
     C.   Tay-Sachs disease
     D.   Niemann-Pick disease

2.   Fig. 61.1 shows a coronal section of the brain.   The path-
     ological changes that are illustrated include
     A.   lissencephaly
     B.   cerebral atrophy
     C.   a diffuse abnormality of the white matter with cavitation
          within the internal capsule and corpus callosum
     D.   a defect from the previous brain biopsy

3.   Fig. 61.2 illustrates some of the microscopic findings in
     this brain.   These changes are diagnostic of
     A.   Tay-Sachs disease
     B.   Krabbe's disease
     C.   Canavan's disease
     D.   Alexander's disease

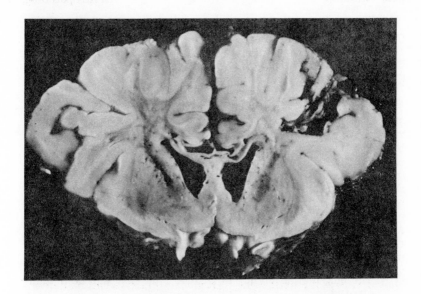

FIG. 61.1: Coronal section of the child's brain.

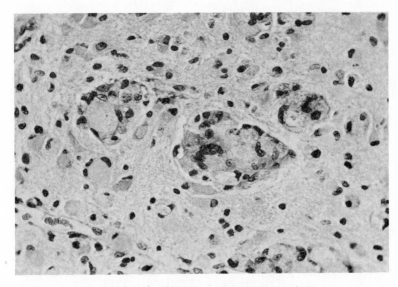

FIG. 61.2: Microscopic section showing the diagnostic histological characteristics of this disorder.

4. The material that accumulates within the macrophages is
    A. a sphingolipid
    B. a ganglioside
    C. galactocerebroside
    D. a normal constituent of myelin

5. Ultrastructurally, the accumulated lipid appears as
    A. membranous cytoplasmic bodies
    B. zebra bodies
    C. multiangular polygonal structures
    D. twisted tubules

6. The enzyme that has been demonstrated to be deficient in
    Krabbe's disease is
    A. sphingomyelinase
    B. galactocerebroside beta-galactosidase
    C. hexosaminidase A
    D. hexosaminidase B

7. The enzyme deficiency in Krabbe's disease can be demon-
    strated in
    A. fibroblasts
    B. brain
    C. leukocytes
    D. amniotic fluid cells

8. In addition to brain, morphological changes characteristic
    of Krabbe's disease have been demonstrated in
    A. the liver
    B. the kidney
    C. peripheral nerves
    D. lymph nodes

9. Another leukodystrophy that is characterized by myelin
    degeneration and accumulation of a sphingolipid is
    A. metachromatic leukodystrophy
    B. Pelizaeus-Merzbacher disease
    C. sulfatide lipidosis
    D. Alexander's disease

10. Histopathological changes characteristic of metachromatic
    leukodystrophy include
    A. Rosenthal fiber deposits
    B. loss of myelin
    C. decreased numbers of oligodendrocytes
    D. deposits of cerebroside sulfate in macrophages and
        neurons

ANSWERS AND DISCUSSION

1. (A) The clinical data are most consistent with a diagnosis
of Krabbe's disease. Although this disease probably "begins"
in utero with the onset of myelination, clinical manifestations
usually become evident between three and six months of age.
This rare disease affects all ethnic groups and both sexes and
is considered to be inherited as an autosomal recessive trait.
Hagberg has divided the clinical course of the disease into three
stages. The first stage is characterized by irritability, excessive crying, febrile episodes, and some stiffness of the
limbs. During the second stage, there is rapid mental and
motor deterioration with hypertonicity, opisthotonic posturing
and seizures. The child becomes decerebrate and blind during
the third and final stage. Death usually occurs before the age
of two years. Examination of the cerebrospinal fluid reveals,
as in the present case, an elevated protein content with a relative increase in albumin and alpha-2-globulin.

In Canavan's disease or spongy degeneration of the white matter, the head becomes enlarged, the patient is hypotonic and
the cerebrospinal fluid protein is not elevated. Patients with
Tay-Sachs disease often display a characteristic exaggerated
startle reflex and have a cherry red spot in the macula. Patients with the infantile form of Niemann-Pick disease have
visceromegaly in addition to the psychomotor retardation. Furthermore, about one-third of them have a cherry red spot in
their macula.

2. (B, C, D) The brain is markedly reduced in size. However,
the gyral pattern is essentially normal and the cortical grey
matter is relatively unaffected. The white matter is reduced
in volume, extremely firm and discolored. The subcortical
"U" fibers or arcuate fibers are less severely involved than
the central white matter. The corpus callosum and the internal capsules show foci of cavitation. The widespread roughly
symmetrical involvement of white matter with relative sparing
of the subcortical "U" fiber is characteristic of a leukodystrophy.
The wedge-shaped defect in the right middle frontal convolution
and underlying white matter is from the previous biopsy.

3. (B) The morphological changes that are illustrated are diagnostic of Krabbe's disease. In this disorder, the white matter contains little myelin but numerous clusters of lipid-laden
macrophages. Formerly, the mononucleated macrophages
were referred to as "epithelioid cells" and the multinucleated
macrophages were termed "globoid cells." Now both types are

commonly designated as globoid cells. These cells are further
characterized by intense red staining with the periodic acid-
Schiff reaction. Oligodendrocytes are severely reduced in number or even absent. The astrocytes show marked proliferation
and are responsible for the rubbery texture of the brain.

4.   (A, C, D) The lipid that accumulates within the macrophages is predominantly galactocerebroside. This sphingo-
lipid is a normal constituent of the myelin sheath. Gangliosides are sphingolipids that contain one or more sialic acid
moieties. They are found predominantly in axon terminals.

5.   (C, D) With the macrophages, the lipid deposits appear
as membrane-bounded accumulations of multiangular polygonal
structures (Fig. 61.3). These may be accompanied by amorphous osmiophilic material. In patients reported by Yunis and
Lee and in a case of ours, there were also numerous longitudinally striated, periodically twisted tubules that had a diameter
of approximately 30 nm. Both the multiangular polygonal structures and the twisted tubules have been obtained when galactocerebroside from patients with Krabbe's disease is injected intracerebrally in young rats. It is not clear why the twisted
tubules have not been encountered more often in the naturally
occurring disease.

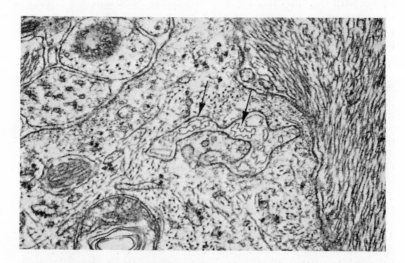

FIG. 61.3:   Electron micrograph showing the ultrastructure of
            the accumulated lipid (arrows). Note the glial fila-
            ments in an astrocyte to the right.

Membranous cytoplasmic bodies are the concentric laminated
deposits of complex lipids found in patients with the GM-1 and
GM-2 gangliosidoses. Zebra bodies are the striated deposits
of lipid found in patients with the mucopolysaccharidoses.

6. (B) The enzyme that has been shown to be deficient in
Krabbe's disease is galactocerebroside beta-galactosidase.
This is a lysosomal enzyme that is responsible for the catabolism of galactocerebroside, a major constituent of myelin.
When myelination begins, the newly formed myelin normally
undergoes rapid turnover. However, in patients with Krabbe's
disease, the deficiency of galactocerebroside beta-galactosidase results in the accumulation of galactocerebroside. This
material accumulates in macrophages and elicits the distinctive
globoid cell reaction. Apparently the accumulation of psycho-
sine results in the death of oligodendrocytes and cessation
of further myelination. Eventually these changes are accompanied by loss of axons.

7. (A, B, C, D) The enzyme deficiency can be demonstrated
in a wide variety of tissues and in blood serum. Assays of
activity in leukocytes and cultured fibroblasts have been used
to make the diagnosis of Krabbe's disease without resorting to
brain biopsy. Amniotic fluid cells obtained by amniocentesis
have been used to establish the diagnosis prenatally.

8. (C) Although the enzyme galactocerebroside beta-galactosidase appears to be deficient throughout the body, morphological changes are found only where myelin is normally present. In the peripheral nerves, the changes are often not conspicuous and certainly not diagnostic by light microscopy. The
characteristic lipid inclusions can be demonstrated by electron
microscopy in the Schwann cells and associated macrophages.
The kidney is known to contain galactocerebroside and might be
expected to show some changes. To date, however, morphological alterations have not been demonstrated by light or electron microscopy in any tissues other than brain and peripheral
nerves.

9. (A, C) Sulfatide lipidosis, otherwise known as metachromatic leukodystrophy, is characterized by myelin degeneration
and the accumulation of galactocerebroside sulfate in the nervous system and a number of visceral organs. This disorder
affects both sexes and has been described in many ethnic groups.
There are at least three variants of which the late infantile
form is the most common. This variant is due to the absence
or marked deficiency of arylsulfatase A. The patient's initial

development is usually normal. The disease usually becomes manifested by a disturbance of motor function between the ages of 12 and 18 months. Progressive deterioration leads to quadriplegia, blindness, deafness and dementia. Death usually occurs during the first or second decades. The adult variant is apparently due to a partial deficiency of arylsulfatase A. Dementia often dominates the clinical picture.

10. (B, C, D) The histopathological features of sulfatide lipidosis or metachromatic leukodystrophy include loss of myelin, decrease in the number of oligodendrocytes and deposits of sulfatide within macrophages and neurons. The lipid deposits are further characterized by periodic acid-Schiff positivity and metachromasia. The Hirsch-Peiffer stain, cresyl violet acidified with acetic acid, produces a distinctive brown color. Peripheral nerves, kidney, liver and gallbladder are also common sites of heavy galactocerebroside sulfate deposition. Because of the known renal involvement, examination of urinary sediment of metachromasia has been utilized as a test for sulfatide lipidosis. Unfortunately, this is an unreliable procedure.

REFERENCES

1. Dulaney JT and Moser H: Sulfatide Lipidosis: Metachromatic Leukodystrophy. In: The Metabolic Basis of Inherited Disease. Stanbury JB, et al. (Eds.). McGraw-Hill Book Co., New York, 1978, pp. 770-809.

2. Hagberg B: Clinical aspects of globoid cell and metachromatic leukodystrophy. Birth Defects: Original Article Series 7:103-112, 1971.

3. Schochet SS Jr., et al.: Krabbe's disease. Acta Neuropath 36:153-160, 1976.

4. Suzuki K and Suzuki Y: Galactosylceramide Lipidosis: Globoid Cell Leukodystrophy. In: The Metabolic Basis of Inherited Disease. Stanbury JB, et al. (Eds.). McGraw-Hill Book Co., New York, 1978, pp. 749-769.

5. Yunis EJ and Lee RE: The morphologic similarities of human and canine globoid leukodystrophy. Amer J Path 85:99-114, 1976.

: :

CASE 62: A 4-1/2-Year-Old Girl with Skeletal Deformities,
          Corneal Clouding and Mental Retardation

CLINICAL DATA

This child was the product of a 36-week gestation. She weighed
4 lbs, 14-1/2 oz at birth and gained weight slowly during the
neonatal period.   She smiled at 4 months, controlled her head
at 5 months, rolled over and transferred objects from hand to
hand at 7 months. At 8 months of age, she was hospitalized
for evaluation of her skeletal deformities and retardation.
Upon admission, she weighed 13 lbs, 4 oz and measured
25-1/2 inches in length. Her head circumference was 17 inches.
Her eyebrows were coarse and thick and there was a gibbus of
her lumbar spine. Both the liver and spleen were enlarged.
She was unable to sit alone or stand with support and displayed
generalized hypotonia with decreased tendon reflexes. A clinical impression of Hurler's disease was confirmed by determination of the urinary mucopolysaccharides.

At the age of 4-1/2 years, the child was admitted to the hospital because of respiratory distress with cyanosis. For several
days, the child had had an upper respiratory infection with
rhinorrhea, cough, and mild fever. Physical examination revealed a markedly cyanotic and unresponsive child with shallow
respirations.   Her pupils were reactive to light but the fundi
could not be visualized because of corneal clouding. There
was generalized hypotonia with decreased deep tendon reflexes
but no pathological reflexes. There was no response to painful
stimuli. The facial features were coarse with thick eyebrows,
hypertelorism and a depressed nasal bridge.   Her tongue was
large and protuberant. Coarse rhonchi and basilar rales were
present.   No heart murmurs were present. The abdomen was
protuberant and both the liver and spleen were enlarged. An
umbilical hernia was present. An x-ray of the chest revealed
cardiomegaly and bilateral lower lobe infiltrates. The child was
digitalized and given oxygen, diuretics and antibiotics. Despite
these measures, the child died on the day following admission.

QUESTIONS

1. Patients with Hurler's disease show urinary excretion of
    A. heparan sulfate only
    B. dermatan sulfate only
    C. keratan sulfate
    D. dermatan sulfate and heparan sulfate

2. Hunter's disease differs from Hurler's disease in that
    there is
    A. urinary excretion of dermatan sulfate and heparan
        sulfate
    B. X-linked recessive inheritance
    C. minimal or no corneal clouding
    D. a longer life span

3. Sanfilippo's disease is characterized by
    A. severe mental retardation
    B. urinary excretion of heparan sulfate only
    C. mild skeletal deformities
    D. cardiomegaly

4. Fig. 62.1 illustrates the appearance of a coronal section
    from this child's brain.   The gross neuropathological
    changes that are commonly encountered in patients with
    Hurler's disease include
    A. thickening and clouding of the leptomeninges
    B. hydrocephalus
    C. "knife-edge atrophy" of the gyri
    D. enlargement of perivascular spaces

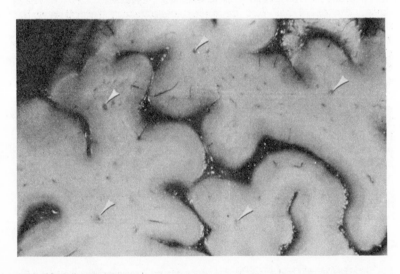

FIG. 62.1: Coronal section of a cerebral hemisphere from this
            child's brain. Note the enlarged perivascular spaces
            (arrows).

5. Fig. 62.2 illustrates the neuronal changes encountered in this child's brain. These changes are
   A. diagnostic of Hurler's disease
   B. indicative of a neuronal storage disease
   C. due to neuronal storage of mucopolysaccharides
   D. due to neuronal storage of gangliosides

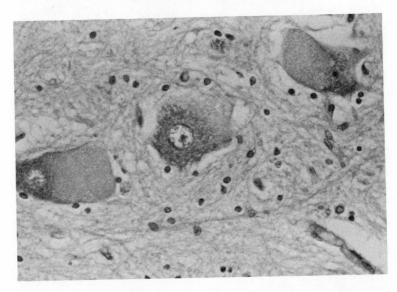

FIG. 62. 2: Microscopic section showing the neuronal alterations observed in this child's brain.

6. Fig. 62.3 illustrates the ultrastructure of the intraneuronal gangliosides in a patient with Hurler's disease. These cytosomes have been described as
   A. zebra bodies
   B. membranous cytoplasmic bodies
   C. microbodies
   D. Lafora bodies

7. Enzyme deficiencies have been described in Hurler's disease. The deficient enzymes are
   A. aryl sulfatase A
   B. galactocerebrosidase
   C. beta-galactosidase
   D. alpha-iduronidase

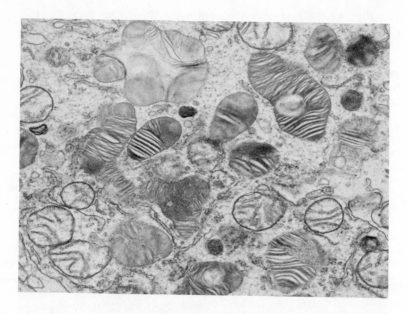

FIG. 62.3: Electron micrograph from a patient with Hurler's disease showing the configuration of the intraneuronal lipid cytosomes.

8. Histological abnormalities observed in the adenohypophysis of patients with Hurler's disease include
    A. vacuolization predominantly of acidophils
    B. vacuolization predominantly of basophils
    C. Crooke's hyalinization
    D. gamma cell hyperplasia

ANSWERS AND DISCUSSION

1. (D) The mucopolysaccharidoses are a group of genetically determined diseases that are characterized by abnormal deposition of mucopolysaccharides in tissues and excretion of mucopolysaccharides. They can be distinguished in part by the nature of the excreted mucopolysaccharide. Hurler's disease and Hunter's disease are characterized by the excretion of both dermatan sulfate and heparan sulfate. Sanfilippo's disease is characterized by the excretion of heparan sulfate only. Maroteaux-Lamy disease is characterized by the excretion of dermatan sulfate only.

Morquio's disease is characterized by the excretion of keratan
sulfate. Mental retardation is associated especially with the
forms of mucopolysaccharidoses in which there is excretion of
heparan sulfate.

2. (B, C, D) Both dermatan sulfate and heparan sulfate are
excreted in the urine by patients with Hurler's disease and with
Hunter's disease. Hunter's disease is somewhat more common
than Hurler's disease and displays similar, but milder, abnormalities. Mental retardation is less pronounced, the lumbar
gibbus does not develop and the patients have a longer life span,
often surviving into the third or fourth decades. In both disorders, death is often due to cardiac involvement which includes
thickening of the valves, endocardium and coronary arteries.
Corneal clouding that is so prominent in Hurler's disease is
generally mild or not present in Hunter's disease. In striking
contrast to the other mucopolysaccharidoses that are inherited
as autosomal recessive traits, Hunter's disease is inherited as
an X-linked recessive trait. Therefore, the disorder is expressed in all males who carry the gene and only in females
who are homozygous.

3. (A, B, C) Sanfilippo's disease is characterized by severe
mental retardation and seizures but mild skeletal and somatic
abnormalities. Cardiac complications and corneal clouding
probably do not occur in this variant of the mucopolysaccharidoses. The mucopolysaccharide excreted in the urine is heparan
sulfate.

4. (A, B, D) The leptomeninges are characteristically thickened due to an accumulation of mucopolysaccharides. When the
brain is fixed, the thickened meninges appear quite cloudy.
Arachnoidal cysts about the foramen of Magendie have been
present in a number of our cases. Dural and ligamentous thickening may cause cervical cord compression. The brains frequently show hydrocephalus that may be quite severe. This has
been attributed to impediment of the cerebrospinal fluid circulation by the thickened leptomeninges. The leptomeningeal thickening extends into the Virchow-Robin spaces, as illustrated in
Fig. 62.1. In some patients, the gyri are mildly narrowed but
not to the degree implied by the expression "knife-edge atrophy."
This designation is generally reserved to describe the very
severe atrophy encountered in cases of Pick's disease.

5. (B, D) The neurons in this patient's brain and spinal cord
were distended by finely granular intracytoplasmic material that
displaced the nucleus and the Nissl granules. Changes of this

nature are indicative of an intraneuronal storage disorder but
are not specific for any particular disease. Although Hurler's
disease is classified as a mucopolysaccharidosis, the material
that accumulates within the neurons is ganglioside. Histochemical procedures do not permit identification of specific
gangliosides. Biochemical data on the ganglioside content of
brains from patients with Hurler's disease are limited and not
without contradiction. The monosialogangliosides GM-2 and
GM-3 are regularly increased whereas GM-1 may be normal
or increased. The elevation in total gangliosides is considerably less, however, than in GM-2 or GM-1 gangliosidoses.

6. (A) By electron microscopy, the ganglioside accumulations
within the cytoplasm of neurons from patients with Hurler's disease typically appear as membrane-bounded, elongated structures
with transverse striations or lamellae. These structures were
named "zebra bodies" by Olszewski. In addition, other cytosomes have irregular lamellae and granular material. Identical
cytosomes have been found in Sanfilippo's disease and Hunter's
disease. Unfortunately, similar configurations can also be
found in GM-1 and GM-2 gangliosidoses. Conversely, membranous cytoplasmic bodies, composed of concentric lamellae
occasionally can be found in Hurler's disease, although they are
typically found in Tay-Sachs disease and generalized gangliosidosis. Thus, one must interpret these various configurations
merely as evidence of ganglioside accumulation but not as diagnostic of specific disorders.

Microbodies or peroxisomes are membrane-bounded osmiophilic structures that are most abundant in kidney and liver and
the sites of various oxidases and catalase. Lafora bodies are
the unbounded intraneuronal accumulations of glucose polymers
that are found in myoclonus epilepsy. These bodies are variable in size and the large ones can be seen by light as well as
electron microscopy.

7. (C, D) Deficiency of beta-galactosidase activity had been
reported in Hurler's disease. This deficiency has also been
demonstrated in generalized gangliosidosis where, in contrast
to Hurler's disease, heparan sulfate and dermatan sulfate do
not accumulate. More recently, the specific enzyme deficiency
in Hurler's disease has been shown to be alpha-iduronidase deficiency.

8. (A) The pituitary glands from patients with Hurler's disease show distinctive widespread vacuolation of the adenohypophyseal cells. The majority of the severely vacuolated cells

appear to be acidophils. These often form acini about a central
lake of colloid. The basophils are less severely vacuolated
and may contain lipid. Ultrastructurally, the lipids resemble
the zebra bodies and granulomembranous bodies found in the
neurons.

REFERENCES

1. Dawson G and Lenn NJ: Polysaccharide Metabolism Dis-
    orders. In: Handbook of Clinical Neurology. Vinken PJ
    and Bruyn GW (Eds.). North-Holland, Amsterdam, 1976,
    Vol. 27, pp. 143-168.

2. Dekaban A and Patton VM: Hurler's and Sanfilippo's
    variants of mucopolysaccharidosis. Cerebral pathology
    and lipid chemistry. Arch Path 91:434-443, 1971.

3. Haust MD: The Genetic Mucopolysaccharidoses (GMS).
    In: International Review of Experimental Pathology.
    Richter GW (Ed.). Academic Press, New York, 1973,
    Vol. 12, pp. 251-313.

4. Legum CP, et al.: The genetic mucopolysaccharidoses
    and mucolipidoses: Review and comment. Adv Pediatr
    22:305-347, 1976.

5. McKusick VA, et al.: The Mucopolysaccharide Storage
    Diseases. In: The Metabolic Basis of Inherited Disease.
    Stanbury JB, et al. (Eds.). McGraw-Hill Book Co.,
    New York, 1978, pp. 1282-1307.

6. Schochet SS Jr., et al.: Pituitary gland in patients with
    Hurler's syndrome. Arch Path 97:96-99, 1974.

: :

CASE 63: A 7-Month-Old Boy with Severe Muscular Weakness, Macroglossia and Cardiomegaly

CLINICAL DATA

This 7-month-old boy was the product of an uncomplicated pregnancy and delivery. At birth he weighed 3000 g. He developed normally during the first four months but subsequently ceased to gain weight, became weaker and lost previously attained motor skills. At the age of 6 months, the child was referred to the university hospital for evaluation.

Examination on admission disclosed a chronically ill-appearing child who weighed 5000 g and measured 65 cm in length. He was unable to raise his head and was barely able to move his arms or legs against gravity. Extraocular muscle movements were normal but sucking and swallowing were impaired. The child had slight macroglossia and moderate hepatomegaly.

A chest x-ray revealed marked cardiomegaly but normal pulmonary vascular markings. An electrocardiogram revealed a normal sinus rhythm and evidence of left ventricular hypertrophy. Urinalysis and hemogram were normal. The serum electrolytes were normal. A fasting glucose level, a glucose tolerance test and the response to epinephrine stimulation were all normal. Serum muscle enzymes showed a mild elevation. Leukocytes were obtained for enzyme assays.

The child's condition continued to deteriorate over the next month. Despite the use of tube feeding, he continued to lose weight. The skeletal muscle weakness became more severe but the bulk of the muscle persisted. Respiration became entirely diaphragmatic and he died of pneumonia. The most striking gross autopsy findings in addition to bronchopneumonia were macroglossia, cardiac hypertrophy and hepatomegaly.

QUESTIONS

1. The clinical data are most consistent with a diagnosis of
   A. Werdnig-Hoffmann disease
   B. endocardial fibroelastosis
   C. Pompe's disease
   D. von Gierke's disease

2. The fasting glucose level is normal and the glucose level
    rises normally after epinephrine stimulation in
    A. Pompe's disease (type II glycogenosis)
    B. type III glycogenosis
    C. type IV glycogenosis
    D. type I glycogenosis

3. Fig. 63.1 is a photograph of a section prepared from the
    deltoid muscle. The photograph illustrates
    A. atrophy of myofibers
    B. vacuolation of myofibers
    C. target fibers
    D. excessive endomysial connective tissue

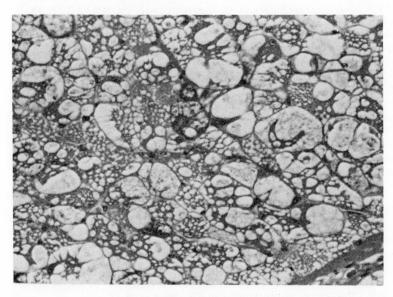

FIG. 63.1: Microscopic section prepared from the deltoid muscle.

4. Sections stained with a periodic acid-Schiff stain showed
    that much of the material within the vacuoles was Schiff
    positive, i.e., stained red. By this procedure, the
    material has been identified specifically as
    A. glycogen
    B. mucopolysaccharide
    C. glycoprotein
    D. none of these

5.   These skeletal muscle findings in an infant are consistent
     with
     A.   von Gierke's disease
     B.   Pompe's disease
     C.   Andersen's disease
     D.   Werdnig-Hoffmann disease

6.   The enzyme deficiency that has been identified in Pompe's
     disease is
     A.   alpha-1, 4-glucosidase
     B.   amylo-1, 6-glucosidase
     C.   glucose 6-phosphatase
     D.   myophosphorylase

7.   The greatest excess of biochemically normal glycogen is
     found in the skeletal muscles in
     A.   type I glycogenosis
     B.   Pompe's disease
     C.   type III glycogenosis
     D.   type IV glycogenosis

8.   Ultrastructurally, the glycogen deposits in muscles from
     patients with Pompe's disease are located in
     A.   the intermyofibrillar spaces
     B.   the sarcoplasmic reticulum
     C.   the T-tubules
     D.   membrane-bounded sacs

9.   Within the central nervous system of patients with Pompe's
     disease, deposits of glycogen are found in
     A.   neurons
     B.   myelin sheaths and oligodendrocytes
     C.   astrocytes
     D.   choroid plexus epithelium

10. The most common of the glycogenoses is
     A.   type I
     B.   type II
     C.   type III
     D.   type IV

ANSWERS AND DISCUSSION

1.   (C) The combination of muscular weakness, hypotonia,
macroglossia, cardiomegaly, and failure to thrive is characteristic of Pompe's disease, the infantile form of type II glycogenosis. The clinical symptoms generally appear within 2-3 months

and death often ensues within 6-8 months from cardiac failure.
Despite the marked skeletal muscle weakness and hypotonia,
the muscles usually retain their normal bulk and are firm to
palpation.   The hepatomegaly is variable in degree and is due
in part to the abnormal glycogen deposition and in part to the
heart failure. Werdnig-Hoffmann disease could account for the
weakness and hypotonia but would not be accompanied by cardiomegaly. Endocardial fibroelastosis would not produce the muscular weakness, hypotonia or macroglossia. Von Gierke's disease, or type I glycogenosis, produces striking hepatomegaly
but is not accompanied by the severe skeletal muscular weakness or the cardiomegaly.

2.   (A) The fasting glucose level is normal and glucose level
rises normally after stimulation with epinephrine in Pompe's
disease.   In type III glycogenosis, the post-prandial glucose
level may be normal but the fasting glucose level is usually low.
Epinephrine fails to elevate the glucose level significantly after
fasting.   In type I and type IV glycogenosis, there is both fasting hypoglycemia and a failure of the glucose level to rise with
epinephrine stimulation.   Type I is further characterized by
ketosis, hyperlipidemia and hyperuricemia.

3.   (B) The myofibers are severely vacuolated and distended
by the vacuolar contents. Some of the vacuoles contain granular material that stains blue with hematoxylin-eosin, while other
vacuoles appear empty due to loss of their contents during pro-
cessing. While there are many causes of vacuolar myopathy,
this degree of alteration is typical of glycogenosis type II or
type III.

4.   (D) The periodic acid-Schiff techniques are not specific for
any particular compound or class of compounds. Periodic acid
is a unique oxidant that forms aldehydes from 1:2 glycols, amino
or alkylamino derivatives of 1:2 glycols or partial oxidation products of 1:2 glycols.   The resulting aldehydes react with de-
colorized Schiff reagent forming the distinctive red compound.
Thus, periodic acid-Schiff staining can result from many compounds, including polysaccharides such as glycogen, mucopolysaccharides, glycoproteins, glycolipids and certain phospho-
lipids.   The elimination of the periodic acid-Schiff staining by pre-
incubation with diastase provides presumptive evident that the
material was glycogen. In Pompe's disease, the glycogen may
be accompanied by mucopolysaccharides, the latter compounds
accounting for the blue color observed with hematoxylin-eosin.

5.   (B) Accumulation of glycogen producing severe vacuolation of muscle fibers in an infant is characteristic of Pompe's disease. In glycogenosis type I, or von Gierke's disease, the muscles are not involved. In glycogenosis type III, or Cori's disease, myopathy develops in the adult rather than the child. In glycogenosis type IV, or Andersen's disease, the abnormal polysaccharide deposits in muscle are less abundant than in Pompe's disease and have a paracrystalline configuration.

6.   (A) Deficiency of alpha-1, 4-glucosidase, or acid maltase, a lysosomal enzyme, has been demonstrated in Pompe's disease. This enzyme is not on the major synthetic or degradative pathways for glycogen. Furthermore, there is an excess of free cytoplasmic, i.e., non-lysosomal glycogen in the tissues from patients with Pompe's disease. Thus, it would appear that the deficiency of acid maltase cannot account for all of the features of this disorder. Nevertheless, assays for acid maltase activity provide the biochemical basis for the diagnosis of glycogenosis type II. Deficiency of amylo-1, 6-glucosidase is found in glycogenosis type III, deficiency of glucose 6-phosphatase is found in glycogenosis type I and a deficiency of myophosphorylase is found in McArdle's disease. A somewhat heterogeneous group of glycogenoses is accompanied by an apparent deficiency of hepatic phosphorylase.

7.   (B) The greatest excess of biochemically normal glycogen is found in Pompe's disease. Normally, muscles contain about 1% glycogen, whereas in Pompe's disease it is increased to about 10%. In glycogenosis type III, the muscle glycogen content may be increased to about 3% but it is biochemically abnormal with short outer chains. In glycogenosis type IV, there is accumulation of an abnormal polysaccharide that is biochemically similar to amylopectin.

8.   (A, D) Ultrastructurally, large quantities of glycogen are found free in the sarcoplasm in the intermyofibrillar spaces. A much smaller quantity is found within the membrane-bounded sacs or lysosomes. In liver, a larger proportion of the glycogen is found within the lysosomes.

9.   (A, C, D) Within the central nervous system of patients with Pompe's disease, intraneuronal deposits of glycogen produce ballooning of nerve cells. These altered cells are most conspicuous in the anterior horns of the spinal cord (Fig. 63.2), the cranial nerve nuclei, the "roof" nuclei of the cerebellum and the basal ganglia. The epithelium of the choroid plexus often contains a great excess of glycogen. The oligodendrocytes and myelin sheaths are normal, but the astrocytes contain mild but definite accumulations of glycogen.

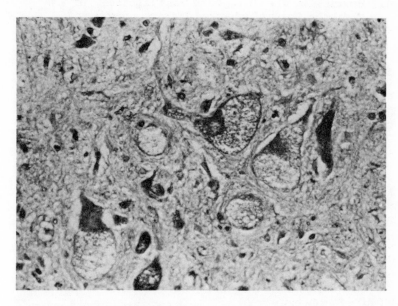

FIG. 63. 2: Microscopic section showing neurons from the anterior horns of the spinal cord.

10. (C) Type III glycogenosis is the most common of the glycogenoses and accounts for about 30% of the cases. Type I was the first of these diseases to be described and is probably the second most common, accounting for about 25% of the cases. Type II is probably the third most common. Type IV glycogenosis is very rare.

REFERENCES

1. Brunberg JA, et al.: Type III glycogenosis. Arch Neurol 25:171-178, 1971.

2. Dreyfus JC: Glycogen Storage Diseases. In: Pathobiology Annual. Ioachim HL (Ed.). Appleton-Century-Crofts, New York, 1974, pp. 289-313.

3. Engel AG, et al.: The spectrum and diagnosis of acid maltase deficiency. Neurology 23:95-106, 1973.

4. Howell RR: The Glycogen Storage Diseases. In: The
    Metabolic Basis of Inherited Disease. Stanbury JB,
    et al. (Eds.). McGraw-Hill Book Co., New York, 1978,
    pp. 137-159.

5. McAdams AJ, et al.: Glycogen storage disease, types I
    to X. Criteria for morphologic diagnosis. Human Path
    5:463-487, 1974.

6. Schochet SS Jr., et al.: Type IV glycogenosis (amylo-
    pectinosis). Arch Path 90:354-363, 1970.

7. Swaiman KF: The Glycogen Storage Diseases. In: Hand-
    book of Clinical Neurology. Vinken PJ and Bruyn GW
    (Eds.). North-Holland, Amsterdam, 1976, Vol. 27,
    pp. 221-239.

: :

CASE 64:   A 17-Year-Old Boy with Dementia and Seizures

CLINICAL DATA

This 17-year-old boy was hospitalized for evaluation of a progressive neurological disorder.   His birth and early development were unremarkable.   The patient appeared to have been
in good health until the age of 13 when he developed grand mal
seizures.   By the age of 15, the seizures had become more
frequent and were no longer controlled by anticonvulsants.   He
became withdrawn and irritable and his school performance
deteriorated. He became progressively more clumsy, dropped
objects from his hands and developed slurred speech. At age
16, myoclonus was first noted.

Examination on admission to the hospital revealed an obtunded,
slender boy with normal vital signs.   The patient was poorly
oriented and would answer only simple questions with slow responses.   The ocular fundi and cranial nerves were normal.
Constant, irregular, jerking limb movements were present. He
could move all extremities upon command but was unable to walk.
The deep tendon reflexes were slightly hyperactive.   Pain perception was intact. The remainder of the physical examination
was noncontributory.

Clinical laboratory studies on blood, urine and cerebrospinal
fluid were all within normal limits.   Electroencephalograms
revealed generalized slowing with periodic spikes that were increased in frequency upon photic stimulation.   Plain skull
x-rays and bilateral carotid arteriograms were unremarkable.
A pneumoencephalogram showed mild ventricular dilatation. A
right frontal lobe brain biopsy was performed to confirm the
clinical impression.

QUESTIONS

1.   The clinical data are consistent with a diagnosis of
     A.   subacute sclerosing panencephalitis
     B.   neuronal ceroid-lipofuscinosis
     C.   progressive myoclonus epilepsy
     D.   juvenile Huntington's chorea

2.   Fig. 64.1 illustrates the histological changes encountered
     in the brain biopsy. These abnormal structures are
     A.   Lafora bodies
     B.   corpora amylacea
     C.   Lewy bodies
     D.   lyssa bodies

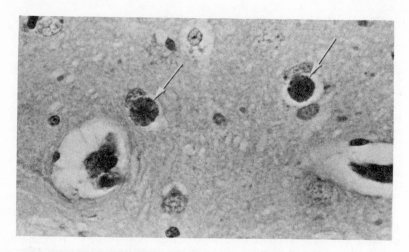

FIG. 64.1: Microscopic section prepared from the brain biopsy specimen. Note the inclusions (arrows).

3. In addition to the Lafora bodies in the central nervous system, "inclusions" or deposits may be found in
    A. the heart
    B. the skeletal muscles
    C. the liver
    D. all of these

4. Fig. 64.2 is an electron micrograph prepared from the biopsy specimen. The picture shows
    A. the intracytoplasmic location of the Lafora body
    B. that Lafora bodies are composed of morphologically normal glycogen
    C. that Lafora bodies are composed of branched fibrils
    D. that Lafora bodies are intralysosomal

5. Chemically, Lafora bodies consist of
    A. sphingolipids
    B. glucose polymers
    C. lipofuscin
    D. gangliosides

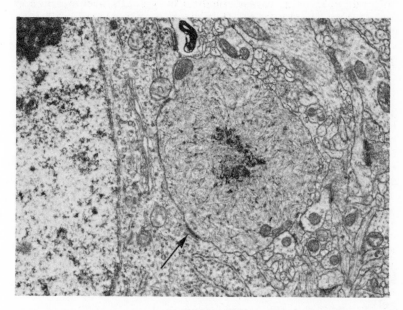

FIG. 64. 2: Electron micrograph prepared from the biopsy specimen showing a Lafora body within a presynaptic
axon terminal. Note the synapse (arrow) and the adjacent neuronal perikaryon to the left.

ANSWERS AND DISCUSSION

1. (C) The clinical data are consistent with a diagnosis of progressive myoclonus epilepsy. This is a rare familial disorder
in which the clinical manifestations usually begins during adolescence.   Frequently, the initial symptoms are generalized seizures that may not be preceded by an aura. Myoclonus develops
within a few years after the onset of the seizures.   The myoclonic jerks are aggravated by any external stimulus and increase in frequency and severity with the passage of time.   The
majority of the patients display personality changes and become
demented.   Ataxia and dysarthria are often observed.   Visual
disturbances are rare and the ocular fundi are virtually always
normal. The usual clinical laboratory studies, including cerebrospinal fluid studies, are normal. Pneumoencephalography
may demonstrate mild ventricular dilatation.   Death ensues
within 5-10 years.

Subacute sclerosing panencephalitis is typically accompanied by
an elevated cerebrospinal fluid protein with elevation of the
gamma globulin. Neuronal ceroid-lipofuscinosis may be difficult to distinguish from progressive myoclonus epilepsy but is
generally accompanied by degenerative changes in the ocular
fundi. Juvenile Huntington's chorea is usually accompanied by
rigidity.

2. (A) The characteristic histological feature of progressive
myoclonus epilepsy is the presence of Lafora bodies. As illustrated, these are spherical intracytoplasmic inclusions that are
found in neuronal perikarya and processes. With hematoxylin-
eosin, they appear as laminated basophilic or amphophilic
spheroids of variable size. The larger Lafora bodies often have
a darker staining core. They stain intensely with the periodic
acid-Schiff techniques. The use of the periodic acid-Schiff
stains will demonstrate many smaller bodies in neuronal processes that are overlooked with hematoxylin-eosin only. The
neurons may contain an increased quantity of lipofuscin. The
Lafora bodies are found throughout the cerebral cortex, within
the basal ganglia and are especially numerous in the substantia
nigra and dentate nucleus. They are also found within Purkinje
cells.

Corpora amylacea have a very similar appearance and staining
reactions but are located within astrocytic processes. For this
reason, they are especially numerous beneath the pia and
ependyma and about blood vessels. They tend to increase in
number with increasing age but are not known to be specifically
associated with any particular disorder. Lewy bodies are laminated, spherical or occasionally elongated, intracytoplasmic inclusions that are found predominantly within pigmented neurons.
They are not stained intensely by the periodic acid-Schiff stain.
They are virtually pathognomonic of Parkinsonism. Lyssa bodies
are now regarded as being identical to Negri bodies and are
found in many but not all cases of rabies. They occur predominantly in Purkinje cells and the pyramidal neurons of the hippocampus.

3. (D) In addition to the Lafora bodies within the central nervous system, patients with progressive myoclonus epilepsy may
have "inclusions" or storage deposits in heart muscle, skeletal
muscle, liver and skin. In the heart, the deposits are relatively
conspicuous and are basophilic with hematoxylin-eosin. They
are intensely stained with the periodic acid-Schiff, the methenamine silver and colloidal iron techniques. In skeletal muscle,

the deposits are often inconspicuous and may be overlooked without ultrastructural studies. In the liver, the deposits appear as ill-defined, hematoxylinophilic masses that are demonstrated somewhat better with the methenamine silver or periodic acid-Schiff techniques.

4. (A, C) The electron micrograph shows a Lafora body within the cytoplasm of a presynaptic axon terminal. The Lafora bodies are found exclusively within the perikarya and processes of neurons. The Lafora bodies are not membrane-bound, i.e., they are not within lysosomes. This can be substantiated histochemically by showing that Lafora bodies do not have acid phosphatase activity. The Lafora bodies are composed of branched fibrils that radiate out from a central core. The fibrils may be accompanied by variable quantities of amorphous, osmiophilic material that is most abundant near the core. Glycogen granules are not present in large numbers.

5. (B) Chemical studies on isolated Lafora bodies have shown that they consist of complex glucose polymers, i.e., polyglucosans. They are accompanied by protein and an acidic anion, probably phosphate. They are chemically similar to corpora amylacea, the storage deposits in type IV glycogenosis, the visceral deposits in progressive myoclonus epilepsy and the material found in basophilic degeneration of the myocardium. The basic biochemical abnormality in progressive myoclonus epilepsy is currently unknown. It has been suggested that all of these fibrillar polyglucosan deposits may be synthesized by reversal of the debranching enzyme system. More recently, it has been suggested that peroxisomes or microbodies are involved in the formation of the polyglucosan deposits encountered in myoclonus epilepsy.

REFERENCES

1. Austin J and Sakai M: Disorders of Glycogen and Related Macromolecules in the Nervous System. In: Handbook of Clinical Neurology. Vinken PJ and Bruyn GW (Eds.). North-Holland, Amsterdam, 1976, Vol. 27, pp. 169-219.

2. Carpenter S, et al.: Lafora's disease: Peroxisomal storage in skeletal muscle. Neurology 24:531-538, 1974.

3. Neville H, et al.: Studies in myoclonus epilepsy (Lafora body form). IV. Skeletal muscle abnormalities. Arch Neurol 30:466-474, 1974.

4. Sakai M, et al.: Studies in myoclonus epilepsy (Lafora body form). Neurology 20:160-176, 1970.

5. Schochet SS Jr.: Neuronal Inclusions. In: The Structure and Function of Nervous Tissue. Bourne GH (Ed.). Academic Press, New York, 1972, Vol. IV, pp. 129-177.

6. Schwarz GA: Lafora's Disease: A Disorder of Carbohydrate Metabolism. In: Scientific Approaches to Clinical Neurology. Goldensohn ES and Appel SH (Eds.). Lea and Febiger, Philadelphia, 1977, pp. 148-159.

7. Yokoi S, et al.: Studies in myoclonus epilepsy (Lafora body form). Arch Neurol 19:15-33, 1968.

: :

CASE 65: A 3-1/2-Year-Old Boy with Seizures and Rapidly
                    Progressive Psychomotor Retardation

CLINICAL DATA

This 3-1/2-year-old boy was the product of an uneventful pregnancy and delivery. His early development was considered
normal; he sat at 6 months and walked at 14 months. Petit mal
seizures were first noted at 29 months of age.   By 34 months
the seizures had increased markedly in frequency and severity.
Generalized seizures began at 37 months.

Examination at 38 months of age revealed an irritable boy who
walked with a wide-based, ataxic gait. Sensation and deep tendon reflexes were normal.   The extraocular movements and
optic fundi were normal. Clinical laboratory studies, including
cerebrospinal fluid studies, were normal. Plain skull x-rays,
carotid arteriograms and a pneumoencephalogram were normal.
An electroencephalogram showed generalized high voltage slow
waves and spike activity.   Nerve conduction velocity was normal.

At 3-1/2 years of age he was readmitted because of seizures,
myoclonus and psychomotor deterioration.   Physical examination revealed an irritable child who could not follow directions
or speak.   Truncal ataxia was pronounced; he could stand but
not walk.   Reflexes were hyperactive and Babinski signs were
present.   Cranial nerve functions were intact.   The ocular
fundi showed retinal atrophy and pigmentary changes. Clinical
laboratory studies were still normal. A right frontal lobe brain
biopsy was performed.

QUESTIONS

1.   The clinical data are consistent with a diagnosis of
     A.   Canavan's disease
     B.   Jansky-Bielschowsky disease
     C.   Tay-Sachs disease
     D.   subacute sclerosing panencephalitis

2.   Clinical laboratory findings not described in the present
     case that have been reported in patients with neuronal
     ceroid-lipofuscinosis include
     A.   hypergranulation of the polymorphonuclear leukocytes
     B.   vacuolization of lymphocytes
     C.   hyperpigmentation of polymorphonuclear leukocyte nuclei
     D.   hyposegmentation of polymorphonuclear leukocyte nuclei

3. Fig. 65.1 illustrates the histological changes encountered
    in the cerebral cortex. These include
    A. the "Schaffer-Spielmeyer process"
    B. intraneuronal accumulation of lipopigments
    C. Lafora bodies
    D. neurofibrillary tangles

4. Fig. 65.2 is an electron micrograph prepared from the
    brain biopsy specimen. Within the cytoplasm of a neuron
    are lipopigment granules having a configuration described
    as
    A. typical lipofuscin granules
    B. fingerprint patterns
    C. curvilinear profiles
    D. membranous cytoplasmic bodies

5. Patients with neuronal ceroid lipofuscinosis may have
    larger, roughly spheroidal aggregates of lipopigments
    (Fig. 65.3) designated as "myoclonus bodies of the pro-
    tein type" in
    A. substantia nigra
    B. locus caeruleus
    C. inferior olivary nucleus
    D. dentate nucleus

6. Patients with neuronal ceroid-lipofuscinosis may have
    extraneural deposits of lipopigments in
    A. skeletal muscle
    B. the myocardium
    C. smooth muscle
    D. the liver

7. A proposed metabolic basis for the neuronal ceroid-
    lipofuscinoses is a genetically determined
    A. aberration in the control of intracellular peri-
        oxidation
    B. enzyme deficiency resulting in the intracellular
        accumulation of GM-2 ganglioside
    C. enzyme deficiency resulting in the intracellular
        accumulation of GM-1 ganglioside
    D. aberration in copper metabolism

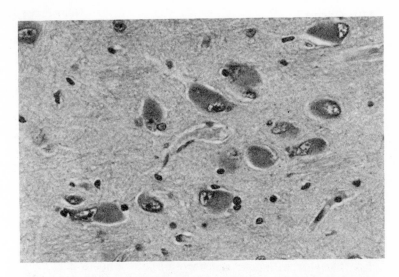

FIG. 65. 1: Microscopic section prepared from the biopsy specimen showing rounded neurons containing accumulated lipopigments.

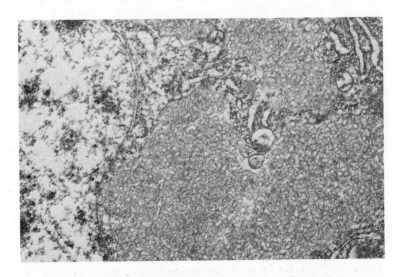

FIG. 65. 2: Electron micrograph prepared from the biopsy specimen showing the configuration of the accumulated
material within the neurons.

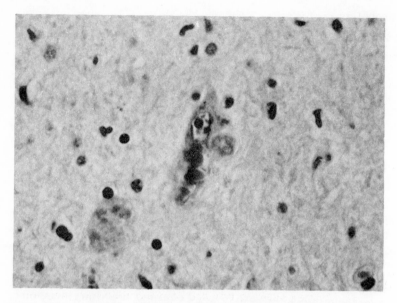

FIG. 65.3: Microscopic section from another patient with neuronal ceroid-lipofuscinosis showing the appearance
of the "myoclonus bodies of the protein type."

ANSWERS AND DISCUSSION

1. (B) The clinical data are consistent with a diagnosis of the
Jansky-Bielschowsky type of neuronal ceroid-lipofuscinosis
(Batten-Vogt syndrome). The terms neuronal ceroid-lipofuscinosis or Batten-Vogt syndrome are applied to a group of metabolic disorders that were formerly regarded, erroneously, as
variants of Tay-Sachs disease and were designated as late infantile, juvenile, and adult amaurotic familial idiocy. These
disorders are characterized by the accumulation of lipopigments
rather than the storage of ganglioside (GM-2 ganglioside), as in
Tay-Sachs disease (infantile amaurotic familial idiocy). Neuronal ceroid-lipofuscinosis shows no ethnic predilection and
generally appears to be inherited as an autosomal recessive
trait. The syndrome can be divided on the basis of clinical
criteria into four relatively distinct, major types. The Jansky-
Bielschowsky type usually begins with seizures between the
ages of 2 and 5 years. The disease progresses rapidly leading
to severe mental and motor retardation. Visual disturbances
often appear only after the patients are severely debilitated.

Cerebellar dysfunction is often prominent. The Spielmeyer-
Sjogren type generally begins somewhat later, between the ages
of 5 and 8 years, and progresses more slowly. Visual disturbances are an important and often initial manifestation. Paralysis may never develop. Kufs' disease is an adult form of
neuronal ceroid-lipofuscinosis that progresses extremely slowly.
The clinical manifestations are dominated by cerebellar and
extrapyramidal signs. Mental deterioration is less severe
than in the other types, blindness is rare and seizures usually
do not occur.

More recently, the Haltia-Santavuori type, an infantile form
characterized by rapid progression and early blindness but
minimal seizures, has been delineated.

Canavan's disease is characterized initially by loss of head control and hypotonia. Later, hyperreflexia and decerebration develop. Seizures occur in less than half of these patients and
head enlargement is often conspicuous.

Patients with Tay-Sachs disease usually have the onset of clinical manifestations at about the age of 6 months. An exaggerated
startle response is a common initial finding. Weakness and
hypotonia are followed by spasticity, deafness and blindness.
A "cherry red spot" can be found in the macula of virtually all
of these patients.

Subacute sclerosing panencephalitis often begins with behavioral
changes and seizures, including myoclonus. Psychomotor retardation, spasticity and blindness follow. The onset of clinical
symptoms is rarely as early as in the present case. The cerebrospinal fluid protein is elevated and shows a marked increase
in gamma globulin.

2.   (A, B) Hypergranulation of the polymorphonuclear leuko-
cytes has been encountered in many patients with the Jansky-
Bielschowsky type and in a few patients with the Spielmeyer-
Sjogren type of neuronal ceroid-lipofuscinosis.   Lymphocytic
vacuolization has been observed commonly in patients with the
Spielmeyer-Sjogren type of neuronal ceroid-lipofuscinosis.
Parents and two-thirds of the unaffected siblings of individuals,
with these disorders also show the same changes.

3.   (A, B) The neurons have rounded contours due to the intracellular accumulation of lipopigments. This alteration in neuronal configuration has been referred to as the "Schaffer-
Spielmeyer process." In the past, it was regarded erroneously

as pathognomonic for the "amaurotic familial idiocies." It
should be interpreted simply as a manifestation of intracellular
accumulation of material and not indicative of a particular disorder or type of material.

In neuronal ceroid-lipofuscinosis, the accumulated lipopigments
consist of lipofuscin and a closely related material, ceroid.
These substances appear as fine brown granules in sections
stained with hematoxylin-eosin. They are intensely stained by
the periodic acid-Schiff reaction and are autofluorescent when
examined with ultraviolet light. They are also stained by the
conventional "fat stains" such as the sudan dyes, by luxol-fast
blue and are acid fast. Although lipofuscin accumulates in many
neurons with advancing age, the quantity of lipopigments seen
in patients with neuronal ceroid-lipofuscinosis is far greater
than normally expected for the patient's age.

4.   (C) The intraneuronal lipopigment granules have an ultrastructural configuration described as curvilinear profiles. In
general, the lipopigment granules in patients with the Jansky-
Bielschowsky type of neuronal ceroid-lipofuscinosis are predominantly of the curvilinear configuration. The granules in
patients with the Spielmeyer-Sjogren type are predominantly of
the fingerprint or typical lipofuscin configurations. These
morphological patterns are apparently not successive stages,
since the configurations do not change from the time of biopsy
to the time of autopsy. In the infantile form of neuronal ceroid-
lipofuscinosis, the accumulated material consists predominantly
of granular osmiophilic material.

5.   (A, B, C, D) Larger, roughly spheroidal aggregates of lipopigment designated as "myoclonus bodies of the protein type" by
Seitelberger are found most commonly in the neurons of the substantia nigra. They may also be found in the thalamus, locus
caeruleus, dentate nucleus and inferior olivary nucleus. Although larger and more conspicuous, they display the same histochemical reactions and have the same ultrastructure as the
smaller lipopigment granules.

6.   (A, B, C, D) The neuronal ceroid-lipofuscinoses are systemic disorders and have excessive amounts of abnormal lipopigments in many different extraneural tissues. These include
skeletal muscle, myocardium, smooth muscle, liver, kidney,
adrenal, thyroid, spleen, lymphocytes and skin. We have found
specimens of peripheral blood lymphocytes, peripheral nerve
and skeletal muscle to be most satisfactory for the morphological

diagnosis of this condition, since the membrane-bounded deposits
of curvilinear profiles (Fig. 65.4) stand in striking contrast to
the normal organelles in these tissues.

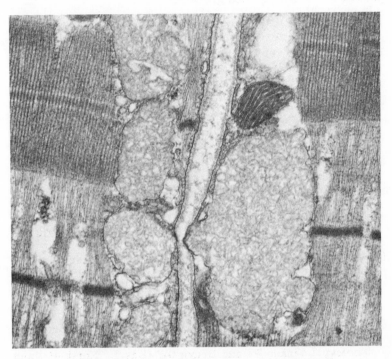

FIG. 65.4: Electron micrograph from another patient with
            Jansky-Bielschowsky type of neuronal ceroid-lipo-
            fuscinosis. The curvilinear profiles are demon-
            strated in a muscle biopsy specimen.

7. (A) Chemical analyses of brain tissue from patients with
neuronal ceroid-lipofuscinoses show no increase in the content
of GM-2 ganglioside as in Tay-Sachs disease or of GM-1 ganglioside as in generalized gangliosidosis. Instead, the tissue contains excessive amounts of two chemically similar lipopigments,
lipofuscin and ceroid. The excessive accumulation of these lipopigments is presumed to result from a genetically determined
aberration in the control of intracellular peroxidation. Peroxidation of polyunsaturated fatty acids produces malonaldehyde and
other active carbonyl compounds. These active compounds

react with the amino groups of proteins, nucleic acids and complex lipids producing non-catabolizable polymers. Thus, a wide
variety of biological molecules, membranes and even organelles
can be inactivated and incorporated into residual bodies which
persist as the lipopigment granules.

REFERENCES

1. Carpenter S, et al.: Specific involvement of muscle,
   nerve and skin in late infantile and juvenile amaurotic
   idiocy. Neurology 22:170-186, 1972.

2. Haltia M, et al.: Infantile type of so-called neuronal
   ceroid-lipofuscinosis. Part 2. Morphological and biochemical studies. J Neurol Sci 18:269-285, 1973.

3. Markesbery WR, et al.: Late-infantile neuronal ceroid-
   lipofuscinosis. An ultrastructural study of lymphocyte
   inclusions. Arch Neurol 33:630-635, 1976.

4. Santavuori P, et al.: Infantile type of so-called neuronal
   ceroid-lipofuscinosis. J Neurol Sci 18:257-267, 1973.

5. Zeman W: The Neuronal Ceroid-Lipofuscinoses. In:
   Progress in Neuropathology. Zimmerman HM (Ed.).
   Grune and Stratton, New York, 1976, Vol. III, pp. 203-
   223.

6. Zeman W, et al.: The Neuronal Ceroid-Lipofuscinoses
   (Batten-Vogt Syndrome). In: Handbook of Clinical Neu-
   rology. Vinken PJ and Bruyn GW (Eds.). North-Holland,
   Amsterdam, 1970, Vol. 10, pp. 588-679.

: :

CASE 66: A Hypotonic Infant with an Abnormally Shaped
          Head, Seizures and Hepatosplenomegaly

CLINICAL DATA

This 3-month-old girl was the product of an uncomplicated pregnancy. At birth, the child was small, hypotonic, hyporeflexic,
and had an Apgar score of 5.   Multiple congenital anomalies,
including an abnormally shaped head, bilateral dislocated hips
and bilateral clubbed feet, were noted. The child developed a
seizure disorder that was treated with phenobarbital. She fed
poorly and required gavage.

At the age of 2 months, she was hospitalized for evaluation of
easy bruisability. Physical examination revealed a small, pale
child with a head circumference of 36.5 cm.   The sagittal suture was widely separated and a large metopic suture was palpable. The anterior fontanelle was unusually large.   The child
had a high, flat forehead and a somewhat flattened occiput. The
ears were low set and the palate was high and arched.   The
child was markedly hypotonic, exhibited no spontaneous movements and only meager withdrawal upon stimulation.   There
was no head control. The eyes did not follow objects and the
pupillary responses were sluggish.   There was a very poor
gag reflex.   Examination of the heart and lungs revealed no
abnormalities. The liver was prominently enlarged and the
tip of the spleen was palpable.

Clinical laboratory studies revealed a hemoglobin of 8.0 g/dl
and a hematocrit of 26%. A white blood cell count and a platelet
count were normal. A partial thromboplastin time was greater
than 150 seconds and prothrombin activity was 14% of normal.
Serum iron was 175 μg/dl and the total iron binding capacity
was 447 μg/dl.   Bilirubin was less than 1 mg/dl but the serum
glutamic oxaloacetic transaminase and lactic dehydrogenase
activities were mildly elevated.   The child was treated with
vitamin K. A liver biopsy was performed, and the specimen
revealed increased deposits of iron in the hepatocytes and
Kupffer cells. A few weeks later, the child developed respiratory difficulties and died.

QUESTIONS

1. The clinical data are consistent with a diagnosis of
    A. Werdnig-Hoffmann disease
    B. Pompe's disease
    C. Zellweger's syndrome
    D. Tay-Sachs disease

2. Commonly encountered clinical laboratory abnormalities in
   patients with Zellweger's syndrome include
   A. elevated caeruloplasmin
   B. elevated serum iron
   C. hypoprothrombinemia
   D. hypoglycemia

3. Figs. 66.1 and 66.2 illustrate the patient's brain. Neuro-
   pathological findings in patients with Zellweger's syndrome
   include
   A. polymicrogyria and/or pachygyria
   B. aqueductal stenosis
   C. subpial siderosis
   D. olivary dysplasia

4. Other conditions in which dysplastic inferior olivary nuclei
   are found include
   A. trisomy 18 (E) syndrome
   B. Dandy-Walker syndrome
   C. lissencephaly
   D. holoprosencephaly

5. Characteristically, visceral lesions encountered in patients
   with Zellweger's syndrome include
   A. oxalate crystals in renal tubules
   B. renal cysts
   C. hepatic fibrosis or cirrhosis
   D. increased iron deposits in liver and bone marrow

6. Ultrastructural abnormalities that have been described in
   hepatocytes from patients with Zellweger's syndrome in-
   clude
   A. absence of peroxisomes
   B. collections of twisted tubules
   C. lipofuscin granules
   D. electron dense mitochondria

ANSWERS AND DISCUSSION

1. (C) The clinical data are consistent with a diagnosis of Zellweger's syndrome. This rare disorder, inherited as an autosomal recessive trait, has been variously interpreted as a developmental defect or a metabolic derangement. Clinical manifestations
are evident from birth and are dominated by profound hypotonia,
hyporeflexia, and weakness. These neurological features are regularly accompanied by a distinctive cranio-facial configuration.

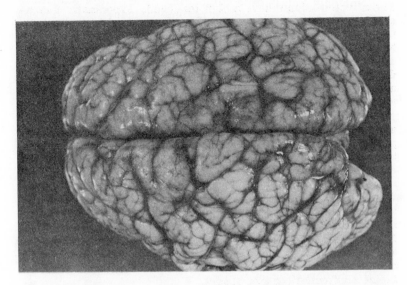

FIG. 66.1: Photograph of the dorsal surface of the brain showing both pachygyria and microgyria.

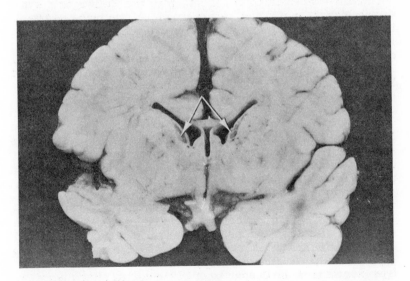

FIG. 66.2: Coronal section of the cerebral hemispheres showing pachygyria, microgyria and subependymal matrix cysts (arrows).

The affected infants have a high forehead, hypoplastic supra-orbital ridges, persistent metopic suture, large anterior fontanelle and a somewhat flattened occiput. In addition, there is hypertelorism, low set, often malformed ears, and a high arched palate. Other skeletal malformations such as campto-dactyly and club feet are common. Hepatomegaly is common and splenomegaly is occasionally present. Cardiac malformations may be present. The children have seizures and feed poorly, often requiring gavage. Cutaneous petechiae, bruises and gastrointestinal hemorrhages are common. Stippled epiphyseal calcifications have been observed in a number of patients when appropriate x-rays are taken. The infants usually die by the sixth month.

Werdnig-Hoffmann disease is also characterized by hypotonia and muscular weakness but lacks the distinctive cranio-facial configuration and hepatomegaly of Zellweger's syndrome. Pompe's disease may produce hypotonia, muscular weakness and hepatomegaly. However, the clinical findings are often dominated by cardiomegaly and heart failure and the cranio-facial malformations are absent.

2. (B, C) Significant, but inconstant, clinical laboratory abnormalities encountered in patients with the Zellweger's syndrome include an elevated serum iron level, an increased total iron binding capacity and hypoprothrombinemia. Hyperbilirubinemia commonly develops but often does not persist. Serum enzyme elevations may be present reflecting hepatic dysfunction. Hyperaminoacidemia and/or aminoaciduria have been described in a few patients. Elevated levels of pipecolic acid, a minor catabolite of lysine, were detected in four patients. The significance of this observation is not clear.

3. (A, D) Brains from patients with Zellweger's syndrome are somewhat heavier than expected for the patient's age and are grossly malformed. Abnormalities of the cerebral cortex are prominent and include aberrant gyral patterns, heterotopias, polymicrogyria and pachygyria. The polymicrogyric cortex is characteristically thickened and contains multiple shallow plications. The pachygyric cortex is even thicker and the surface is smooth. Generally, microgyria and pachygyria are regarded as manifestations of aberrant or arrested neuronal migration. More recently, studies have suggested that microgyria results from necrosis of the deeper layer of the cortex after migration has been completed. The thalamus and basal ganglia are essentially normal. The white matter generally shows pallor of myelin staining and a small amount of sudanophilic lipid in

macrophages and glial cells, especially in periventricular regions. The deep white matter contains an increased number of fibrillary astrocytes. The ventricular system is often mildly enlarged. Subependymal matrix cysts are often present (Fig. 66.2). The cerebellar cortex is often dysplastic and may contain heterotopias. The inferior olivary nuclei are dysplastic and have simplified convolutions (Fig. 66.3).

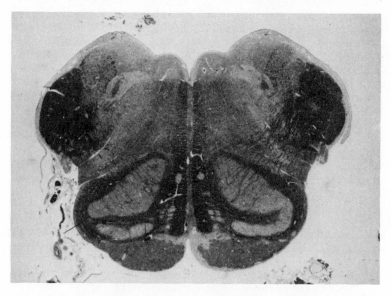

FIG. 66.3: Macrosection of the brain stem showing the malformed inferior olivary nuclei.

4. (A, B, C) Dysplastic inferior olivary nuclei are found in several other disorders. Several authors have described dysplasia of the inferior olivary nuclei as constant findings in the lissencephaly-pachygyria group of malformations and in brains from individuals with the trisomy 18 (E) syndrome. It is also a common finding in patients with the Dandy-Walker malformation. Patients with holoprosencephaly have agenesis or hypoplasia of the corticospinal tracts. The olives thus have an unusually ventral position and are very prominent. Nevertheless, they are not dysplastic.

5. (B, C, D) Characteristically, visceral lesions are found in the kidneys and liver. The kidneys contain multiple small

subcortical cysts. The liver shows fibrosis or cirrhosis and
excessive deposits of iron in both the hepatocytes and Kupffer
cells.   The bone marrow also contains an excess of stainable
iron.   Other visceral lesions that have been reported occasionally include hypoplasia of the thymus and hyperplasia of the
pancreatic islets.

6.   (A, D) Only a few specimens from patients with Zellweger's
syndrome have been studied by electron microscopy.   Goldfischer, et al., reported peroxisomes to be absent from hepatocytes and renal tubular cells.   They also described electron
dense mitochondria in hepatocytes and cortical astrocytes.   Biochemically and histochemically, they demonstrated a defect in
electron transport proximal to the cytochromes.   Thus, these
authors regard Zellweger's syndrome as a metabolic disorder
rather than a malformation, as suggested by Volpe and Adams.

Membrane-bounded collections of twisted tubules in hepatocytes are a characteristic ultrastructural feature of Gaucher's
disease.   The tubules are composed of the non-degradable glucocerebroside.   Lipofuscin granules are normally present in
hepatocytes.

REFERENCES

1.   Danks DM, et al.: Cerebro-hepato-renal syndrome of Zell-
     weger. J Ped 86:382-387, 1975.

2.   Goldfischer S, et al.: Peroxisomal and mitochondrial de-
     fects in the cerebro-hepato-renal syndrome. Science 182:
     62-64, 1973.

3.   Opitz JM, et al.: The Zellweger syndrome (cerebro-hepato-
     renal syndrome). Birth Defects: Original Article Series
     5:144-158, 1969.

4.   Patton RG, et al.: Cerebro-hepato-renal syndrome of Zell-
     weger. Amer J Dis Child 124:840-844, 1972.

5.   Richman DP, et al.: Cerebral microgyria in a 27-week
     fetus: An architectonic and topographic analysis. J Neuro-
     path Exp Neurol 33:374-384, 1974.

6.   Volpe JJ and Adams RD: Cerebro-hepato-renal syndrome
     of Zellweger. An inherited disorder of neuronal migration.
     Acta Neuropath 20:175-198, 1972.

: :: :

CASE 67: A Middle-Aged Man with Progressive Memory
              Loss, Disorientation and Poor Judgment

CLINICAL DATA

This 52-year-old man was admitted to the hospital for evaluation
of slowly progressive memory loss, disorientation and poor
judgment.

On examination, the patient was found to be severely demented,
agitated and hostile. His speech was impaired. His pupils were
small but reacted normally to light. There was a full range of
extraocular movements. Muscle tone was increased, a fine
resting tremor was present and the patient's gait was impaired.
The deep tendon reflexes were brisk. Grasp and snout reflexes
could be elicited.

A lumbar puncture yielded clear, colorless cerebrospinal fluid
under normal pressure. There was 1 white blood cell per cmm,
the glucose content was 75 mg/dl and the protein content was
59 mg/dl. Blood glucose level, thyroid function tests and a serological test for syphilis were normal. An electroencephalogram was abnormal with diffuse slowing. Plain skull x-rays
and an isotopic brain scan were normal. A pneumoencephalogram revealed cerebral atrophy with a dilated ventricular system. The patient was discharged to a custodial care facility.
Six months later, he died.

QUESTIONS

1. Based on the clinical data and general statistical informa-
    tion, the most appropriate clinical diagnosis in the present
    case would be
    A. Alzheimer's disease
    B. Pick's disease
    C. Huntington's chorea
    D. arteriosclerotic dementia

2. Grossly discernible changes characteristically encountered
    in the brain from patients with Alzheimer's disease include
    A. diffuse cerebral cortical atrophy
    B. prominent striatal atrophy
    C. multiple lacunar infarcts
    D. hydrocephalus ex vacuo

3. Histopathological changes characteristic of Alzheimer's disease include
    A. spheroidal inclusions within the cytoplasm of neurons
    B. neurofibrillary tangles confined to the hippocampus
    C. numerous senile plaques and neurofibrillary tangles scattered throughout the cortex and in certain nuclear structures
    D. granulovacuolar degeneration involving a relatively large number of pyramidal cells in the hippocampus

4. Neurofibrillary tangles are
    A. commonly encountered in Purkinje cells
    B. argentophilic
    C. composed of skeins of twisted tubules or bifilar helices
    D. found only in patients with Alzheimer's disease and in elderly non-demented patients

5. Exact counterparts of the naturally occurring Alzheimer's neurofibrillary tangles have been produced experimentally by the use of
    A. aluminum compounds
    B. vincristine
    C. colchicine
    D. none of these

6. Senile plaques are
    A. composed in part of degenerated neurites
    B. commonly found in the white matter
    C. not detectable in sections stained with hematoxylin-eosin
    D. composed in part of amyloid

7. Hirano bodies are
    A. encountered most often in the hippocampi
    B. eosinophilic spindle- or spheroidal-shaped bodies
    C. found only in man
    D. derived from Alzheimer's neurofibrillary tangles

8. Gross alterations characteristic of Pick's disease include
    A. severe, so-called "knife-edge" atrophy
    B. severe atrophy of the posterior three-fifths of the superior temporal gyrus
    C. relative preservation of the pre- and postcentral gyri
    D. atrophy of the striatum

9. The histological findings characteristic of Pick's disease include
   A. argentophilic spheroids in the cytoplasm of neurons
   B. Lewy bodies
   C. Lafora bodies
   D. granulovacuolar degeneration

ANSWERS AND DISCUSSION

1. (A) Alzheimer's disease is the most appropriate clinical diagnosis for this patient. The dementias, disorders that produce a decline or deterioration in intellectual function, are common clinical problems, especially among older individuals. It has been estimated that 4.5% of persons over the age of 65 have moderate to severe dementia. Obviously many others are affected to a lesser degree. Younger individuals, often between 45 and 60, who become demented, are frequently described as having presenile dementia, whereas older individuals, over 60, who become demented, are often described as having senile dementia. Many authors now regard this distinction on the basis of age as arbitrary and invalid. At least 70% of the cases of dementia, both presenile and senile, are due to Alzheimer's disease. In addition to progressive deterioration of intellectual function, patients with Alzheimer's disease often show spatial disorientation, agnosia, aphasia and apraxia. Motor dysfunction and rigidity are frequently present and some of the patients have myoclonic jerks. Both sexes are affected approximately equally and a considerable number of cases are familial.

Pick's disease is a very rare cause of dementia but generally regarded as clinically indistinguishable from Alzheimer's disease. Some workers claim, however, that the electroencephalogram is more apt to be normal in Pick's disease and diffusely abnormal in Alzheimer's disease.

Huntington's chorea may produce a profound dementia; however, it is usually accompanied by choreiform movements. A familial history usually can be elicited.

Arteriosclerosis with associated encephalomalacia is a major cause of neurological deficits but is probably a rare cause of dementia. Most patients diagnosed clinically as having arteriosclerotic dementia are found to have Alzheimer's disease when appropriate pathological studies are carried out.

2. (A, D) The grossly discernible alterations in brains from patients with Alzheimer's disease are manifestations of atrophy.

Reduction in brain weight may range from moderate to marked
and tends to be more pronounced in those patients whose clinical manifestations began at a relatively early age, i.e., more
marked in patients with "presenile dementia." The cerebral
cortical atrophy is usually diffuse but, as in the present case
(Fig. 67.1), may be somewhat more severe in the frontal and
temporal lobes than in the parietal and occipital lobes. The
hippocampal formations may be severely affected. In association with the cerebral atrophy, there is enlargement of the
ventricular system, so-called hydrocephalus ex vacuo (Fig.
67.2). The basal ganglia are also involved by the cerebral
atrophy, but pronounced atrophy of the striatum (the caudate
nucleus and the putamen) is characteristically associated with
Huntington's chorea and can also be seen in some cases of
Pick's disease.

3. (C, D) The histopathology of Alzheimer's disease is somewhat complicated since the morphological changes are quanti-
tatively and topographically, rather than qualitatively, different
from those seen in elderly but non-demented patients. The most
significant morphological findings are numerous senile plaques
and neurofibrillary tangles (Fig. 67.3). In both elderly non-
demented patients and patients with Alzheimer's disease, neurofibrillary tangles may be found in the hippocampi. However,
neurofibrillary tangles are far more numerous and widespread
in the isocortex from patients with Alzheimer's disease. Similarly, senile plaques occur in both elderly non-demented patients
and patients with Alzheimer's disease but are far more numerous and widespread in patients with Alzheimer's disease.
Granulovacuolar degeneration is encountered predominantly in
the pyramidal cells of the hippocampi. Patients with Alzheimer's
disease usually have more extensive granulovacuolar degeneration than elderly non-demented patients or patients with other
neurological disorders. Hirano bodies are commonly encountered in the hippocampi of patients with Alzheimer's disease.
However, these spindle- or spheroidal-shaped structures are
nonspecific and found in a number of different conditions. The
neurons often contain increased quantities of lipofuscin but this
is a nonspecific, often age-related alteration.

4. (B, C) In addition to elderly individuals and patients with
Alzheimer's disease, neurofibrillary tangles are found regularly
in patients with postencephalitic parkinsonism, progressive supra-
nuclear palsy, the parkinsonism dementia complex and in older
adults with Down's syndrome.

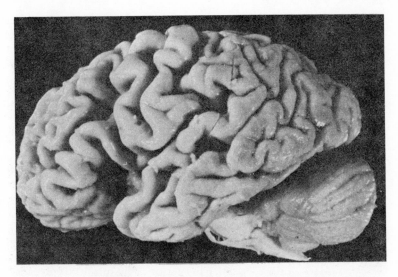

FIG. 67.1: Photograph of the brain from this patient with Alzheimer's disease. Note the diffuse atrophy that is slightly more severe in the frontal and temporal lobes.

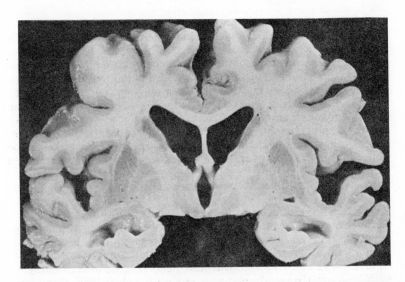

FIG. 67.2: Coronal section of the cerebral hemispheres. Note the cortical atrophy and the hydrocephalus ex vacuo.

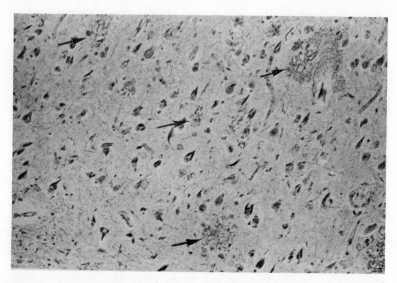

FIG. 67.3: Microscopic section stained with the Bodian silver stain, prepared from this patient's cortex. Note the numerous neurofibrillary tangles and senile plaques (arrows).

They have been described occasionally in patients with Pick's disease, Kufs' disease, amyotrophic lateral sclerosis, idiopathic parkinsonism and tuberous sclerosis. The topographic distribution of the neurofibrillary tangles varies among these conditions. The neurofibrillary tangles are found throughout the cerebral cortex in patients with Alzheimer's disease. In elderly non-demented individuals, the neurofibrillary tangles are most numerous in the hippocampi and may be sparse or even absent elsewhere in the cortex. In postencephalitic parkinsonism, the brain stem nuclei are maximally affected. Certain neurons, such as the Purkinje cells, are almost invariably unaffected regardless of the disease process.

Neurofibrillary tangles in the cortex are usually triangular or flame-shaped (Fig. 67.4), whereas those in the basal ganglia, hypothalamus and brain stem are more commonly globose. These variations in shape are probably due merely to the configuration of the involved neurons. The tangles stain weakly with hematoxylin-eosin and periodic acid-Schiff techniques but are intensely argentophilic. The neurofibrillary tangles are

also congophilic and birefringent in polarized light. These latter properties are due to the regular orientation of the components and do not reflect the presence of amyloid.

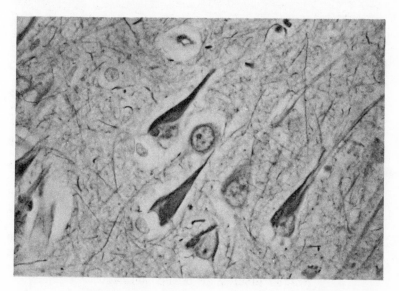

FIG. 67. 4: Microscopic section stained with the Bodian silver
stain, showing the usual triangular or flame-shaped
neurofibrillary tangles.

Ultrastructurally, the Alzheimer's neurofibrillary tangles appear as skeins of abnormal twisted tubules (Fig. 67.5). These
have a maximal diameter of 20 nm and at intervals of about 80
nm, narrow to a diameter of about 10 nm. Originally and again
more recently, it has been suggested that these structures are
bifilar helices rather than twisted tubules. The morphogenesis
of these twisted tubules or bifilar helices and their relation to
the normal neuronal fibrous proteins is currently unsettled.

5.   (D) Aluminum compounds and various mitotic spindle inhibitors, such as colchicine and vincristine, produce intraneuronal tangles that resemble the Alzheimer's neurofibrillary
tangles by light microscopy. However, ultrastructurally they
are composed of skeins of thin filaments rather than the distinctive twisted tubules and cannot be regarded as counterparts of
the Alzheimer's neurofibrillary tangles. The experimental tangles are probably derived from reassembled microtubule
proteins.

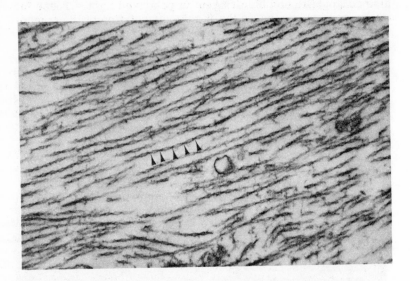

FIG. 67.5: Electron micrograph showing the ultrastructure of the Alzheimer's neurofibrillary tangles. Note the periodic constrictions (arrowheads) along the twisted tubules or bifilar helices.

6. (A, D) Senile plaques are most numerous in patients with Alzheimer's disease but are also found in association with other neurological diseases and in elderly individuals without specific neurological disorders. They have also been reported in various species of old animals. Senile plaques can be found throughout the cerebral cortex but may be especially abundant in the hippocampi. The cerebellar cortex and spinal cord are rarely affected and white matter is uninvolved. The number and distribution of senile plaques does not always coincide with the number and distribution of neurofibrillary tangles.

Senile plaques are indistinctly stained with hematoxylin-eosin, are better demonstrated with periodic acid-Schiff or trichrome techniques and are best demonstrated with various silver stains. Senile plaques contain clusters of degenerating neurites and amyloid in the extracellular space between the neurites and in the center of the plaque. The so-called mature plaques also contain microglial cells and reactive astrocytes. Eventually the neurites and reactive cells disappear and only the amyloid deposits persist. The factors responsible for causing the neurites to degenerate and for initiating formation of the plaques are currently unknown.

7.   (A, B) Hirano bodies are spindle- or spheroidal-shaped
bodies that are encountered most often in the hippocampi. Occasionally they have been observed in the cerebrum, cerebellum, brain stem and spinal cord. These bodies are eosinophilic
but are more conspicuous when stained red with one of the trichrome techniques or purple with phosphotungstic acid-hematoxylin. They are composed of highly organized complex arrays
of filaments. Their ultrastructural appearance varies with the
plane of section. They may appear as a lattice work of inter-
secting filaments, as rows of punctate densities closely applied
to filaments or as broad feathery fibrils. Most Hirano bodies
appear to rise in degenerating neurites. Hirano bodies are regularly found in patients with Alzheimer's disease but are also
encountered in patients with the amyotrophic lateral sclerosis -
parkinsonism dementia complex, sporadic amyotrophic lateral
sclerosis, Pick's disease and in elderly individuals without specific neurological disorders. They have also been seen in various animals. Hirano bodies are interpreted as a nonspecific
manifestation of neuronal degeneration. They do not appear to
be derived from the Alzheimer's neurofibrillary tangles.

8.   (A, C, D) Although clinically indistinguishable, Pick's and
Alzheimer's diseases are quite different pathologically. Grossly,
Pick's disease is characterized by very severe gyral atrophy
that is often described as "knife-edge" atrophy (Fig. 67.6).
The atrophy usually shows a lobar distribution with maximal
involvement of the frontal and temporal lobes and minimal involvement of the occipital lobes. Certain areas are typically
preserved and stand out in striking contrast to the adjacent
atrophic areas. The preserved areas include the posterior
three-fifths of the superior temporal gyri, the precentral gyri,
the postcentral gyri and the transverse gyri. Many of the
brains show marked atrophy of the basal ganglia; maximal in
the caudate nuclei and moderate in the putamina and pallida.

9.   (A) The characteristic histological findings in Pick's disease are the so-called Pick bodies. These are globular intracytoplasmic inclusions that are most readily demonstrated in
the pyramidal neurons of the hippocampi and in the small neurons of the dentate fascia. Elsewhere in the cortex they are
most abundant at the margins of the atrophic lobes. The Pick
bodies appear as homogeneous basophilic spheroids in sections
stained with hematoxylin-eosin, but they are more conspicuous and
characteristically demonstrated as argentophilic spheroids in
sections stained with various silver techniques (Fig. 67.7).

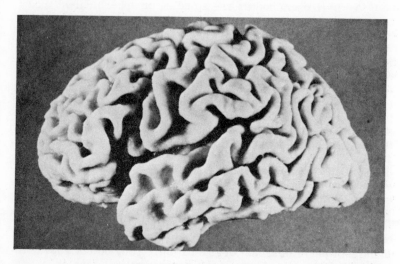

FIG. 67.6: Photograph of the brain from a patient with Pick's disease. Note the very severe knife-edge atrophy and the relative preservation of the precentral gyrus, the postcentral gyrus and the posterior portion of the superior temporal gyrus.

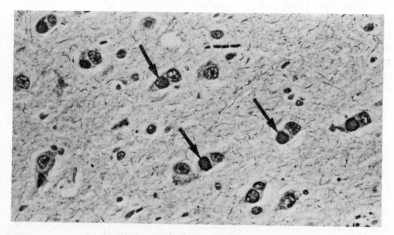

FIG. 67.7: Microscopic section, stained with the Bodian silver stain, from a patient with Pick's disease. Note the argentophilic intracytoplasmic inclusions (arrows) in the pyramidal neurons of the hippocampus.

The atrophic cortex shows marked neuronal loss and severe gliosis. A variable, but usually small, number of senile plaques and neurofibrillary tangles also may be present. Ultrastructurally, the Pick bodies consist of unbounded intracytoplasmic aggregates of twisted tubules, smooth microtubules or neurofilaments. The Pick bodies appear to be a particular type of neuronal reaction that results in the aggregation of any available neuronal fibrous proteins. Similar appearing argentophilic spheroids in primates with experimental kuru are composed of aggregates of smooth microtubules.

REFERENCES

1. Katzman R: The prevalence and malignancy of Alzheimer's disease. Arch Neurol 33:217-218, 1976.

2. Poser CM: The presenile dementias. JAMA 233:81-84, 1975.

3. Schochet SS Jr., et al.: Neurofibrillary tangles in patients with Down's syndrome. A light and electron microscopic study. Acta Neuropath 23:342-346, 1973.

4. Schochet SS Jr. and McCormick WF: Ultrastructure of Hirano bodies. Acta Neuropath 21:50-60, 1972.

5. Terry RD: Dementia: A brief and selective review. Arch Neurol 33:1-4, 1976.

6. Tomlinson BE and Henderson G: Some Quantitative Cerebral Findings in Normal and Demented Old People. In: Neurobiology of Aging. Terry RD and Gershon S (Eds.). Raven Press, New York, 1976, pp. 183-204.

7. Wisniewski HM and Terry RD: Neuropathology of the Aging Brain. In: Neurobiology of Aging. Terry RD and Gershon S (Eds.). Raven Press, New York, 1976, pp. 265-280.

: :

CASE 68: A 61-Year-Old Woman with Rapidly Progressive
          Dementia

CLINICAL DATA

This 61-year-old woman was hospitalized for evaluation of a
rapidly progressive neurological disorder. Over the past six
months, the patient had displayed progressive memory loss
and personality changes. Previously she was a fastidious
housekeeper but had become slovenly in her housework and
personal care. She was no longer able to cook because of the
memory loss. Her gait had become unsteady over the past
three months and she would hold onto walls and furniture for
support. She had suffered several falls without significant injury. Her speech had become slow and repetitive over the past
two months.

On admission, she appeared chronically ill but her vital signs
were normal. She was withdrawn and her recent memory and
recall were severely impaired. Her speech was slow and halt-
ing. Her gait was wide-based and unsteady. The cranial nerves
were intact. There was no papilledema or optic atrophy. Muscle strength appeared to be normal. Finger to nose testing
elicited an intention tremor. Myoclonic jerks were precipitated
by sudden movements, noises or lights. The deep tendon reflexes were hyperactive and Babinski signs were present bilaterally. The sensory examination was within normal limits.

Routine laboratory studies, including a serological test for syphilis, were normal. A lumbar puncture yielded clear spinal fluid
under normal pressure, containing 0-1 cell/cmm and 44 mg/dl
of protein. Skull and chest x-rays were normal. An electroencephalogram was abnormal with diffuse slow wave activity
most pronounced over the temporal areas. A radioisotopic
brain scan was normal. A pneumoencephalogram revealed mild
ventricular dilatation. A brain biopsy was performed to confirm the clinical impression.

QUESTIONS

1.   The clinical data are most consistent with a diagnosis of
     A. Alzheimer's disease
     B. Jakob-Creutzfeldt disease
     C. Pick's disease
     D. Huntington's chorea

2. The histological characteristics of Jakob-Creutzfeldt disease include
   A. loss of neurons
   B. astrocytosis
   C. status spongiosus
   D. neurofibrillary tangles

3. Ultrastructural studies have shown the vacuoles to be located in
   A. neuronal perikarya
   B. terminal axons and dendrites
   C. myelin sheaths
   D. astrocytes

4. The transmissible spongioform encephalopathies that affect man include
   A. Jakob-Creutzfeldt disease
   B. kuru
   C. scrapie
   D. Canavan's disease

ANSWERS AND DISCUSSION

1. (B) The clinical data are consistent with a diagnosis of Jakob-Creutzfeldt disease. This is an uncommon cause of dementia, yet one that is being diagnosed with increasing frequency. The disorder usually becomes apparent clinically between the ages of 40 and 60 and affects both sexes equally. Familial cases, apparently transmitted as an autosomal dominant trait, have been reported. The full range of clinical manifestations has not been clearly delineated. The disease is generally characterized by rapidly progressive dementia, prominent behavioral changes, pyramidal tract involvement, cerebellar dysfunction and myoclonus. Lower motor neuron involvement and sensory abnormalities are infrequent. Late in the course of the disease, the patients may become mute. Death usually ensues after 9 to 18 months. Electroencephalographic abnormalities are found in the majority of cases, initially appearing as diffuse or focal slowing and later as paroxysms of sharp waves or spikes. The cerebrospinal fluid shows minimal abnormalities, at most consisting of mild elevation in the protein content. Pneumoencephalograph usually reveals mild ventricular dilatation.

One of the major clinical diagnostic problems is distinguishing Jakob-Creutzfeldt disease from Alzheimer's disease with myoclonus. Some workers feel that the distinction can be made by electroencephalography. The course of Jakob-Creutzfeldt disease is generally much more rapid than Alzheimer's disease.

2.   (A, B, C) The histological characteristics of Jakob-Creutz-feldt disease, like the clinical manifestations, are currently in the process of being delineated more precisely.   The dominant histological features, as illustrated in the biopsy specimen from the present case (Fig. 68.1), consist of neuronal loss, astrocytosis and widespread vacuolation. The neuronal loss is often patchy. Small clusters of microglial cells may be encountered about the debris from dead neurons. Excess lipofuscin is found in the majority of the remaining neurons and a few have eccentric nuclei and chromatolytic cytoplasm. Astrocytic proliferation is generally pronounced and may be seen even in areas with little or no neuronal degeneration. One of the most conspicuous features is widespread vacuolation or status spongiosus. By light microscopy, the vacuoles appear to be within the neurons and the neuropil. Unusual cases have been reported that contain senile plaques in the cerebrum and kuru plaques within the cerebellum, in addition to the other histological features.

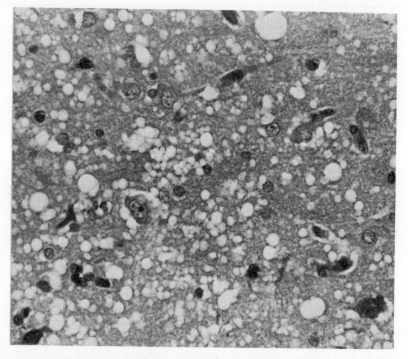

FIG. 68. 1: Microscopic section of the biopsy specimen from the present case.

3. (A, B, D) Electron microscopic studies on biopsy specimens from patients of Jakob-Creutzfeldt disease have shown
the vacuoles in a variety of structures. These include neuronal
perikarya, axons, dendrites and astrocytes. In some instances,
herniated, swollen neuronal or astrocytic cytoplasm appeared
as vacuoles by light microscopy. Significantly, the extracellular space is not enlarged.

4. (A, B) The transmissible spongiform encephalopathies are
slow or chronic viral infections. They share the common features of being transmissible by inoculation with infected tissue,
of having protracted incubation periods and of producing neuronal
degeneration, astrocytosis and status spongiosus. Kuru was the
first of these diseases to be transmitted from man to primates.
This disorder is found among the natives of eastern New Guinea.
Women and children of both sexes are involved predominantly.
The disease is characterized by ataxia, tremor, emotional
lability and mild dementia. The illness leads to death within a
year. The histopathological changes within the nervous system
consist of neuronal degeneration, intense astrocytosis and mild
vacuolation of the neuropil. Distinctive stellate plaques of amyloid, the so-called kuru plaques, are found in the cerebellum of
about half the patients and elsewhere in the brain of occasional
patients. The disease has been transmitted to primates by various routes of inoculation. The incubation periods, initially 18
to 38 months, have been reduced to about one year in subsequent
passages. Natural transmission among the affected natives is
thought to be due to contamination with infected tissues during
ritualistic endocannibalism.

During the original studies on the histopathology of kuru, similarities with Jakob-Creutzfeldt disease were noted. After the
successful transmission of kuru to primates, similar attempts
were made with tissue from patients with Jakob-Creutzfeldt disease. The disease developed in the primates 11 to 14 months
after inoculation. In contrast to kuru, subsequent transmissions
have not further reduced the incubation period. Although im-
practical as a routine diagnostic procedure, it would appear that
transmission of the disease to primates is currently the most
accurate way to diagnose Jakob-Creutzfeldt disease. Recently,
the disease has been transmitted to mice and guinea pigs. The
transmissible agent has not been fully characterized.

Scrapie is another transmissible spongiform encephalopathy.
However, the natural disease occurs in sheep rather than man.

REFERENCES

1. Kirschbaum WR: Jakob-Creutzfeldt disease. American Elsevier, New York, 1968.

2. Lampert PW, et al.: Subacute spongiform virus encephalopathies. Amer J Path 68:626-646, 1972.

3. Masters CL and Richardson EP Jr: Subacute spongiform encephalopathy (Creutzfeldt-Jakob disease). The nature and progression of spongiform change. Brain 101:333-344, 1978.

4. Roos R, et al.: The clinical characteristics of transmissible Creutzfeldt-Jakob disease. Brain 96:1-20, 1973.

: :

CASE 69: A 55-Year-Old Man with Slowly Progressive
                Difficulty Walking

CLINICAL DATA

This 55-year-old man experienced the insidious onset of a right
foot drop. Over the next year, his gait deteriorated further and
he had difficulty walking, even with a cane.   He also noticed
mild weakness in his hands.   He had no pain, abnormal sen-
sations, cranial nerve symptoms or sphincter dysfunction.

On physical examination, he appeared well-nourished and in no
acute distress.   All cranial nerve functions were intact and the
ocular fundi appeared normal.   There was marked weakness
with mild atrophy of the distal leg muscles and moderate weakness of the proximal leg muscles.   The arm and hand muscles
were mildly weak and showed mild atrophy.   The deep tendon
reflexes, especially at the ankles and knees, were hyperactive.
Babinski signs were present. Sensory examination disclosed
no abnormalities.

Routine laboratory studies, including a serological test for
syphilis, were normal.   Electromyography of random muscles
revealed some "giant" motor units and numerous abnormal resting potentials.   A lumbar puncture yielded cerebrospinal fluid
with a normal cell, glucose and protein content.   A brain scan,
cervical spine x-rays and a myelogram were normal.

A biopsy of the gastrocnemius was performed.

QUESTIONS

1.   The clinical data are most consistent with a diagnosis of
      A.   polymyositis
      B.   carcinomatous neuropathy
      C.   amyotrophic lateral sclerosis
      D.   cervical spondylosis

2.   Fig. 69.1 is a photograph of a frozen section stained by the
      NADH-TR technique, prepared from the gastrocnemius
      biopsy specimen.   The section shows
      A.   changes that are diagnostic of amyotrophic lateral
            sclerosis
      B.   histopathological features of denervation
      C.   selective atrophy of type 2 myofibers
      D.   "ragged-red" fibers

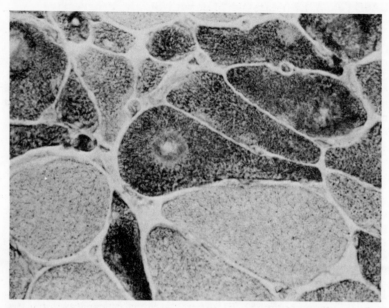

FIG. 69.1: Frozen section stained with the NADH-TR technique
prepared from the gastrocnemius biopsy specimen.

3. A sural nerve biopsy specimen from a patient with amyo-
    trophic lateral sclerosis would be expected to show
    A. histologically normal peripheral nerve
    B. segmental demyelination
    C. axonal atrophy
    D. onion bulb formations

4. Neuropathological features of sporadic amyotrophic lateral
    sclerosis include
    A. degeneration of the corticospinal tracts
    B. atrophy of the ventral roots of the spinal cord
    C. atrophy of the dorsal roots of the spinal cord
    D. loss of motor neurons

5. Familial amyotrophic lateral sclerosis is characterized by
    A. autosomal dominant inheritance
    B. degeneration of the corticospinal tracts
    C. demyelination of the posterior columns
    D. atrophy of the ventral roots of the spinal cord

6. Guamanian amyotrophic lateral sclerosis is characterized
    by
    A. degeneration of the corticospinal tracts
    B. Lewy bodies in the substantia nigra
    C. abundant neurofibrillary tangles
    D. loss of motor neurons

ANSWERS AND DISCUSSION

1. (C) The clinical data are most consistent with a diagnosis
of amyotrophic lateral sclerosis. The common, sporadic form
has a prevalence of about 4-6 per 100,000 and predominantly
affects individuals between the ages of 40 and 70.   Men are
afflicted nearly twice as often as women.   The clinical manifestations result from a combination of lower motor neuron
degeneration and varying degrees of corticobulbar and corticospinal tract degeneration.   Weakness, affecting distal limb
muscles, is the most common initial manifestation.   This is
generally accompanied by atrophy and fasciculations.   With
progression of the disease, quadriplegia and bulbar paralysis
may eventually develop. The course of the disease is invariably
progressive, and many of the patients die within 3-5 years.
Involvement of the respiratory muscles and pneumonia are
frequently the causes of death.

The motor manifestations may be accompanied by cramps, or
even paresthesias, but there are no objective sensory losses.
Impairment of sphincter control is uncommon and disorders of
eye movement are rare.

2.   (B) The muscle biopsy specimen shows histopathological
features of denervation. These changes are common to most
denervating processes and are not specifically diagnostic of
amyotrophic lateral sclerosis. The most significant feature
is the presence of small angular myofibers of both major fiber
types. The atrophic fibers may be scattered individually or
aggregated in either small or large groups, i.e., whole fascicles. Very severely atrophic myofibers may be reduced to
clusters or "knots" of pycnotic nuclei.

It is important to note that the mere presence of scattered atrophic myofibers is not acceptable evidence of denervation. Both
fiber types must be shown to be involved. With the NADH-
tetrazolium reductase reactions, all denervated myofibers, regardless of type, tend to stain relatively dark.   Accurate
identification of the fiber types is best accomplished by the use
of the ATPase reactions.

Another finding characteristic of denervating processes is the presence of target fibers. These are distinctive-appearing, three-zoned myofibers that are best seen in frozen sections stained by the modified trichrome or NADH-TR techniques, and in paraffin-embedded sections stained by the trichrome or phosphotungstic acid-hematoxylin techniques. The central zone is pale, devoid of cross-striations and deficient in most enzymatic activity. Ultrastructurally, the myofilaments and Z-discs are in total disarray, and mitochondria are severely reduced in number. The intermediate zone is darkly stained and shows enhanced oxidative enzyme activity. Ultrastructurally, this zone is characterized by mildly disarrayed myofilaments and Z-discs, numerous mitochondria and abundant profiles of sarcoplasmic reticulum. The outer zone is formed by the nearly normal staining and structured periphery of the myofiber. The target fibers are predominantly type 1 myofibers. The change has been variously interpreted as the direct consequence of denervation or as a manifestation of reinnervation of a previously denervated myofiber.

Another feature of denervating processes is fiber-type grouping. This results from reinnervation of a group of previously denervated myofibers by axonal sprouts from an intact neuron. It is manifested by the presence of relatively large groups of myofibers of a single fiber type. This finding is less common in patients with amyotrophic lateral sclerosis than in certain other denervating disorders. It was not seen in the present specimen.

Selective atrophy of the type 2 myofibers results in the presence of uniformly scattered, small, angular myofibers. It is a common and relatively nonspecific finding in muscle biopsy specimens. It occurs in association with disuse, neoplasia, collagen vascular diseases, myasthenia, etc. The precise pathogenesis of this phenomenon is unknown.

3. (A) The sural nerve is a predominantly sensory nerve with a small number of autonomic fibers. In a patient with amyotrophic lateral sclerosis, a motor neuron disease, the sural nerve would be expected to be histologically normal.

4. (A, B, D) The most conspicuous histopathological changes in the central nervous system of individuals with amyotrophic lateral sclerosis are degeneration of the corticospinal tracts and atrophy of the ventral roots of the spinal cord (Fig. 69.2). The dorsal roots are generally well-preserved. The anterior horns of the spinal cord show a reduction in the number of motor neurons. The loss of neurons is most conspicuous and

best evaluated in the cervical and lumbar enlargements, where these cells are normally most numerous. Among the cranial nerve nuclei, the hypoglossal nucleus is usually the most severely affected and shows the greatest loss of neurons. The remaining motor neurons show a variety of changes that are neither especially conspicuous nor pathognomonic for sporadic amyotrophic lateral sclerosis. Various types of small acidophilic intracytoplasmic inclusions may be present in neuronal perikarya. Proximal axons are often enlarged and filled with skeins of neurofilaments. Some of the neurons appear atrophic. Rarely, neurons show chromatolysis or even appear to be undergoing neuronophagia. Both the anterior horns and the cranial nerve nuclei show varying degrees of gliosis.

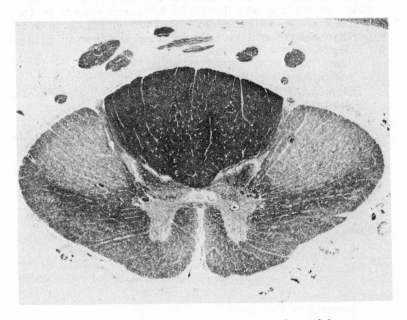

FIG. 69. 2: Macroscopic section of the spinal cord from a patient with sporadic amyotrophic lateral sclerosis.

5. (A, B, C, D) About 5% of cases of amyotrophic lateral sclerosis appear to be familial and inherited as an autosomal dominant trait with equal involvement of the sexes. The disease is otherwise indistinguishable clinically from the sporadic form of amyotrophic lateral sclerosis. In addition to the usual histopathological characteristics, about one-half of these cases show

demyelination of the posterior columns and spinocerebellar tracts, and degeneration of Clarke's column. Some also show neurofibrillary tangles in anterior horn motor neurons.

6.   (A, C, D) Another variety of amyotrophic lateral sclerosis accounts for 5-10% of all deaths among the adult natives on Guam. Men are affected more commonly than women. The average age of onset is earlier, and the survival is longer, than with sporadic amyotrophic lateral sclerosis. Both a genetic basis and environmental factors have been implicated by various authors. In addition to the usual histopathological features of amyotrophic lateral sclerosis, these patients have numerous neurofibrillary tangles distributed widely in the brain, and even among the motor neurons of the spinal cord. Previously, the disease was thought to be linked closely to the parkinsonism-dementia complex that is also prevalent in Guam. These diseases are now generally regarded as separate entities.

REFERENCES

1.   Bobowick AR and Brody JA: Epidemiology of motor-neuron diseases. N Eng J Med 288:1047-1055, 1973.

2.   Hirano A: Progress in the Pathology of Motor Neuron Disease. In: Progress in Neuropathology. Zimmerman HM (Ed.). Grune and Stratton, New York, 1973, Vol. II, pp. 181-215.

3.   Mulder DW: Motor Neuron Diseases. In: Peripheral Neuropathy. Dyck PJ, et al. (Eds.). W.B. Saunders Co., Philadelphia, 1975, Vol. 2, pp. 759-770.

: :

CASE 70: A 64-Year-Old Man with Tremor and Rigidity

CLINICAL DATA

This 64-year-old man had a six-year history of progressive tremor and rigidity. He was hospitalized for treatment of an enlarged prostate.

Neurological examination revealed an elderly-appearing man with slow speech and mild dementia. His face was "mask-like" and he drooled occasionally. There was marked tremor at rest in both hands and mild tremor at rest in the legs. Cogwheel rigidity was evident in his neck and all four limbs. His posture was stooped and he walked with a shuffling gait. Following a prostatectomy, the patient developed bronchopneumonia and died.

QUESTIONS

1. This patient's underlying neurological disorder was
    A. essential tremor
    B. parkinsonism
    C. pseudobulbar palsy
    D. Alzheimer's disease

2. Gross pathological features of parkinsonism include
    A. depigmentation of the substantia nigra
    B. pigmentation of the globus pallidus
    C. atrophy of the brain stem
    D. lacunar infarcts in the basal ganglia

3. Characteristic histological features of parkinsonism include
    A. Lewy bodies
    B. degeneration of pigmented brain stem neurons
    C. Marinesco bodies
    D. neurofibrillary tangles in brain stem neurons

4. A parkinsonism-like syndrome can result from intoxication with
    A. lead
    B. carbon monoxide
    C. manganese
    D. phenothiazines

5. A biochemical lesion common to most forms of parkinson-
   ism is a deficiency of
   A. GABA in the striatum
   B. tyrosine hydroxylase in the striatum
   C. dopamine in the striatum
   D. pyridoxine in the striatum

6. Neuromelanin in the substantia nigra differs from cutaneous
   melanin in several respects. Neuromelanin is
   A. synthesized on melanosomes
   B. produced by the action of tyrosinase
   C. not found in albinos
   D. synthesized by peroxidation of catecholamines
      associated with lipofuscin

7. Huntington's chorea is characterized by
   A. dementia
   B. progressive choriform movements
   C. atrophy of the caudate nucleus
   D. necrosis of the globus pallidus

ANSWERS AND DISCUSSION

1. (B) This patient's underlying neurological disorder was
idiopathic parkinsonism. This is a relatively common disease
with an estimated prevalence of 100-150 cases per 100,000
population. The clinical manifestations usually become apparent
during the fifth to seventh decades. The usual initial symptom
is tremor at rest. The tremor most commonly affects the
hands, arms and legs, diminishes upon voluntary movement
and stops during sleep. Rarely, the tremor may be unilateral.
Rigidity is probably the second most common manifestation and
one that contributes significantly to the patient's disability. The
patients often have postural instability and an abnormal shuffling
gait. They may be stooped and take small steps that become
progressively more rapid, so-called "festination." An important
clinical feature that is often overlooked is impairment of mental
function. This has been found in 50 to 70% of the patients.
Snout, sucking and hyperactive jaw reflexes can be elicited in
some of the cases with dementia. Sialorrhea, or drooling, is
a common finding and is due to impaired swallowing. Speech
may be quite abnormal.

In a dwindling number of patients, the parkinsonism is considered
to be a late sequela of encephalitis, especially encephalitis
lethargica. The clinical manifestations in these patients with
postencephalitic parkinsonism include more pronounced evidence
of autonomic dysfunction and, occasionally, oculogyric crises.

Essential tremor is a rare disorder characterized by trembling of the affected parts of the body.   In contrast to parkinsonism, there is no associated rigidity, bradykinesia, postural abnormality, etc. Alzheimer's disease is dominated by the dementia with an only minor component of extrapyramidal dysfunction. Pseudobulbar palsy is weakness of muscles supplied by the medulla, usually as a result of bilateral cerebral lesions. The syndrome often includes emotional lability.

2.   (A, C) The most obvious gross pathological feature of parkinsonism is depigmentation of the substantia nigra and, to a lesser extent, the locus caeruleus.   In Fig. 70.1, a brain stem with normally pigmented substantia nigra (top) is compared with the brain stem and depigmented substantia nigra from the present case (bottom).

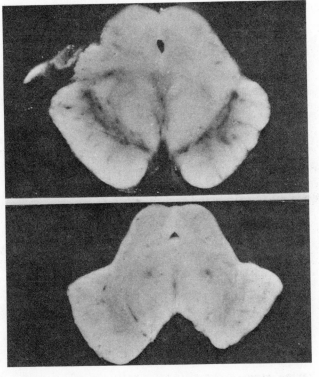

FIG. 70. 1: Transverse section of the brain stem from a control (top) is compared with the brain stem from the present case (bottom).

A very common, although less conspicuous change, is atrophy of the brain stem and the cerebral cortex. Within the cerebrum, the frontal lobes tend to be involved most severely. Some of the earlier workers stressed perivascular degeneration in the basal ganglia. These changes appear to be lacunar infarcts that are more closely associated with hypertension and cerebral arteriosclerosis than with parkinsonism. Gross pigmentation of the globus pallidus is one of the characteristics of Haller-vorden-Spatz disease.

3. (A, B, D) The most significant histological feature of parkinsonism is the degeneration of pigmented neurons in the brain stem. This change is most conspicuous in the zona compacta of the substantia nigra. The number of pigmented neurons is reduced and melanin is often found free in the neuropil and within macrophages as a result of the neuronal breakdown. A variable number of the remaining neurons contain laminated intracytoplasmic inclusions, the so-called Lewy bodies (Fig. 70.2).

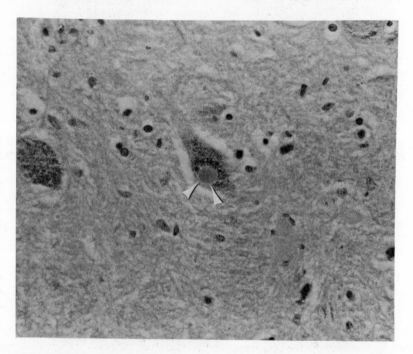

FIG. 70.2: Microscopic section of the substantia nigra showing a Lewy body (arrows) in the cytoplasm of a pigmented neuron.

These may be single or multiple, spherical or vermiform. They stain red with hematoxylin-eosin and blue or green with the trichrome stains. Histochemical studies have indicated the presence of protein and complex lipids such as sphingomyelin. Ultrastructurally, the Lewy bodies appear as unbounded, laminated structures containing a central core and one or more peripheral zones. The central core contains thin filaments that form linear or circular profiles. The outer zones contain radially oriented thicker filaments. These inclusions are characteristic of idiopathic parkinsonism. However, their origin and relation to the underlying biochemical lesions is unclear. Lewy bodies can also be found in the locus caeruleus, dorsal motor nucleus of the vagus and occasionally in various other brain stem neurons. In patients with postencephalitis parkinsonism, the brain stem neurons characteristically contain neurofibrillary tangles rather than Lewy bodies. In both types of parkinsonism, occasional dystrophic axons can be found in the pigmented brain stem nuclei.

Marinesco bodies are intranuclear inclusions that are found in the pigmented neurons of the substantia nigra, locus caeruleus and dorsal motor nucleus of the vagus. These inclusions increase in number with increasing age but are not associated with any specific disorder.

4. (B, C, D) A parkinsonism-like syndrome can result from various intoxications. Among the causative agents are carbon monoxide, manganese and phenothiazines. The parkinsonism-like syndrome observed in manganese miners and in carbon monoxide poisoning has been attributed to degeneration of neurons in the substantia nigra. The phenothiazines probably produce the syndrome by their effect on the striatum.

5. (C) A biochemical lesion common to most forms of parkinsonism is a deficiency of dopamine in the striatum. This deficiency is generally due to degeneration of dopamine synthesizing neurons that have their perikarya in the substantia nigra and their axonal terminals in the striatum. The degree of dopamine deficiency in the striatum roughly correlates with the degree of neuronal loss from the substantia nigra. The underlying cause for the degeneration of brain stem neurons in the common, so-called idiopathic type of parkinsonism is completely unknown. The Lewy bodies probably should be regarded as morphological indicators of this particular type of neuronal degeneration. Parkinsonism is treated by the administration of L-dopa rather than dopamine, since the latter compound is excluded by the blood brain barrier. The specific neurons responsible for the decarboxylation of L-dopa in patients with parkinsonism have not been identified with certainty.

The parkinsonism-like syndrome produced by the phenothiazines is probably due to blocking of post-synaptic receptors in the striatum rather than a dopamine deficiency.

6.   (D) Neuromelanin differs in several respects from cutaneous melanin.   Neuromelanin appears to be formed by the peroxidation of catecholamines that are sequestered onto lipofuscin granules.   Melanosomes and tyrosinase are not involved in its synthesis.   The substantia nigra is normally pigmented in albinos.

7.   (A, B, C) Huntington's chorea is a severe degenerative disease with a prevalence of about 5-10 cases per 100,000 population.   The disease is inherited as an autosomal dominant trait with complete penetrance.   The clinical manifestations usually do not become evident until after the age of 30 and consist predominantly of progressive choreiform movements and dementia. The disease is ordinarily fatal in about 15 years; however, suicide is rather common among affected individuals.   The gross pathological features consist of diffuse cortical atrophy and severe atrophy of the head of the caudate nucleus.   Microscopically, there is preferential loss of small neurons and gliosis in the caudate nucleus and putamen. The claustrum and pallidum also show some atrophy.   The cerebral cortex shows loss of neurons especially from the deeper layers of the frontal and parietal lobes.   The biochemical basis for Huntington's chorea is unsettled; abnormalities of catecholamine metabolism, deficiency of gamma aminobutyric acid (GABA), and abnormal neuronal proteins have been reported.

REFERENCES

1.   Alter M and Myrianthopoulos N: Chronic Progressive Hereditary Chorea of Huntington. In: Scientific Approaches to Clinical Neurology. Goldensohn ES and Appel SH (Eds.). Lea and Febiger, Philadelphia, 1977, pp. 1091-1108.

2.   Fahn S and Duffy P: Parkinson's Disease. In: Scientific Approaches to Clinical Neurology. Goldensohn ES and Appel SH (Eds.). Lea and Febiger, Philadelphia, 1977, pp. 1119-1158.

3.   Martin WE, et al.: Parkinson's disease. Neurology 23: 783-790, 1973.

4. McDowell FH and Markham CH: Recent Advances in
    Parkinsonism. F.A. Davis Co., Philadelphia, 1971.

5. Stahl W and Swanson PD: Biochemical abnormalities in
    Huntington's chorea brains. Neurology 24:813-819,
    1974.

6. Turner B: Pathology of Paralysis Agitans. In: Handbook
    of Clinical Neurology. Vinken PJ and Bruyn GW (Eds.).
    North-Holland, Amsterdam, 1968, Vol. 6, pp. 212-217.

: :

DIAGNOSES: CASE STUDIES

1: Duchenne muscular dystrophy
2: Polymyositis
3: Hypokalemic periodic paralysis
4: Werdnig-Hoffmann disease
5: Myotonic dystrophy
6: Kearns-Shy syndrome
7: Myasthenia gravis
8: Arsenical neuropathy
9: Guillain-Barre disease
10: Charcot-Marie-Tooth disease
11: Amyloid neuropathy
12: Giant axonal neuropathy
13: Arnold-Chiari malformation
14: Dandy-Walker malformation
15: Holoprosencephaly
16: Subependymal matrix hemorrhage
17: Kernicterus
18: Subdural hematoma
19: Coup-contrecoup lesions
20: Gunshot wound
21: Wernicke's encephalopathy
22: Carbon monoxide poisoning
23: Methanol poisoning
24: Reye's syndrome
25: Group B streptococcal meningitis
26: Pneumococcal meningitis
27: Abscess
28: Tuberculous meningitis
29: Aspergillosis
30: Cryptococcosis
31: Toxoplasmosis
32: Cysticercosis
33: Herpes simplex encephalitis
34: Cytomegalovirus infection
35: Rubella
36: Subacute sclerosing panencephalitis
37: Progressive multifocal leukoencephalopathy
38: Multiple sclerosis
39: Temporal arteritis
40: Cerebral infarct

41:   Brain stem hemorrhage
42:   Aneurysms
43:   Angiomas
44:   Vein of Galen aneurysm
45:   Leukemia
46:   Metastatic carcinoma
47:   Glioblastoma
48:   Cerebellar astrocytoma
49:   Brain stem glioma
50:   Ependymoma
51:   Medulloblastoma
52:   Microglioma
53:   Angioblastic meningioma
54:   Acoustic nerve tumor
55:   Germinoma
56:   Craniopharyngioma
57:   von Recklinghausen's disease
58:   Tuberous sclerosis
59:   Sturge-Weber disease
60:   Tay-Sachs disease
61:   Krabbe's disease
62:   Hurler's disease
63:   Pompe's disease
64:   Myoclonus epilepsy
65:   Neuronal ceroid-lipofuscinosis
66:   Zellweger's syndrome
67:   Alzheimer's disease
68:   Jakob-Creutzfeldt disease
69:   Amyotrophic lateral sclerosis
70:   Parkinsonism

Index

INDEX

POST-TEST

MULTIPLE CHOICE

1. Histological features expected in a muscle biopsy specimen
    from a young boy with Duchenne muscular dystrophy
    include
    A. degenerating myofibers
    B. target fibers
    C. perifascicular atrophy
    D. increased endomysial connective tissue

2. Histological features that would be sought in a muscle
    biopsy specimen from a patient with polymyositis include
    A. target fibers
    B. perifascicular atrophy
    C. myofiber degeneration and myophagocytosis
    D. "ragged-red" fibers

3. The most characteristic histopathological change in a
    muscle biopsy specimen from a patient with hypokalemic
    periodic paralysis is
    A. perifascicular atrophy
    B. nemaline rods
    C. internal nuclei
    D. vacuolated myofibers

4. Muscle biopsy specimens from patients with Werdnig-
    Hoffmann disease typically show
    A. atrophic myofibers that are both type 1 and type 2
    B. atrophic myofibers that are exclusively type 1
    C. myriads of central nuclei
    D. hypertrophied type 1 myofibers

5. Muscle biopsy specimens from individuals with myotonic
    dystrophy characteristically show
    A. numerous internal nuclei
    B. ring fibers
    C. preferential atrophy of type 1 myofibers
    D. "ragged-red" fibers

6. Infants with myotonic dystrophy have
    A. a mother affected with myotonic dystrophy
    B. a father affected with myotonic dystrophy
    C. difficulty sucking and swallowing
    D. myotonia

7. So-called "ragged-red" fibers result from the presence
    of collections of
    A. nemaline rods
    B. abnormal mitochondria
    C. abnormal glycogen
    D. lipofuscin

8. Nerve biopsy specimens from individuals with arsenical
    neuropathy typically show
    A. amyloid deposits
    B. axonal degeneration
    C. onion bulbs
    D. Renaut corpuscles

9. Onion bulbs may be prominent in peripheral nerve biopsy
    specimens from patients with
    A. Dejerine-Sottas disease
    B. hypertrophic Charcot-Marie-Tooth disease
    C. Refsum's disease
    D. amyotrophic lateral sclerosis

10. Peripheral nerve biopsy specimens from patients with
     Guillain-Barre disease characteristically show
     A. segmental demyelination
     B. perivascular inflammatory cell infiltrates
     C. selective degeneration of large myelinated fibers
     D. giant axonal enlargements

11. Giant axonal neuropathy may result from
     A. a rare hereditary disease of childhood
     B. "glue-sniffing"
     C. occupational exposure to methyl butyl ketone
     D. occupational exposure to n-hexane

12. Endoneurial deposits of amyloid may be seen in patients
     with
     A. hereditary amyloid neuropathy
     B. myeloma
     C. primary amyloidosis
     D. secondary amyloidosis

13. Infants with a meningomyelocele characteristically have
    an associated
    A. Arnold-Chiari malformation
    B. spina bifida occulta
    C. hypotelorism
    D. enlargement of the posterior fossa

14. Components of the Arnold-Chiari malformation include
    A. elongated tongues of cerebellar tissue
    B. elongated medulla with "Z-shaped" cervico-
       medullary junction
    C. elongation of the pons
    D. "keel-shaped" mesencephalic tectum

15. Infants with the Dandy-Walker malformation have
    A. a malformed "keel-shaped" mesencephalic tectum
    B. a posterior fossa cyst composed of ependyma and
       leptomeninges
    C. aqueductal stenosis
    D. an enlarged head with an abnormally high inion

16. Holoprosencephaly is commonly found in infants with
    A. cyclopia
    B. cebocephaly
    C. bilateral, lateral cleft lips
    D. hypertelorism

17. Subependymal matrix hemorrhages
    A. usually occur in premature infants
    B. result from mechanical obstetrical trauma
    C. follow periventricular leukomalacia
    D. may be the source of subarachnoid blood

18. Conditions that predispose to the development of
    kernicterus or bilirubin encephalopathy include
    A. immaturity
    B. Rh and ABO incompatibilities
    C. anoxia
    D. alkalosis

19. Subdural hematomas are especially common in individuals
    who have a history of
    A. alcoholism
    B. epilepsy
    C. hypertension
    D. sickle cell anemia

20. The immediate cause of death in an individual with a
     supratentorial mass lesion such as a subdural hema-
     toma, is frequently
     A. subfalcial (cingulate) herniation
     B. uncal herniation
     C. secondary brain stem (Duret) hemorrhage
     D. compression or kinking of the internal carotid
         arteries

21. A massive contrecoup injury in a patient with a minimal
     coup injury is most apt to result from
     A. sudden deceleration of the head as from a fall
     B. sudden acceleration of the head as from a blow
         with a hammer
     C. crushing as from being driven over by an automobile
     D. a penetrating missile

22. The size of a wound track produced by a bullet passing
     through the brain is influenced most by
     A. tumbling of the bullet
     B. yaw
     C. mass of the bullet
     D. velocity of the bullet

23. Lesions in addition to the wound track itself that are
     commonly encountered with bullet wounds of the head
     are
     A. orbital roof fractures
     B. uncal contusions
     C. tonsillar contusions
     D. tears of the corpus callosum

24. Lesions due to Wernicke's encephalopathy are encountered
     in the
     A. mammillary bodies
     B. periaqueductal grey matter
     C. subthalamic nuclei
     D. optic tracts

25. Leigh's disease is due to
     A. thiamine deficiency
     B. the presence of a thiaminase
     C. the presence of a glycoprotein that inhibits ATP-
         thiamine pyrophosphate phosphotransferase
     D. the presence of a glycoprotein that inhibits the for-
         mation of thiamine diphosphate

26. Conditions other than Wernicke's encephalopathy that are encountered <u>most</u> frequently among alcoholic patients include
   A. cerebellar vermal atrophy
   B. Marchiafava-Bignami disease
   C. periventricular leukomalacia
   D. central pontine myelinolysis

27. Delayed deaths due to certain intoxications are commonly characterized by the presence of pallidal necrosis. These agents include
   A. methanol
   B. carbon monoxide
   C. cyanide
   D. ethylene glycol

28. Individuals who die acutely from carbon monoxide intoxication show
   A. necrosis of cardiac muscle
   B. cherry-red colored skin, mucous membranes and blood
   C. a blue-green discoloration of the brain
   D. pallidal necrosis

29. Bilateral putamenal necrosis is characteristically seen in delayed deaths from
   A. cyanide intoxication
   B. ethylene glycol intoxication
   C. methanol intoxication
   D. hydrogen sulfide intoxication

30. Pathological alterations that may be seen in Reye's syndrome include
   A. microvesicular lipid deposition in the liver
   B. hepatic glycogen depletion
   C. cerebral edema
   D. Cowdry type A intranuclear inclusions in oligo-dendrocytes

31. Agents that commonly cause meningitis in the neonatal period include
   A. Hemophilus influenzae
   B. Neisseria meningitidis
   C. Escherichia coli
   D. group B beta hemolytic streptococci

32. Circumstances that predispose to the development of
    pneumococcal meningitis include
    A. alcoholism
    B. arteriovenous malformations
    C. splenectomy during adulthood
    D. head trauma

33. Conditions that predispose to the development of brain
    abscesses include
    A. bronchiectasis
    B. congenital heart disease
    C. ear and paranasal sinus infections
    D. diverticulitis

34. Deaths from brain abscesses are due most often to
    A. ventriculitis
    B. meningitis
    C. destruction of vital centers
    D. herniations

35. Cerebrospinal fluid from a patient with tuberculous
    meningitis typically shows
    A. a pleocytosis with a predominance of lymphocytes
    B. a pleocytosis with a predominance of neutrophils
    C. an elevated protein content
    D. a moderately reduced glucose content

36. Tuberculous meningitis may produce
    A. a thick exudate that is especially abundant at the
       base of the brain
    B. occlusive vasculitis
    C. obstructive hydrocephalus
    D. dolichoectasia of the basilar artery

37. Opportunistic mycotic infections are most commonly
    due to
    A. Blastomyces dermatitidis
    B. Cryptococcus neoformans
    C. Aspergillus species
    D. Candida species

38. Fungal infections that are characterized by hyphae in
    tissue include
    A. candidiasis
    B. mucormycosis
    C. aspergillosis
    D. cryptococcosis

39. Toxoplasmosis may be acquired by
    A. transplacental passage
    B. consumption of undercooked meat
    C. ingestion of cat feces
    D. ingestion of sheep feces

40. Cysticercosis is due to parasitism by the larval form
    of
    A. Taenia solium
    B. Entamoeba histolytica
    C. Toxocara canis
    D. Nosema cuniculi

41. A hemorrhagic meningoencephalitis characteristically
    results from infection with
    A. Naegleria fowleri
    B. Entamoeba histolytica
    C. Toxocara canis
    D. Nosema cuniculi

42. Gross neuropathological changes typically encountered
    in adults with encephalitis due to herpes simplex type 1
    include
    A. hemorrhagic necrosis of the inferior and medial
       aspect of the frontal lobes
    B. hemorrhagic necrosis of the medial aspect of the
       temporal lobes
    C. hemorrhagic necrosis of the basis pontis
    D. hemorrhagic necrosis of the lateral portions of the
       corpus callosum

43. Disseminated herpes simplex and herpes simplex
    encephalitis in neonates is caused
    A. most commonly by type 1 herpes simplex virus
    B. most commonly by type 2 herpes simplex virus
    C. most commonly by type 3 herpes simplex virus
    D. equally as often by type 1 and 2 herpes simplex virus

44. Virus can be isolated readily from the cerebrospinal fluid
    of patients with
    A. herpes simplex type 1 encephalitis
    B. herpes simplex type 2 encephalitis
    C. mumps meningoencephalitis
    D. St. Louis encephalitis

45. Cytomegalovirus infections produce
     A. enlarged cells with only nuclear inclusions
     B. enlarged cells with only cytoplasmic inclusions
     C. enlarged cells with nuclear and cytoplasmic
         inclusions
     D. microglial nodules

46. Lesions typically encountered in the congenital rubella
     syndrome include
     A. congenital heart defects
     B. microcephaly
     C. cataracts
     D. colobomas

47. Histological findings in brains from children with sub-
     acute sclerosing panencephalitis typically include
     A. perivascular mineralization
     B. intranuclear inclusions
     C. distension of neuronal perikarya
     D. demyelination

48. Viruses that have been identified in brain tissue from
     patients with progressive multifocal leukoencephalopathy
     include
     A. an SV40-like virus
     B. the JC virus
     C. the BK virus
     D. the EB virus

49. In patients with progressive multifocal leukoencephalo-
     pathy, papovavirus particles are demonstrated most
     often in the nuclei of
     A. astrocytes
     B. oligodendrocytes
     C. neurons
     D. ependymal cells

50. In multiple sclerosis, foci of demyelination are commonly
     located
     A. in the optic nerves
     B. about the angles of the lateral ventricles
     C. in the spinal cord
     D. in the brachial and lumbar plexi

51. Devic's disease is generally regarded as a variant of
    multiple sclerosis with involvement predominantly of
    the
    A. cerebellum and spinal cord
    B. cerebellum and optic pathways
    C. spinal cord and optic pathways
    D. peripheral nerves and optic pathways

52. Temporal arteritis is characterized histologically by
    A. transmural fibrinoid necrosis
    B. abundant eosinophils in the inflammatory cell
       infiltrate
    C. fragmentation of the internal elastic lamina
    D. granulomatous inflammation with giant cells

53. Infarcts resulting from embolization are typically
    A. anemic infarcts
    B. hemorrhagic infarcts
    C. border zone infarcts
    D. multiple infarcts

54. Depending on the presence or absence of atherosclerosis,
    previous carotid thrombosis and vascular anomalies, a
    carotid artery thrombosis may produce
    A. no cerebral infarction
    B. infarction in the distribution of the ipsilateral
       anterior and middle cerebral arteries
    C. infarction in the distribution of the contralateral
       middle and anterior cerebral arteries
    D. infarction in the basis pontis

55. Olivary hypertrophy is
    A. a form of transneuronal degeneration
    B. secondary to accumulation of lipofuscin in the neurons
       of the inferior olivary nuclei
    C. encountered in association with the Wallenberg
       syndrome
    D. a lesion that results from destruction of the dento-
       rubro-olivary tract

56. The most common cause of hemorrhage in the pons is
    A. hypertension
    B. rupture of a basilar artery aneurysm
    C. caudal displacement of the brain stem secondary to a
       supratentorial mass lesion
    D. rupture of a pontine angioma

57. The prevalence of saccular aneurysms among all patients coming to autopsy is about
    A. less than 2%
    B. 2 to 3%
    C. 5 to 7%
    D. greater than 10%

58. Saccular aneurysms occur most commonly on the
    A. anterior cerebral arteries
    B. middle cerebral arteries
    C. posterior cerebral arteries
    D. basilar artery

59. Compared to unruptured saccular aneurysms, ruptured saccular aneurysms tend to be
    A. smaller
    B. equal in size
    C. larger
    D. much larger, so-called "giant" aneurysms

60. The type of angioma encountered most commonly among all patients coming to autopsy is
    A. arteriovenous
    B. venous
    C. cavernous
    D. varix

61. The type of angioma most apt to produce neurological complications is
    A. arteriovenous
    B. venous
    C. cavernous
    D. varix

62. Complications of a vein of Galen aneurysm include
    A. congestive heart failure
    B. intracranial hemorrhage
    C. hydrocephalus
    D. pulsatile exophthalmos

63. Cerebral lesions that have an increased prevalence among patients with leukemia include
    A. Charcot-Bouchard aneurysms
    B. lobar hemorrhages
    C. mycotic infections
    D. progressive multifocal leukoencephalopathy

64. The chemotherapeutic agent most apt to produce a peripheral neuropathy is
    A. nitrogen mustard
    B. methotrexate
    C. vincristine
    D. cyclophosphamide

65. The most common sources of meningeal carcinomatosis are
    A. lung carcinoma
    B. breast carcinoma
    C. pancreatic carcinoma
    D. prostatic carcinoma

66. The cerebrospinal fluid from a patient with meningeal carcinomatosis typically has
    A. an elevated glucose content
    B. a reduced glucose content
    C. an elevated protein content
    D. a reduced protein content

67. Glioblastomas
    A. occur more commonly in men than women
    B. arise most often in the occipital lobes
    C. frequently metastasize extracranially
    D. are characterized histologically by areas of necrosis surrounded by pseudopalisades

68. A cystic cerebellar neoplasm in a child is most apt to be
    A. an ependymoma
    B. an astrocytoma
    C. a hemangioblastoma
    D. a medulloblastoma

69. In children, foci of glioblastoma are found most commonly in
    A. optic nerve gliomas
    B. diencephalic gliomas
    C. pontine gliomas
    D. cerebellar astrocytomas

70. Myxopapillary ependymomas are found typically
    A. in the lateral ventricles
    B. in the cerebello-pontine angles
    C. within syringomyelic cavities
    D. in the conus medullaris and filum terminale

71. Histological characteristics of medulloblastomas include
     the presence of
     A. perivascular pseudorosettes
     B. Homer Wright rosettes
     C. Flexner-Wintersteiner rosettes
     D. cells with hyperchromatic nuclei and scanty cyto-
         plasm

72. "Cerebellar sarcomas" are
     A. desmoplastic medulloblastomas
     B. arachnoidal sarcomas of the posterior fossa
     C. a form of meningeal carcinomatosis
     D. malignant hemangioblastomas

73. So-called "microgliomas" are
     A. lymphoreticular neoplasms that arise in the central
         nervous system
     B. more common in immunosuppressed individuals
     C. a form of plasmacytoma
     D. encountered predominantly during the first decade

74. Meningiomas
     A. occur somewhat more often in men than in women
     B. may be encountered within the ventricular system
     C. invade the adjacent neural parenchyma
     D. occur equally as often at all ages

75. Acoustic neurinomas
     A. arise from the cochlear branch of the eighth nerve
     B. arise from the vestibular branch of the eighth nerve
     C. often develop in the internal auditory meatus
     D. are neurofibromas

76. "Ectopic pinealomas" are
     A. germinomas of the hypothalamic region
     B. derived from ectopic pinealocytes
     C. histologically similar to seminomas
     D. found predominantly in elderly women

77. Craniopharyngiomas are
     A. more apt to be calcified in adults than in children
     B. more common than pituitary adenomas
     C. usually at least partially cystic
     D. apt to induce gliosis and Rosenthal fiber formation
         in the adjacent neural parenchyma

78. Hemangioblastomas
    A. arise most often in the cerebellum
    B. may be a component of the von Hippel-Lindau syndrome
    C. are the most common cystic or partially cystic tumor of the cerebellum
    D. occur most often in young children

79. Neoplasms thought to be derived from Schwann cells include
    A. acoustic neurinomas
    B. traumatic neuromas
    C. neurofibromas
    D. esthesioneuroblastomas

80. Findings considered highly suggestive or diagnostic of von Recklinghausen's disease include
    A. six or more cafe-au-lait spots, each more than 2 cm in diameter
    B. bilateral acoustic neurinomas
    C. a plexiform neurofibroma
    D. a single peripheral neurilemoma

81. Tay-Sachs disease is attributed to a deficiency of
    A. hexosaminidase A activity
    B. galactocerebrosidase activity
    C. glucocerebrosidase activity
    D. alpha-iduronidase activity

82. Common cutaneous manifestations of tuberous sclerosis include
    A. a "port-wine" nevus
    B. adenoma sebaceum
    C. hypopigmented leaf-shaped macule
    D. Morton's neuroma

83. Manifestations of Sturge-Weber disease include
    A. a "port-wine" nevus of the face
    B. epilepsy
    C. mental retardation
    D. glaucoma

84. Pathologic findings in Sturge-Weber disease include
    A. cortical neuroglial hamartomas
    B. leptomeningeal venous angioma
    C. calcospherites in the superficial layer of the cerebral cortex
    D. subependymal giant cell astrocytomas

85. Characteristics of Tay-Sachs disease include
    A. occurrence predominantly among Sephardic Jews
    B. development of a "cherry-red" spot in the macula
    C. an exaggerated startle response
    D. hepatosplenomegaly

86. Neuropathological features of Krabbe's disease include
    A. a paucity of myelin and focal cavitation in the cerebral white matter
    B. perivascular accumulations of globoid cells
    C. subpial, perivascular and subependymal deposits of Rosenthal fibers
    D. distension of neurons by galactocerebroside

87. The death of oligodendrocytes in Krabbe's disease has been attributed to the toxic effect of
    A. sphingosine
    B. galactocerebroside
    C. psychosine
    D. sphingomyelin

88. Peripheral nerves are involved in
    A. Krabbe's disease
    B. metachromatic leukodystrophy
    C. Alexander's disease
    D. Canavan's disease

89. Neuropathologic findings in Hurler's disease include
    A. distension of neurons by mucopolysaccharides
    B. distension of neurons by gangliosides
    C. thickened leptomeninges
    D. widened perivascular spaces

90. Hurler's disease is attributed to a deficiency of
    A. aryl sulfatase A activity
    B. galactocerebrosidase activity
    C. alpha-iduronidase activity
    D. heparan sulfatase activity

91. Pompe's disease is characterized by
    A. weak, hypotonic skeletal muscles
    B. cardiomegaly
    C. cirrhosis
    D. deficiency of acid maltase activity

92. Inclusions composed of polyglucosans include
    A. Marinesco bodies
    B. Lafora bodies
    C. Lewy bodies
    D. corpora amylacea

93. Characteristics of the Jansky-Bielschowsky form of
    neuronal ceroid-lipofuscinosis include
    A. early onset of seizures
    B. early onset of visual disturbances
    C. megabarencephaly
    D. a "cherry-red" spot

94. Pathological features of Zellweger's syndrome include
    A. polymicrogyria and/or pachygyria
    B. subependymal matrix cysts
    C. malformation of the inferior olives
    D. status marmoratus

95. Histopathological findings indicative of Alzheimer's dis-
    ease include
    A. neurofibrillary tangles in numerous cortical neurons
    B. numerous senile plaques
    C. granulovacuolar degeneration
    D. Marinesco bodies

96. Pathological features characteristic of Pick's disease
    include
    A. "knife-edge" atrophy of cortical gyri
    B. neurofibrillary tangles in cortical neurons
    C. argentophilic spheroids in cortical neurons
    D. atrophy of ventral spinal roots

97. Pathological findings in the cerebral cortex from patients
    with Jakob-Creutzfeldt disease include
    A. spongiform degeneration
    B. numerous neurofibrillary tangles
    C. numerous neuritic plaques
    D. astrocytosis

98. Pathological findings in patients with sporadic amyotro-
    phic lateral sclerosis include
    A. neurogenic atrophy of skeletal muscle
    B. degeneration of the corticospinal tracts
    C. degeneration of the posterior columns
    D. atrophy of the dorsal roots

99. Pathological features of idiopathic parkinsonism include
    A. depigmentation of the substantia nigra
    B. Lewy bodies in pigmented neurons
    C. Marinesco bodies in the substantia nigra
    D. neurofibrillary tangles in the striatum

100. The most conspicuous gross pathological finding in Hunt-
     ington's chorea is
     A. pigmentation of the globus pallidus
     B. depigmentation of the substantia nigra
     C. atrophy of the caudate nucleus
     D. cavitation in the putamen

ANSWER KEY

The authors have made every effort to thoroughly verify the answers to the questions which appear on the preceding pages. However, as in any text, some inaccuracies and ambiguities may occur; therefore, if in doubt, please consult standard references.

THE PUBLISHER

1. A, D	35. A, C, D	69. C
2. B, C	36. A, B, C	70. D
3. D	37. C, D	71. B, D
4. A, D	38. B, C	72. A
5. A, B, C	39. A, B, C	73. A, B
6. A, C	40. A	74. B
7. B	41. A	75. B, C
8. B	42. A, B	76. A, C
9. A, B, C	43. B	77. C, D
10. A, B	44. B, C	78. A, B
11. A, B, C, D	45. C, D	79. A, C
12. A, B, C	46. A, B, C	80. A, B, C
13. A	47. B, D	81. A
14. A, B, C, D	48. A, B	82. B, C
15. B, D	49. B	83. A, B, C, D
16. A, B, C	50. A, B, C	84. B, C
17. A, D	51. C	85. B, C
18. A, B, C	52. C, D	86. A, B
19. A, B	53. B, D	87. C
20. C	54. A, B, C	88. A, B
21. A	55. A, D	89. B, C, D
22. D	56. C	90. C
23. A, B, C	57. C	91. A, B, D
24. A, B	58. B	92. B, D
25. C	59. C	93. A
26. A, B, D	60. B	94. A, B, C
27. B, C	61. A	95. A, B, C
28. B	62. A, C	96. A, C
29. C	63. B, C, D	97. A, D
30. A, B, C	64. C	98. A, B
31. C, D	65. A, B	99. A, B
32. A, D	66. B, C	100. C
33. A, B, C	67. A, D	
34. D	68. B